Plant Power

Laurel Dewey

Here is calm so deep, grasses cease waving...
Wonderful how completely everything in
wild nature fits into us,
as if truly part and parent of us.
The sun shines not on us, but in us.
The rivers flow not past, but through us,
thrilling, tingling, vibrating every fiber and
cell of the substance of our bodies,
making them glide and sing.

John Muir

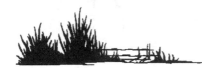 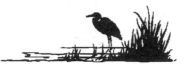

Also by Laurel Dewey

THE HUMOROUS HERBALIST—
A Practical Guide to Leaves, Flowers, Roots, Barks & Other
Neat Stuff (1996)

PLANT POWER

The Humorous Herbalist's Guide To Finding, Growing, Gathering & Using

30 Great Medicinal Herbs

Laurel Dewey

Illustrations
Jack Jones

10 9 8 7 6 5 4 3 2 1

ISBN 1-884820-37-9

Libary of of Congress Catalog Card No. 99-94569

ATN/Safe Goods
P.O. Box 36
East Canaan, CT, 06024
For additional copies of this book, call (860) 824-5301

Manufactured in the United States of America.

CONTENTS

~ CHARTS ~

~ TERMINOLOGY ~

~ BIBLIOGRAPHY ~

~ HERBAL RESOURCES ~

~ INDEX ~

~ PAGES FOR NOTES ~

Dedication

This book is dedicated to:

Mom & Dad

Thank you for always encouraging me to use
my full potential.
I may have been a late bloomer, but I've almost outlived those
Brontë sisters.

Granny

Thank you for teaching me one of life's most important
lessons:
"No one can make you look stupid unless you allow it."
I know you're listening.

"Unk"

Thank you for insisting that I write what makes me happy.
I'm finally following that advice.

*To all the herbalists & natural healers
that have lived and are yet to be born.*

Thank you for being willing to travel the road less taken.
It's not always easy, but it has a much better view.

Acknowledgements

No book is written without the assistance of others.
Many thanks to Jack Jones for the illustrations, Richard D. Burns
and Mark Dodge for the layout, Amy Lawrence for the creativity,
M&D Editing for "tightening it up,"
John Duvall for the great formulas, Ken Kuhns and
the Peach Valley CSA Farm for the education and memorable
lunches, Pat Noel for giving a little herb column a big chance and to
the many herbalists, wildcrafters and teachers along the way who
helped give life to this book.

While I encourage readers to take more responsibility for their health and well-being, this book should not be considered a replacement for intelligent medical advice. At various times in our lives, we all need a qualified perspective from someone who can discuss the various treatments available for any number of health problems and concerns. That qualified perspective may come from a medical doctor, a naturopathic physician, a traditional Chinese medical doctor, an acupuncturist, a reflexologist or a skilled herbalist. The options are out there and I advise everyone to take advantage of them.

While this book may help you on your journey, it is not meant to take the place of any physician or holistic professional. This book is also not intended to treat, diagnose or prescribe. The information presented within these pages is meant to educate, enlighten and inform. Pregnant or nursing women should always consult a doctor or qualified holistic professional before using herbal therapy.

And then the day came
when the risk
to remain tight in a bud
was more painful than the risk
it took to blossom.

Anais Nin

INTRODUCTION

$\mathcal{A}$ few weeks after the release of my first book, *The Humorous Herbalist*, people started asking me when I was going to write my *next* book. "My *next* book?!" was my usual reply. I was still recovering from the long, solitary hours spent writing and editing hundreds of pages. The thought of delving into another tome to herbal healing was the last thing on my mind.

But that didn't mean I wasn't willing to at least *think* about the idea. For two years I considered various ideas that would entice readers. As with *The Humorous Herbalist,* I wanted to write a book that *I* would want to read. It would have to be reader-friendly—never complicated and always infused with humor and interesting information to keep people turning the pages.

But there would also have to be something more—something I wasn't yet able to put my finger on.

During this two year period, I wasn't spending every waking hour dreaming up the next herbal offering. Nearly every month of the year, I traveled from coast to coast attending alternative health shows, book conventions and herbal symposiums. I lectured and taught herb classes that included everyone from 10 year olds to senior citizens. I had the opportunity to meet many people and I began to notice things that bothered me.

There seemed to be a desire by many practitioners in alternative medicine to create an aura of mystery when discussing the use of herbs. This "mystery" only served to separate "those who have the knowledge" from "those in search of the knowledge." What, in my opinion, should be an open exchange of age-old information, had turned into a kind of elitist mentality by many in the alternative health field.

For centuries, herbal medicine belonged to the people. There was an intuitive bridge between the plants and the people. Granted, most of those people lived in the backwoods and distant valleys of the world where the mind was allowed to connect to the voice of nature. But there was always a willingness by everyone to share the healing knowledge— to pass it down as one generation's gift to the other. There were no "rights" or patents to the herbs because everyone knew that you "can't patent nature."

But then science entered the picture. Researchers were tripping over themselves in an attempt to isolate what they loved to refer to as "active compounds" in herbs. By isolating these supposed "active ingredients," and then manipulating them in a lab, they could produce a standardized herbal product deemed "better than nature itself." And since science was able to alter the herb's natural form, they were now finally able to "patent nature." Product labels were filled with multi-syllabic words that no one but clinical herbalists and lab researchers understood. Nevertheless, the public was enticed to try the products, always with the promise of fast, reliable, "guaranteed" results. In one fell swoop, science entered the herbal world with the same mindset that existed in the drug industry.

And that, my friends, is when I started getting upset.

The fact that scientists had the nerve to state that "isolated compounds" were better than the whole, synergistic miracle that nature created was a tremendous disservice to the public in my opinion. In their quest to identify, test and label chemical compounds within plants, science missed the most important aspect of herbal medicine. The whole plant has an inner mind that is so vast and miraculous that it defies the narrow definitions any person can give it. Plants in their whole state, adapt to the body's needs *at that specific time* and then work with the body to cleanse, nourish and rebuild whatever needs to be restored. Herbs absolutely have an inner knowing that directs them wherever they need to go. Every part of that herb—including the so-called "insignificant elements"—has a reason for being there. Leave any of those compounds out of the herb and it quickly becomes less than its original form. While I realize that it is science's job to conduct extensive studies and report back with cold, hard facts, there are some things in the plant world that defy scientific analysis. Herbs can sometimes be unpredictable—the minute you think you've got them pigeonholed, they suddenly reveal another side you never knew existed.

I came to this conclusion one day when I was standing amidst a glorious stand of aspen trees in the mountains of western Colorado. In the stillness of that moment, with only the wind to whisper through the leaves, a most amazing thing happened. I suddenly realized the noble power that filled every living thing in that forest. These are not just one dimensional beings dropped upon the earth in some accidental manner. The trees and plants are sentient beings with an intelligence all their own. To understand that intelligence takes years of walking quietly alone through meadows and forests. Once you discover it for yourself, only then do you realize that that Divine spirit is lost when it ends up under a microscope.

And that's when I knew what I needed to write about in my next book.

It would be about people returning to the land. It would encourage everyone to take a greater responsibilty for knowing what was growing in their own backyard and if those plants would make good medicine. It would imbue readers with a desire to become more self-sufficient—to grow and learn to use medicinal herbs that could help themselves and those they love. More than anything, perhaps readers would feel the gentle pull of their ancestors who lived in synergy with nature and had the common sense necessary to survive in harmony with the seasons.

The mysteries of herbal medicine are not found in the basic knowledge and understanding of plants, but rather in the overwhelming vastness of what nature offers. When you fully comprehend that a tree or plant has the innate power to heal the body, you set your feet on the right path. When you realize that same tree or plant has the wisdom to heal both mind and spirit, your life is changed forever.

May this book set you on that path.

Laurel Dewey
May 1999

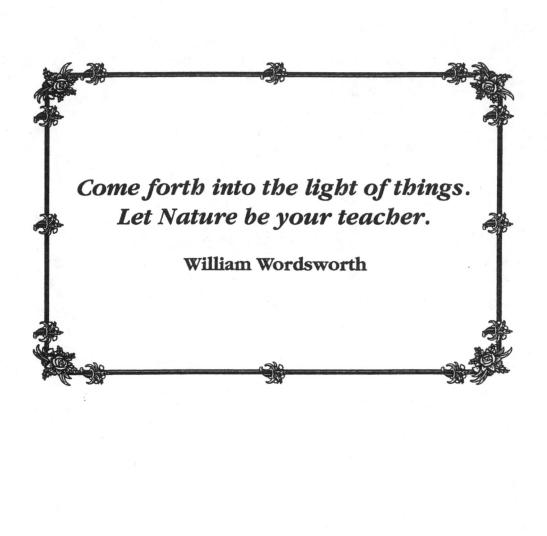

Come forth into the light of things.
Let Nature be your teacher.

William Wordsworth

The Basics

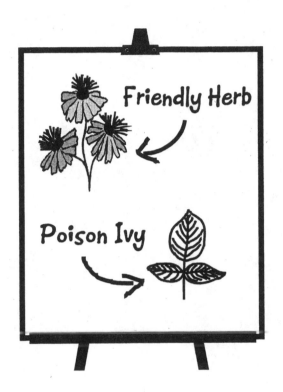

~

Chapter 1

WHAT QUESTIONS SHOULD I BE ASKING MYSELF?

Before you bring out the shovel or raid the local nursery for plants and seeds, there are seven questions you need to ask yourself. Your answers will help determine the exact type of herb garden you want and need.

1. What specific medicinal herbs would I love to have at my fingertips?

Perhaps you have read about a particular medicinal herb that has intrigued you. Maybe there are a few popular herbal remedies you have purchased on a regular basis from your local health food store that you'd like to try to grow. Whichever herbs you choose, pick plants that you know you will use. I have seen many herb gardens filled with medicinal herbs that are never harvested. As you are choosing those herbs, don't forget to ask yourself...

2. Will these herbs be compatible with the region where I live?

You may love to have a certain tree or shrub in your backyard, but that plant may or may not flourish where you live. This is not to say that you can't "break the rules" and cultivate some herbs that normally would not be found naturally growing in your area. However, if you are starting to grow medicinal herbs (or any herbs, for that matter), it is always best to make life easy and select herbs that match your region's individual growing conditions. For example, some herbs that flourish in the high mountains at 9000 feet would never make it through two days in the direct, hot desert sun. Seed/plant catalogs often provide appropriate regional "zones" when describing both live plants and seeds. If you can't find that kind of information in the catalog, ask the catalog representative for more specific zone information for the plants you would like to grow.

Also, it is important to consider your region's particular growing season. Someone living in southern California where the temperatures usually don't dip below freezing obviously enjoy a year-long growing season. However, another person living in northern Montana has a shorter frost-free growing season which can often last a few months. Since some herbs need 60 to 90 days to fully mature, those living in areas where there are shorter growing seasons might only get to appreciate their ready-to-use herbal garden for a few weeks before the first frost damages the crop. This factor would lead you to then ask yourself....

3. Should I purchase seeds and plant from "scratch" or should I buy established seedlings and/or full-grown herbs?

This question can apply to everyone, no matter the region where you reside. For those who live in regions that have shorter growing seasons, buying established plants is often preferred over seeds so that you can enjoy the plants for a longer period of time. For the herb novice who might be concerned with planting seeds, purchasing established seedlings/live plants for your first garden tends to make one feel more confident and less likely to be disappointed. Some herbs must be purchased in live plant form since they are either difficult to start from seed (such as rosemary) or are sterile (such as true peppermint). You might want a few herbs that are not readily available at your local nursery or through your favorite plant catalog in a "live plant" form. If this is the case, buying the seeds is your only option. If the herb is considered "easy" to "moderately easy" to grow from seed, consider starting the seedlings indoors in a temperature-controlled environment at least six weeks before the typical "last frost."

If you are fortunate to have a greenhouse, you can get a head start on your seeds and offer your plants months of life no matter where you live. The backyard herbalist should seriously consider another important point that is often overlooked when it comes to choosing herbs. And that is making sure that you grow enough of the herb to serve your individual or family needs. A lovely little carpet of chickweed is fine, but if you intend to make the famous chickweed skin salve, you will need a whole lot more than a little carpet. On the other hand, one aspen or poplar tree is quite sufficient to provide you with all the necessary buds and bark you will ever desire. But, wait! Before you start buying up dozens of herb seed packets and/or pots of seedlings and plants, ask yourself....

4. How much available space do I have to work with?

Your eyes may be bigger than your backyard! In other words, you might want to include 20 herbs in your garden but you realistically only have space for a maximum of ten. Cramming herbs on top of each other can cause stunted plant growth as well as an uneven design scheme that looks more like a "bunch of weeds" rather than a tailored herb garden. It is important to always allow adequate spacing between plants. Not only will spacing look more pleasing to the eye but that extra six inches to a foot of space gives the herb "spreading room." Anyone who has planted herbs that fall into the mint family can fully appreciate these words of wisdom and warning. You might start out with three spearmint plants, but within two years—thanks to the underground root runners—you can easily have dozens of new spearmint plants all vying for their place in the sun. If you don't have enough space for all the plants you would like to grow, consider placing some of those in containers. (Chapter 6 deals with container gardening and what plants work best in this medium).

So you can get a better idea of what your herb garden will look like, draw a diagram outlining where you want to place the herbs, always allowing sufficient space between plants. If you want to get artistic with your backyard garden, you might want to plant your herbs within ovals, squares or crosses. Many of the English herb gardens from centuries past and even today are designed in intricate patterns that are pleasing to the eye as well as functional. If artistry is something you are interested in pursuing, you will want to categorize your herbs not only by color but by size. In other words, plants such as rosemary, sage and thyme can work well as low hedges if they are routinely manicured and shaped. Good ground cover herbs include cleavers (lady's bedstraw) and chickweed. If you want to make a dramatic statement and include tall, striking herbs, consider mullein, fennel, marshmallow and even stinging nettle. (Mind you, if you do choose nettle, you'll likely be *receiving* dramatic statements from visitors).

When selecting your proposed growing site, take sun, shade and wind into consideration. There should be a combination of sun and shade and a protection from wind since steady or heavy gusts of wind can stunt plant growth as well as blow off top soil. When choosing a particular herb, check to see how much sun or shade it requires. This will help determine where it should be placed in your garden. As important as where you place your plant is what you put your plant in. Which brings us to the question....

5. *What kind of soil do my herbs need?*

While it is true that most herbs can grow in the poorest of soils, the following adage usually holds true: *the better the soil composition, the healthier the herb*. This is not to say that herbs require a tremendous amount of fertilizer. Too much fertilizer tends to affect their natural growth. Unless you are fortunate to have a rich supply of healthy soil, you will probably need to bring in what is called "amendments" to enrich the planting ground. However, before bringing in just any ol' amendments, consider the pH of your soil (i.e., the acid/alkaline balance). Some herbs thrive in acid soil while others require a more alkaline environment. I will delve further into this soil subject in Chapter 2.

The bottom line is that many herbs can be grown in soil that is not consistent with what they prefer. In other words, acid soil loving herbs can sometimes make it in alkaline soil environments. However, the resulting plant may not be as striking or as medicinally active as you would wish. While you are contemplating the soil, don't forget to ask yourself...

6. *How much water do my herbs need?*

Many herbs, such as spearmint and cleavers, require a regular supply of water. Some herbalists make a point to plant their minty herbs under or near a dripping hose line to ensure a steady drip of water. Herbs like watercress not only need water, they need to be swimming in it 24 hours a day! Then there are plants such as rosemary, sage and thyme that require intermittent watering and actually flourish when they are allowed to almost dry out. If your garden has only one faucet source for your hose, try to plant the water-loving herbs close to the faucet to save yourself extra steps. If you happen to have a creek or natural spring running through your property, take advantage of it and place those water-craving herbs (such as watercress) in that area. Conversely, don't plant herbs that require little water in that area since it could stunt their growth due to root rot.

After you have answered these six questions, take a deep breath and ask yourself one more question...

7. *How much time do I have to commit to my herb garden?*

Once established, your average herb garden requires little upkeep, except for the requisite weeding and watering. However, obviously the more plants you have, the more attention you may need to pay to their continued growth. The bulk of your time will be spent in the initial seeding and/or sowing of established seedlings and plants. Consider including a high percentage of perennial medicinal plants into your garden or annuals that tend to re-seed themselves each season. That way, you can depend on seeing these faithful friends return year after year.

A medicinal herb garden is not just for visual enjoyment but also for harvesting. Once you determine what you want to do with your various herbs (i.e., making a tea, a tincture or a healing salve), you will be better able to decide how much time you will need to dedicate to your garden.

Remember to mark your planting rows with the name and/or seed packet photo of the herb! You may think you will remember what you put in the ground, but believe me, two months later it will be a distant memory!

Chapter 2

~

Is My Soil Satisfactory?

The nice thing about growing herbs is that most plants don't need special soil or fertilizers to help them grow. When you find herbs in their natural habitat, the soil is often rocky, parched and lacking in richness compared to the pampered beds of flowers found in front yards.

However, truly poor soil can yield poor, stunted herbs. What you are looking for in your soil is good aeration, crumbly to the touch and well drained so that water does not pool for hours on top. Use a shovel to dig into the dirt about ten inches deep. Is it easy to do or is it like chiseling stone? If it is the latter, you need to add some natural additives to make the dirt more pliable. Turn over the dirt. Is it dark and easily crumbled or does it rock to and fro like a granite boulder? If it resembles that boulder, you will want to add more soil conditioners to the ground. Some of the better conditioners are peat moss, sawdust and compost which should make up one-quarter to one-third of the soil volume. Don't 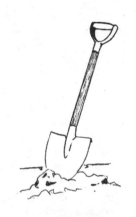 overdo on the compost thinking that "more is better." Too much compost can burn tender herbal plants as well as produce smaller varieties.

One herbalist I know swears that leaves are the best way to amend any kind of soil. According to her, leaves loosen up clay soil and tighten up sandy soil. I've tried using leaves and it seems to help but I also can't resist throwing in a little compost here and there. As always, if you want to purchase soil amendments, always try to locate those that are organic.

AFTER ADDING THE CONDITIONERS...

Once you have blended in your soil conditioners, you might want to check the pH level of your dirt. The pH measures the acid or alkaline content of the soil. The scale runs from 0 at the acid end to 14 for excessively alkaline. Most culinary and medicinal herbs flourish in a neutral pH soil which falls into the 6.0 to 7.5 range. Some herbs might require more acid or alkaline to encourage their growth. For specific acid or alkaline requirements, check the backs of plant seed packets or ask your nursery for their opinion. Your local nursery most likely sells an at-home pH kit that allows you to verify the acid/alkaline balance of your soil. Soil tests may also be available through your Agricultural Extension Service. The cost is either free or minimal. You can usually locate the Agricultural Extension Service by looking in the front of your telephone book under the "Government" heading and then looking under either the "county" or "state" listing.

If your backyard soil turns out to be on the overly acid side, try mixing five pounds of agricultural limestone for every 100 square feet of planting area. This should raise the pH by 1/2 to 1 point. Wood ashes can also create a more alkaline environment but don't go overboard with them since they can sometimes turn the soil too alkaline. If overly alkaline soil is your problem, add three pounds of iron sulfate for every 100 square feet of soil. This should lower the pH by 1/2 to 1 point.

Want to make an all-natural, homemade, nutritious, herbal "manure" for your herb garden?

This herbal "manure" is anti-fungal (the comfrey), a natural insecticide (the tansy) and supplies a high dose of nitrogen (stinging nettle) to the soil which helps green things grow faster. Best of all, it is easy to make!

Tightly pack equal parts fresh tansy flowers and stems, fresh comfrey leaves and stems and fresh nettle leaves and stems (wear gloves so you don't get stung!) into a cleaned out garbage can. Cover with water at least twice the volume. Cover and situate the garbage can so that it has full sun for at least four hours each day. Stir the mixture daily. The point is to literally let this concoction rot which takes about one or two weeks. The smellier and more pungent, the better. However, your neighbors may not take to that notion. After the liquid is sufficiently pungent, pour directly onto plants or dilute it half and half if you can't stand the smell. I must tell you that the aroma tends to linger for up to two days after pouring it on the plants. The fragrance is reminiscent of a sewage plant backing up which can cause a whole new set of problems if you live in close proximity to neighbors who don't appreciate your organic approach to gardening. I can tell you I have had to fib on a few occasions when bemused neighbors came knocking on my door, asking if I had reported the sewage problem to the city. After assuring them that all was taken care of, I rinsed down the smelly plants with just enough water to mask the strong odor but not enough to wash it away. While this homemade "manure" might not be pleasant to pour it will certainly help produce a healthier and happier herbal garden.

SOIL OF CLAY?

If soupy, lumpy, water-logged clay soil is your problem, you will have to add more amendments such as sawdust, peat moss and dried leaves to the ground. Good drainage is a must for all types of soil, but of paramount concern with the clay variety. Since clay holds water longer, root shoots become soaked with moisture and have a difficult time spreading underground as well as securely anchoring into the earth. One of the only herbs that is an exception to the heavy clay rule is watercress. Watercress demands a 24 hour supply of water and thrives in muddy places such as riverbanks, streams and ponds where the *addition* of clay helps to hold moisture for longer periods of time.

MATCH SOIL TO HERB

Always check to make sure if certain herbs require a specific type of soil. For example, sage and mullein do well in a dry, "undemanding" soil while nettles, lemon balm and spearmint need moist, rich soil to propagate healthy plants. The chart at the end of each herb chapter titled "The Dirt On..." states the specific kind of soil each herb needs.

Once your soil is in good shape and sufficiently tilled to promote adequate aeration, you are ready to start planting!

You Gotta Get Some Earthworms!

Although they are slimy to the touch, earthworms are your herb garden's best friend. Worms live to eat…and eat and eat and eat. In fact, some researcher with far too much time on his hands discovered that the average group of earthworms pass more than 50 tons of materials per acre through their little bodies. That "material" is called "castings" which contain twice the calcium, two and a half times the magnesium, five times the nitrates, seven times the phosphorus and eleven times the potassium of topsoil.

Best of all, earthworms love each other, which creates more and more workers to produce more and more castings. Ain't nature grand?

Should I Try Cover Cropping?

If your soil looks as if it has played its last song, maybe you should consider what is called "cover crops." Another term for this is "green manures." Cover crops/green manures are specific plants grown to improve the soil's mineral count, allow more aeration in compacted soils and fortify the resulting garden with massive amounts of vitamins and minerals.

Cover crops are also valuable since they cut the amount of compost or fertilizer normally needed. There are certain plants that work best as cover crops due to their innate mineral content or their ability to attract nutrients into the soil.

There are a host of plants that can work as cover crops. Using the herbs specifically mentioned in this book, they include burdock, black mustard, fennel, yellow dock (any dock will do actually), red clover and alfalfa. Burdock, yellow dock, red clover and alfalfa have a tendency to take over a yard. While this might be a problem for some gardeners, those who love medicinals consider it a blessing.

The point of cover cropping is to broadcast one type of seed over a large area with the intention of tilling it into the soil before or after it goes to seed. During this process, the deep tap roots and mineral-rich elements within the aerial parts merge into the ground, giving your garden a nutritious head start for the planting season.

Alfalfa is often mentioned when it comes to green manures. This cow-loving herb needs well-drained soil that is not too acid, falling somewhere between 6 and 7.5 on the pH scale. Alfalfa is considered a high-protein perennial crop that requires a full year of growth before being tilled under. It is worth the wait since research has shown a year-old stand of alfalfa can supply up to 200 pounds of nitrogen in addition to plenty of organic material per acre. Science has proven that alfalfa—as well as other plants in the legume family such as peas, beans and vetch—is able to host a unique kind of bacteria on the nodules of their roots called "rhizobia." The bacteria has the enviable ability to attract nitrogen in the air and "fix" it into the soil. One of the ways to ensure this "nitrogen fixing" ability is to coat the seed with something called an "inoculant" which is a specific strain of nitrogen-fixing bacteria suited for that particular seed. As the seeds sprout and mature, the bacteria enter the root hairs, grab the nitrogen from the air and bring it down to "fix" on the nodules of the root hairs. Inoculants can be purchased at nurseries or through seed catalogs. Make sure you match the right inoculant with the right seed. For more thorough instructions on how to use inoculants, read the directions provided on each bag.

To benefit from crop cover plants, it is a good idea to rotate them throughout your garden. Split your planting area in half and plant herbs on one side and the cover crop of your choice on the other. The following year, after tilling under the cover crop, reverse the plan.

You can turn over your cover crop with a shovel if the area in question is small enough and you've got energy to spare. Personally, I prefer the use of a rear-mounted rotary tiller since it makes a lot of noise and produces a lovely mulch as it eats and turns its way through the rows. If you don't own a rotary tiller, they can often be rented for the day.

Unless you wish to build up a storehouse of organic material in your soil, it is always best to turn over your cover crop while its leaves are still tender. If you wait until the cover crop goes to seed before turning it under, you will add rich organic humus to your land. However, you may also end up with a yearly supply of that cover crop since it will think it's a weed and act accordingly. If you plow it under after it goes to seed, wait eight to ten weeks before planting your herb garden. If you turn it under while it is still young, you can plant your medicinals in about two weeks.

~

Chapter 3

"CAN WE FINALLY PLANT SOMETHING?"

*Y*ou will probably choose either seeds or seedlings/plants for your herb garden. When purchasing seeds and live plants, it is important to find a nursery or catalog company that is established and reputable. *Johnny's Selected Seeds* in Albion, Maine has a wide variety of medicinal seed varieties for both the backyard and commercial grower. No matter what seed catalog you choose, it is imperative that you know not only the common name of the herb but the botanical Latin name as well. **Using the Latin botanical name when ordering your seeds or plants is very important when you are dealing with medicinal herbs.** For example, there are many types of medicinal echinacea, including *Echinacea angustifolia, Echinacea purpurea* and *Echinacea pallida*. While some herbalists like to combine all three echinacea species in their herbal formulas, others always choose their favorite individual species. For this reason, simply asking for "echinacea" results in the inevitable response, "Which one?" Another great example is the herb thyme. The herb seed catalog *The Thyme Garden* features over 60 varieties of this venerable herb, including camphor thyme, lavender thyme, pinewood thyme and lime thyme. If you call these folks up and say you want to buy a packet of thyme seed, you're obviously going to have to be more specific.

WATCH FOR THE DATE STAMP!

Seed packets should be stamped with the current year which ensures a certain amount of germination guarantee. If you buy last year's seed packets hoping to save a few dollars you might end up with a lower germination rate. While seeds are usually viable for up to five years (as long as they are stored in either airtight glass jars or sealed brown bags), the germination rate will decrease with each passing year.

WHAT'S A HYBRID AND WHY SHOULD I CARE?

A hybrid is a cross-pollinated plant that shares the characteristics of two different species of the same plant. Hybrids can occur in laboratories or naturally in the garden when two separate varieties of a plant are planted close to one another. For example, you might have *Echinacea angustifolia* growing alongside *Echinacea purpurea*. If the wind is right, the two could cross-pollinate and create a hybrid echinacea that blends the two plants into one. Sounds great, you say? Well, think again. The resulting hybrid seed is only good for one season of growth. After that, the hybrid plant is either sterile (non seed bearing) or bears seeds that are not true to type. In other words, when the hybrid seeds mature, the plants may be stunted or deformed in some way. Hybrids have a built in dependency factor—meaning that you, the grower, must depend upon the seed company each year to supply you with more seeds.

Hybrid seeds are often chemically treated to prevent disease. Those hybrid seeds that are manufactured in labs often lack the nutritional value of their open-pollinated (non-hybrid) seed counterparts. However, over the last 50 years, the public has been led to believe that hybrid seeds are the way to go when you want big, beautiful, bodacious plants in your garden. Many seed companies brag about their hybrids, boasting about the plant's wonderful uniform shape, large fruit or vibrant colors.

While bigger seems to equal better to some people, gardening purists shun anything that smacks of seed manipulation. There are many hybrid vegetable seeds on the market. Fortunately, there are currently only a handful of hybrid herb seeds. Thank goodness for small favors. Medicinal herb gardens are not meant to be filled with flashy, "sexy" plants that defy the laws of nature. On the whole, a functional medicinal herb garden should look like rows of cultivated weeds.

I mention this subject simply for those who may be unaware of this gardening trend and to encourage gardeners (those who love herbs as well as those who adore their vegetables) to support the small seed companies who dedicate themselves to open-pollinated or "Heirloom" seed varieties which are true to the plants that grew hundreds of years ago and which will always produce a viable seed. The "faster, better, quicker" approach, in my opinion, does not belong in the herb or vegetable garden.

The word "hybrid" is not always easily visible on seed packets. However, when you see an "x" in the plant's botanical name, this is an indication that it is indeed a hybrid variety. Each catalog will have its own coding for hybrids which could be anything from an "x" to a "•." Look for a symbols box in front of the catalog to determine what coding is used. When you see words like "open-pollinated" or "heirloom," you are assured of non-hybrid seeds. When in doubt, you can always call or write the company and ask if they include hybrid seeds in their herb selections.

SHOULD I PRE-SOAK MY SEEDS?

Pre-soaking seeds can often help when germination is difficult. Unfortunately this method is not as effective for small seeds (such as yarrow or mullein) or seeds that are light and almost feathery to the touch. The reason is that these types of seeds tend to clump up in the water and become almost impossible to separate for planting.

However, larger seeds such as alfalfa and red clover may benefit greatly from eight to ten hours of pre-soaking. Place the seeds in small bowls of lukewarm water since cold water can "shock" the seeds and delay or prevent germination. Some herbal purists only use bottled spring water or tap water that has been run through a purifier to prevent additives such as chlorine in the city tap water from soaking into their seeds. If you want to do this, make sure you warm the water slightly so the seeds are not chilled. Remember to slip the seed packet under each bowl so you will remember which seeds go with which packet. Cover with a dishcloth or newspaper to keep pets and bugs out of the bowl. After eight to ten hours, strain the water from the seeds and plant them while they are still water-soaked.

Adding one or two drops of liquid kelp fertilizer to each bowl of water gives the seeds an extra boost of vitamins and, some say, encourages healthier growth of the plant. Liquid kelp fertilizer can be found at many garden nurseries as well as health food stores in the seed sprouting department. One effective brand I like is the *Sproutman's Kelp Fertilizer* which is made by The Sprout House in Ramona, California.

THE SECRETS TO SUCCESSFUL SEEDING

When you start growing medicinal herbs, you will quickly learn a new word: stratifying. It is also referred to as "pre-chilling" in some catalogs. Some medicinal herbs such as arnica, wintergreen, mullein, marshmallow, echinacea angustifolia and St. John's wort—to name only a few—germinate best when placed in a pot or flat, moistened with water and then allowed to chill at around 35 to 40 degrees Fahrenheit. How long does the plant need to chill? That depends entirely on the specific seed. For an herb such as mullein, you may only need to chill the pot or flat of seeds for one or two days. However, wintergreen needs to be chilled a minimum of 60 days, with some seeds requiring 120 days before they will germinate. There are always exceptions to the rule. Some herbs that supposedly have strict guidelines, such as I indicated, decide to sprout no matter what the conditions. That's the mystery and sometimes the frustration of Mother Nature.

TO COVER OR NOT TO COVER

If seeds haven't germinated fast enough for you in the past, maybe it's because you are dowsing them with too much dirt. As a general rule, large seeds need to be covered with a sprinkling of soil while small seeds should be scattered onto the soil, then pressed firmly into the dirt. As always, there are exceptions to

17

this rule. Some large seeds, such as garden sage should not be covered in dirt since they need plenty of light to germinate. Your best bet is to check the individual seed packet for each herb and note any special light or dark requirements. Some of the major seed catalogs such as *Johnny's Selected Seeds* give a great deal of information under each medicinal herb heading, including light, soil, and germination time. Another seed company catalog, *Horizon Herbs*, also goes into great detail on how to plant their seeds as well as important things to consider.

LIGHT VERSUS DARKNESS

Grow lights are gaining more popularity, especially when you need to start seeds two or three months in advance in colder climates. Available in full spectrum, glass tubing, grow lights mimic natural sunlight which "tricks" the seed into germinating in an artificial environment. The mistake some people make with grow lights is that they assume that if 16 hours of artificial light speeds the growth of their seeds and/or seedlings, round the clock artificial light will make them grow even faster. The fact is that all plants need a certain amount of darkness during the germination process. Thus, make sure your seeds get about five to seven hours of continuous darkness each day.

There are some seeds that actually require darkness in order to germinate. Fennel, horehound and blue violet are a few herbs that germinate best in darkness. To achieve this, you can actually place your growing flat under a bed or couch or simply cover it with a towel or piece of burlap. However, check the flat daily to see if any of the seeds have germinated. **When one of them has germinated, the flat can be placed in indirect light**. Many novice herb growers have mistakenly kept the flat in darkness, expecting all of the seeds to germinate. Unfortunately, what happens is that by the time the last seeds germinate the first seedlings are dying from lack of light.

KEEP THAT TEMPERATURE LEVEL

Excluding the seeds that require pre-chilling, most seeds need a steady temperature of 70 to 85 degrees F. to germinate. After sprouting, it is best for the temperature to be a constant 60 to 65 degrees F. Basil, for example, flourishes in direct sun and germinates best when the temperature is a constant 70 to 75 degrees F. Never expose your seeds to sharp drops in low temperatures—such as from 70 degrees F. to a chilly 45 degrees F.—since this will shock them and lessen your chances for successful germination.

DON'T OVER WATER!

The tendency for some gardeners is to over water their seeds in hopes of making them grow faster. Drowning seeds in water is never a good idea and may cause the seeds to lose contact with the soil. Additionally, once your seeds turn into seedlings, do not douse them with too much water since their delicate bodies will quickly absorb every bit of water and literally become waterlogged. Once this happens, seedlings quickly droop and die.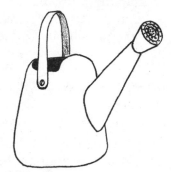

The only exceptions to this "do not drown seeds" rule is the wild edible, salad plant/herb, watercress. Watercress, as its name implies, needs to be swimming in water. In fact, watercress grows best when it's *under* water, such as in stream beds and ponds. Herbs in the mint family—spearmint, peppermint, catnip and lemon balm—also require moist (but *not* soggy!) soil to germinate as well as a steady stream of daily water to ensure steady and healthy growth.

For all other seeds, gently mist them with lukewarm water—cold water tends to "stun" the seeds and shuts off their desire to sprout. Never let the soil completely dry out or germination will stop completely.

GETTING A JUMP ON MOTHER NATURE

Depending upon how involved you want to get in the seeding process, there are several variables that can help guarantee greater germination as well as speed the initial growth of seedlings.

If you live in a climate where you have less than 90 frost-free days, you will need to start your seeds indoors under controlled lighting and heating conditions in order to see your herbs reach maturity. A greenhouse is an ideal answer for those living in areas where summer months are short-lived. (If a greenhouse is impractical for you, consider container planting for some of your herbs which is discussed in-depth in Chapter 6).

If you do not know what the individual herb seedlings look like, you should plant the seeds in a sterile soil mix specifically blended for seed trays. "Sterile" soil simply means that the dirt has been sifted and is free of stray seeds or roots that might appear in addition to the seeds you plant. It is best not to mix compost into the sterile soil mix since compost often has other plants (i.e., seeds) blended in which can cause plant identification confusion during germination when your seeds sprout along with the seeds hidden within the compost.

Frankly, I'm not a big lover of sterile, store-bought soil since it is devoid of nutrients which young seedlings need for a healthy start. I much prefer to bring home several six-gallon sized pails of rich, moist, "quakie" dirt (soil that grows under wild aspen trees) and start my seeds in that medium. However—and this is a *big* "however"—if you do not have any idea what your herb seedlings are supposed to look like, non-sterile soil will often produce not just your seeds but whatever other seeds happened to be hanging out in the soil at the time you collected it. Since you won't be able to identify which is your seedling and which is some wild thing, you'll be too afraid to pick any of it out of the dirt. The result is that the wild seedlings can, in turn, crowd out your herb seedlings and then you're back to square one. The answer to this dilemma: until you can tell the difference between what you planted and what is volunteering in the soil, stick with the store-bought, sterile mix.

CELLS & FLATS

You can plant your herbs in plastic flats in rows of two or three depending upon the size of the seed. However, some herb farmers prefer to use individual plastic "cells" which nestle in the flat. Cells are simply individual compartments with a drainage slit at the bottom that accommodate one to three seeds. Large seeds need a larger cell while smaller seeds can handle a smaller cell. Typically, nurseries and seed catalogs sell 72 cell trays (which is a very small cell for small seeds), 38 cell trays and 24 cell trays. While you will obviously be able to get more seeds in the 72 cell tray, there is not a lot of room for growth once the seed germinates. This means you will need to transplant the seedling sooner or you will have a mish-mash of roots protruding beneath the cell and getting criss-crossed with roots from nearby cells. Using a cell tray also allows you to literally "pop" the individual seedling out of its cell and plop it into the ground when it is time to transplant it.

A "FASTER" PLANT

Whether you choose to use plain dirt flats or flats with cell trays, one way to speed up germination of your seeds is to cover them with a clear plastic raised dome. Plastic raised domes can be bought through seed catalogs as well as your nursery. These tough, resilient domes, hold in both moisture and heat, much like a mini-greenhouse effect. The result of using a dome means that germination of seeds is between 20 and 40 percent faster. Other advantages of plastic domes include reducing the need to water the seeds due to the artificially created humid environment.

FIGHTING BUGS WITH BUGS

The first time somebody told me to buy a box of bugs in order to get rid of some ferocious garden pests, I thought they were a few stacks short of a full pancake breakfast. The idea of introducing still more annoying flying creatures into my garden was foreign to my sensibilities. But when it was explained to me that there are "beneficial insects" that live to devour such pests as aphids, whiteflies, grasshoppers, mites and much more, my interest was piqued.

Since I run screaming from anything with the words "chemical" on the can, the idea of letting nature do its thing was intriguing. I started researching this "bug eats bug" phenomenon and discovered some odd little facts. Robert Kourik writes in his book *Designing and Maintaining Your Edible Landscape Naturally* that if we didn't have the natural balance of predatory and parasitic insects, "we would be over our heads in a mass of bugs." Kourik states that "In one year, a single adult aphid, left unchecked by nature's ecological controls, would bury the earth a mile deep in new aphids!" After sitting back and visualizing that horrid sight, I decided I'd give it the ol' herbal try.

Here is the way beneficial insects work. First, there are two kinds of beneficial insects: "predators" and "parasites." Predator insects spend their entire lives eating other insects. Parasite insects, on the other hand, deposit an egg within the targeted insect (or host) from which a larva emerges that, in turn, eats the host's innards. Lovely, eh?

In order for both predators and parasites to have enough energy to destroy their targets, they typically require plenty of nectar, pollen and sap. In other words, they can't survive on bugs alone. This is something to consider when you decide to use beneficial insects in your yard.

Some predator and parasite insects that I have had good luck using include: ladybird beetles or ladybugs (various varieties eat aphids, mealybugs, armored scales and mites), green lacewings (loves aphids, mealybugs, scale, whiteflies and mites), tachinid flies (a parasite of many grasshoppers, beetles, sawflies and caterpillars) and dragonflies (which feast on small flying insects including the pesky mosquito).

There are many more predator and parasite insects available through either local or mail order suppliers. If you purchase your bugs through the postal service, they will be sent by overnight mail and must be released in your yard as indicated on the box. Some insects require release within 48 hours of receipt while others can last for weeks if kept under the proper conditions.

For myself, fighting bugs with bugs has introduced me to a whole new world. It has also given me a new respect for the "good" bugs of the world. I now have a greater understanding of nature's checks and balances as I sit and watch in amazement as my store-bought insects consume those nasty destructive creatures with glee. Consider it just another form of free garden entertainment.

When using plastic domes over your flats, DO NOT leave the flat in direct sunlight. Two things will happen: first, the seeds will become too hot and a white or green mold can develop in the dirt. Secondly, while the plastic domes are durable, the extreme heat will eventually crack and break the dome's surface. Indirect sunlight is your best bet to ensure controlled heat within the unit and many seasons of use from your plastic domes.

Plastic wrap can be used in place of factory-made plastic domes. However, plastic wrap has a tendency to sink in the middle so you will have to tape it tightly to the sides of the flat to create a taut surface. Since plastic wrap will not "rise up," you will need to remove it sooner than you would the raised plastic domes, when the seedlings begin pressing against the surface of the plastic wrap.

Some growers suggest using sheets of glass in lieu of plastic domes. However, glass is expensive, creates a greater amount of heat under the flat and is not very practical since it is so easy to break. In addition, it is far too easy to cut your fingers, hands and arms on the sharp edges of the glass.

TRANSPLANTING—WHEN & HOW

Seedlings can be safely transplanted into larger growing containers or outside (when the freeze warnings have passed) once they have two pairs of leaves and/or are at least two inches in height.

Transplanting is best done in the evening after the sun has set. Transplanting during the day under the hot sun can dry out tender seedlings, making their transfer more tenuous. If you are able to do your transplanting after sunset, your seedlings will have at least eight hours of cool, evening temperatures to perk back to life before the morning sun beats down on them.

It is always best to "harden off" your herbs outside before transplanting. Hardening off means to set the seed flat outside in partial shade—*never in direct sunlight*—for two or three hours each day to get them accustomed to the less protected outside world. This can be done two or three days in advance of transplanting. Herbs that are hardened off first before transplanting tend to suffer less shock. If you lose a few seedlings during this process, don't get too upset with yourself. Chances are, those seedlings were too weak to survive the transplant in the first place.

How To Make A Cheap, Mineral-rich Water For Your Indoor & Outdoor Plants

Don't discard the water after boiling eggs. When the water is lukewarm, pour it into the soil around the main stem of the herb. The eggshell releases minerals into the water that will give your seeds and full grown plants a natural boost!

> ## *PAY ATTENTION TO THE WILD ONES*
>
> When you find an herb in the wild, you might think that it didn't take any special soil, lighting, temperature or treatment for it to grow. But think again. Nature has its own rules for wild plants. For example, plants that require plenty of moisture and shade generally will not be found in dry, sun-filled wastelands. Many of the so-called "rules" for successful seed cultivation are partly due to watching the plant in the wild. If a cultivated, garden herb needs to have a certain temperature to germinate, for instance, it is a good bet that it's wild counterpart happens to live in that exact environment and requires the same conditions. When you are out in meadows, forests or along stream beds, pay close attention to the plants that are growing in these areas. Look around the area and see what other herbs are growing around them. After you become more aware of what grows where, you will start to see similarities when it comes to poor soil versus rich soil and full sun versus partial shade. Once you learn the tendencies of specific herbs, you will be better able to judge the likelihood of finding it based upon the places it enjoys growing. For example, cleavers is typically found growing in shady, moist soil in often densely forested areas. Knowing this, you wouldn't head out to the middle of the parched desert in search of cleavers.

Stop watering your seedlings for two days before the transplant. Watered seedlings are difficult to handle since the protective dirt tends to break apart, leaving you with a fragile, dangling seedling that has nothing to support it.

Try to handle the seedlings as little as possible since the salt from body perspiration has been known to wilt a tender leaf in minutes. Gently dig them out of their seed flat with a spoon or trowel, making sure you dig deep enough to unearth the myriad of roots that are forming. If you are using seed flats that have individual seed cells, you can easily pop the seedlings out from the bottom of the cell.

Be sure to water your herbs well after transplanting but don't saturate the soil with too much water. Gently pat down the earth around the seedling's root to ensure that the roots are firmly sunk into the ground.

Remember to have garden "name tags" ready to place into the ground so you will know what you have planted. Old popsicle sticks make good markers. Write the names of each herb with one of those permanent ink pens that won't fade or run when it rains.

DIRECT SEEDING

If you live in climates that aren't prone to seasonal freeze warnings, direct seeding into the garden may be your best bet. Aside from the herb seeds that require special care (such as stratifying/pre-chilling), the rest can easily be sown into the warm soil with no problems. You will still need to identify what soil works best for each herb seed and how much light is needed for the seeds to germinate. One of the mistakes I used to make when direct sowing outdoors was burying every single seed I planted. I soon learned that many herb seeds enjoy a light dusting of soil over them. However, simply broadcasting a handful of seeds into a field, wishing them luck and walking away doesn't always work either. If a strong wind comes up a day or two after you've cast your seed onto the soil, those little fellows could be blown in a variety of directions. What I like to do with small seeds that require light (chickweed, red clover and spearmint to name a few), is broadcast a handful down a row and then walk over them, which presses them into the ground while still allowing a certain amount of light to hit them. Remember to thin the seedlings once they are two to three inches tall to allow plants plenty of "elbow room" to grow.

GIVE YOUR GARDEN A TEA BREAK

Are you troubled by poor soil?

Do you want to strengthen seedlings and help them to become more disease-resistant?

Of course you do! And I have three great garden teas that can do wonders for your herbs.

The first one is dandelion. The fresh flowers from this prolific weed can be used to help establish seedlings and/or plants to draw up the necessary nutrients it needs from the soil. Dandelion tea can also help remedy the deficiencies inherent in poor soil. To make the tea, place four to five handfuls of fresh dandelion flowers in a large cook pot. Cover with one gallon of water and gently heat without boiling. Turn off the heat and cover the pot, allowing the mixture to sit eight to ten hours. Strain the flowers heads and pour the liquid around the base of each plant. Remember to ONLY use dandelion flowers that have not been sprayed with pesticides.

The second terrific tea is chamomile. Two handfuls of chamomile flowers should be soaked in one gallon of cold water for three days. Cover and stir the mixture occasionally. Spray or water seedlings with the full strength tea to prevent many plant maladies such as damping off disease (a destrutive fungus that attacks seedlings, forcing them to flop over and die).

The third garden tea is made from oak bark. This mighty tea is thought to encourage a strong, lush growth pattern as well as deter disease such as rot and mildew. Additionally oak bark tea also infuses plants with a built-in tolerance to drought as well as encourages a hearty seed production. To make this magnificent oak bark tea, place one cup of dried bark for every one cup of water into a large cook pot. Bring the mixture just to a boil and then remove from the heat. Keep the mixture covered and store in a dark, cool area for three to four weeks. When it is ready, the solution can be sprayed or poured undiluted over herbs every seven to ten days. For stubborn or lackluster looking herbs, you can use the oak bark tea mixture several days in a row, with a 10 day break interval.

CAN I DIRECT SEED ALL SEEDS AT THE SAME TIME?

Another mistake I made when I was just starting out with herb gardens was thinking that all herb seeds were planted in the spring. After wasting a lot of time and money on seeds, I discovered that some seeds are best sown in the fall for a spring arrival. Often, these are plants that require stratification (pre-chilling) time in order to germinate. As always, there are exceptions to this rule. For example, it is best to plant mullein seeds in late fall since the seed needs cold temperatures to sprout. However, I have broken all the rules and scattered mullein seed on the ground in late spring and early summer and had some minor success. The only problem is that those late spring/early summer seedlings never matured as well as the ones planted in late fall.

CHOOSING ESTABLISHED PLANTS INSTEAD OF SEEDS

For those of you who fear your thumb is anything but green, choosing established herb plants over seeds might be your best bet. Some medicinal herbs such as true peppermint can only be garnered from the plant since the herb is sterile and reproduces by root runners only. Other herbs such as rosemary and rose hips require a demanding set of criteria to grow and should be bought as established plants unless you love gardening challenges.

When choosing your herb seedlings or fully grown plants from the nursery, only purchase the plants that have healthy leaves, flowers and stems. If the plant looks droopy, has brown or dried leaves underneath or looks as though it could be the "runt" of the litter, pass it by and find a stronger looking plant.

ROOT CUTTINGS

Root cuttings are another option over seeds in some cases. It generally works best with herbs that have large or well established roots. The only exception to this rule are herbs that have long tap roots such as anise. Unfortunately, they don't transplant very well and those that do make it, have to be treated like precious gems in order to flourish. I've had the best luck with herbs that send out new growth from spreading roots. Spearmint, horehound and watercress are three good examples. To plant a root cutting, you'll need to dig up the herb you want (remember, only choose herbs that are healthy and show signs of strong growth) and shake off the dirt. Look for sections two to four inches in length that have at least one bud present. Cut these sections at horizontal angles and space them two to four inches apart in your garden. Cover them with one inch of soil, gently packing the earth on top of them. Water the area thoroughly without allowing it to become too muddy. The soil must remain continually moist for any growth to occur.

The best time to plant root cuttings is in early to late spring, especially if you live in climates that have short growing seasons. If you live where the sun shines and the snow doesn't fall, make sure you plant root cuttings during periods of the year when there will be steady daytime temperatures above 70^0 F. and evening temperatures that do not fall below 50^0 F.

GIVE YOUR HERBS A BUDDY TO BOND WITH IN THE GARDEN

The term "companion planting" means choosing groupings of plants that assist each other in growth and development. While there are those who consider this more "hooey" than science, I have found it to be helpful in many cases. For example, fennel is generally disliked by most garden plants and, therefore, should be given a nice little spot all to itself. However, planting yarrow or stinging nettle next to herbs that have natural volatile oils (such as spearmint and lemon balm) tend to increase those aromatic oils. For more specifics on companion planting, check the chart at the end of each chapter to determine the compatibility of different herbs.

Once your herbs take off and mature into healthy specimens, it will be time to harvest your crop, dry the plants and collect seeds for next season.

NATURAL & GENTLE PEST CONTROL FOR YOUR PLANTS

Since you will be using your herb garden for medicinal purposes, you do not want to use any chemical pesticides on your plants. Here are seven natural solutions that really work to rid your plants of whiteflies, aphids, snails and many more destructive intruders.

• In a 32 oz. squirt bottle that has a large spray opening, place one pinch of cayenne pepper for every 8 oz. of warm water. Shake the bottle vigorously and spray herbs from a distance of approximately three to four feet. Allow the cayenne to softly filter down onto the plant as opposed to clumping up on it. Bugs hate cayenne and many herbs love it. Some herb growers swear that occasional use of cayenne spray encourages herbs to grow faster and larger.

• Dr. Bronner's Liquid Peppermint Soap (available at most health food stores) can be diluted one-half teaspoon to two gallons of warm water and misted on plants to repel aphids and other bothersome garden critters. Since the soap is biodegradable, it will not harm your soil. You will need to follow through with this soapy treatment every other day for optimum effectiveness. Of course, if it rains, you will have to reapply the soap after each downpour.

• Place one to three tablespoons *each* of powdered kelp, cayenne powder and biodegradable soap (once again, I use Dr. Bronner's brand) into one gallon of water. Shake vigorously, then lavishly pour or spray on plants. I've had good success using this method to rid my plants of whiteflies.

• While on the subject of whiteflies, try this unusual but very effective deterrent. Hang or tack a bright shiny canary yellow plastic plate directly one inch above or to the side of each affected plant. Lightly spray the surface of the yellow plate with an inexpensive brand of cooking spray. The plate should not be dripping with the oil, but it should be sufficiently covered. For some unknown reason, whiteflies absolutely adore bright yellow and drive headlong into the plate, pasting themselves into the oil. To be effective, once a day I suggest you wipe away the trapped whiteflies and spray another coat of cooking oil on the plate. It is not a 100 percent solution for whiteflies, but it definitely puts a dent in their progress. For really stubborn whitefly problems, I recommend using both the kelp/cayenne/soap mixture along with the yellow plates.

• Strong teas—double or triple strength—of thyme or rosemary make aromatic sprays that help repel flies and general insects without affecting beneficial bugs.

• One cup of feverfew flower heads can be ground into a fine powder and soaked overnight in a gallon of water. The next day, add two tablespoons of a biodegradable liquid soap, shake the jug vigorously and spray or pour on plants to combat an array of nasty flying and crawling pests that seek to damage your herbs.

• Colloidal silver helps prevent fungus from growing on plants. Place one or two droppers of colloidal silver in a quart of warm water and spray on herbs. This treatment needs to be done daily if plants are chronically prone to fungus.

Chapter 4

WHAT DO I DO WITH ALL THIS STUFF?

~

HARVESTING, DRYING & SEED COLLECTING

Just as there is a better way to plant your seeds, there is also a preferable method for harvesting, drying and collecting seed from your fully grown herbs.

HARVESTING

When herbs are harvested correctly, you can almost guarantee greater potency of the plant and, often times, better taste. Cutting leaves, stems and flowers allows your herbs to flourish and actually stimulates new growth.

Leaves are always best picked *before* the herb flowers to ensure tenderness. After flowering, leaves often become tough and lacking in the taste department. The optimum time of day for gathering leaves is early morning, after the dew has evaporated but before the sun becomes too hot. Pick herbs only on sunny, dry days since moisture-laden plants are at risk for forming molds. If you wish to harvest the entire plant, always make sure there are at least two sets of leaves left on the stem. This way, the herb can keep growing, allowing you to possibly obtain another cutting before the plant becomes dormant for fall or winter. Scissors are preferred over using your hands since you can get a cleaner cut. When you cut the leaf, slice it diagonally. This method often promotes faster recovery of the herb and tends to generate renewed growth.

Flowers should be harvested when they are at their fullest and/or most colorful. Discard flowers that have brown edges or turned up petals. Some herbs, such as St. John's wort, are at their most medicinally active when there are both flowers *and* buds present on the plant. Other herb favorites, such as calendula, produce a bevy of flowers from one plant and are actually "activated" to bloom more frequently when flower heads are picked.

Roots of perennials (plants that live and bear fruit and seeds for many years before dying) are best dug up in the autumn since that is the time the energy of the plant is concentrated in the ground. The second best time to dig up roots is early spring—i.e., March or April, depending upon when the ground thaws out. However, once leaves, buds and flowers begin appearing on the herb, the healing energy has left the root and is involved in the maturing process of the aerial parts of the plant. Because of this, the root is lacking in healing energy at this time. Does this mean that if you need a root in the middle of summer from a particular perennial herb, it won't do it's job? No, it just won't have the same high potency it has in autumn or early spring.

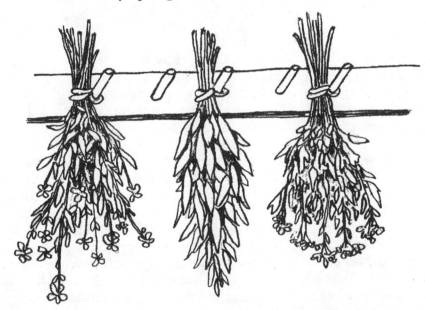

Roots of annual herbs (plants that have one year of life before going to seed and dying) are at their medicinal best when they are harvested before the plant flowers. If gathered after the flowering, the annual's root is less active.

Roots of biennial herbs (plants that establish a good root system the first year, flower and/or bear fruit the second year and then die) should be gathered in autumn of the *first* year after the foliage has fallen. If you gather a biennial herb's roots in the second year of life when the plant is bearing seeds, flowers and/or fruits, the root tends to be tougher and lacking in medicinal power.

Barks of trees are typically harvested in early to late spring. It is at this time when it is the easiest to release the inner bark (which is what you are after) from the rough outside protective bark. However, I have harvested bark as late as mid-summer and, aside from having a bit more difficulty separating the inner bark, it has worked out just fine. To harvest bark, **use only the branches of trees, NOT the trunk**. Improper harvesting of tree trunks by overly enthusiastic herbalists has lead to the early death of many trees.

The only exception to this rule is if you happen upon a recently fallen tree in the woods. "Recently fallen" is defined as a tree that still has some sap running through it. This could be due to the fact that it did not completely separate from its roots when it fell. By the way, I don't encourage the practice of using your body or a bulldozer to knock down trees that are leaning over simply because you think they are "ready to die." Many of these "leaning" trees still have years of life in them. If you find a tree that is leaning over and dead as a doornail, pass it up since you will not be able to harvest anything off of it. To harvest the trunk bark off recently fallen trees, use either a sharp, pointed knife for bark that is not too thick and hard or a small, sharpened hatchet for tree trunks that are more dense and difficult to remove. Make a horizontal cut approximately six inches around the diameter of the trunk and then match that cut one foot above it. Cut two horizontal line cuts to connect the horizontal cuts, thus forming a square. Cut or pry the square section away from the trunk of the tree. This is what you are going to work with. Peel, cut, chisel or slice the outer bark away from the inner layer of bark (which is the active medicinal part that you will keep). Discard all of the outer bark since it contains too many tannins which are terribly bitter and far too astringent for the body. If you can, try to peel the inner bark off the outer bark in strips, which makes the drying process easier.

The inner bark of the branches can be harvested from recently fallen or standing trees. Choose branches that still have life coursing through them and do not break. For large branches, repeat the harvesting process mentioned above for recently fallen trees. For smaller branches, use a knife or, better yet, garden snippers, slicing the branches off with a diagonal cut. Personally, unless I really need the bark, I don't bother with small branches since the energy I exert in the harvest is far greater than the amount of inner bark I am able to gather.

If you attempt to harvest trunk bark (from recently fallen trees) or branch bark at the wrong time of year (late summer or fall), chances are you'll find that it is either too difficult to pry the inner bark from the outer bark or that there is hardly any inner bark left to peel.

Fruits should be harvested when they are ripe. However, not all fruits are harvested during the summer. Rose hips mature in late fall, often after one or two light snow showers which tend to seal in their sweet taste.

The gummy resin/sap/pitch of a tree is best obtained in the early morning or after sunset when it is more solid. If you live in snowy climates, sap is often easy to remove when the thermometer dips below freezing. Look for natural scars on the tree where the sap is present. If you cannot find any natural cut on the trunk that is within reach, you can hammer a four inch nail halfway into the trunk of the tree and then immediately remove it. Within 24 hours, you should see sap dripping from where the nail entered the tree trunk. Use this process only as a final option. If I can't harvest sufficient sap from a tree, I just keep walking and searching until I discover a tree which is naturally scarred and producing sap.

DRYING

Many herbalists feel that certain herbs work best for medicinal purposes when they are used fresh. However, circumstances and climate often dictate that some of your herbal bounty will need to be dried and stored for later use.

Before you dry your plants, DO NOT rinse them with water to get rid of dirt or bugs. This tends to darken the dried plant, promote mold and sometimes reduce its inherent medicinal value. (The only exception to this "no rinse" rule is when you harvest roots). For the same reason, do not pick plants for drying out of the garden or the wild after a rain storm. Allow all moisture to naturally evaporate before cutting the plants. If you are concerned about dirt and bugs, you can occasionally shake your herbs as they are drying.

To dry leaves, gather a bunch of stems, tie securely at one end with string or a rubber band and suspend upside down in a dust-free, warm, non-humid environment. Leaves can also be dried separately in a screened, air dryer. However, they have a tendency to curl and not be as tasty as leaves hung upside down. One of the theories for this is that when the stems are hung upside down, the volatile oils within the stem and leaves are forced downward which enhances the flavor and texture of the dried leaf. Once the stem of leaves is dry—it should easily break apart between your fingers—the leaves are ready to be stripped from their stem and stored. (For proper storage, see Chapter Five).

Flowers are also best dried suspended upside down. Some larger flower heads such as yarrow can be picked off the plant individually and allowed to air dry on parchment paper or a clean cloth. Newspaper is not a good idea since the dye used in the ink has a chemical base.

Roots should be cleaned immediately with cool water. Cut off any small side shoots and then slice the root in half lengthwise. Larger roots, such as burdock which has a taproot that can extend two or three feet, can be cut into three inch sections and then split in half. If the root is fat, you might want to cut it into four lengthwise slices to speed the drying process. Roots are best dried on parchment paper or on a clean cloth and out of direct sunlight. *This is very important* since direct sunlight will sap all of the inherent volatile oils within the root. Roots can also be dried in a slow oven between 100 and 120 degrees F. Crack the oven door a few inches to make sure the roots are not trapped in the heat. Remember that this is not an Olympic race—roots need to be given as much time as they need to dry, with as low a temperature as possible. Roots are ready to be stored when they are hard, brittle and, if small enough, easily broken.

Barks are easy to dry, especially if they have been pulled off in narrow strips instead of chunks. Some people go to the trouble of threading wire or string through a series of them (ala a string of popcorn) and hanging them in a ventilated, shady area to dry. You can do this but it takes considerable time and patience. Usually I just lay the strips of bark on paper towels or in my screened air dryer. In three or four days, they are ready to break into smaller pieces and store in airtight glass jars.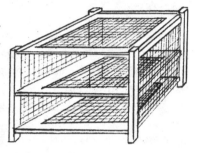

Most fruits are at their medicinal peak when they are eaten fresh. Drying can sap up to half their healing value. That's not to say that dried fruits are worthless. I'm just not sure how much dried fruit you'd have to eat in order to get any medicinal benefit. Some fruits, such as rose hips, should have the seeds painstakingly removed first before drying. (You can read more in-depth information about rose hips in chapter 28). Others, such as cherries, need only to have their single stone removed before drying. Your best bet as far as retaining the most medicinal punch from fruits is to discover good recipes where the fresh fruit is made into an *uncooked* jam or spread. I say uncooked because, once again, cooking really reduces the healing advantage of any fruit. (In the rose hips chapter, there is a recipe for "jam" made from the uncooked hips. I'm sure it could be adapted to any fruit within reason).

A FEW RULES OF THE GAME

Don't allow plants to over dry or they will lose their medicinal potency, odor and taste. Never place any part of an herb in direct sunlight to dry since it will vastly reduce the natural oil content in the plant which, in turn, limits its healing benefit. Additionally, keep your drying area free from excess humidity since this can attract mold to the herbs. Also, do your best to keep dust or fumes from cars or appliances away from the herbs. For this reason, kitchens and garages are not your best choices.

Attics and basements make good drying areas if they are clean and relatively dust free. If you simply cannot find an adequate place to dry the herbs, consider investing in or making a mesh covered housing unit for your herbs which will prevent most dust and airborne debris from getting on the plants. Mesh covered units will *not*, however, insulate them from airborne fumes.

GRAB THOSE SEEDS!

Seeds are the foundation to next year's crop. In some cases, such as with anise, fennel and fenugreek, the seed is actually the medicinal part of the plant.

You may not have to depend completely upon your local nursery or herb catalog for your favorite seeds if you know how to gather them properly. Seeds can be hidden in pods, flower heads, or as in the case of rose hips, in the actual herbal healing fruit. Wait until the herb is in the last stages of development to collect its seeds. If you pick a plant too early for its seed, you will stop the growth process and, thus, its seed development.

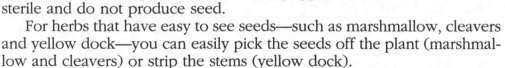

For small seeds that are difficult to collect, suspend a handful of branches with flower heads/pods/fruits attached, upside down and enclose in a paper bag. Secure the paper bag around the top of the stem with a string or rubber band. Allow the plant to dry in an enclosed, dry, non-humid environment, shaking the bag every now and then to help dislodge trapped seeds. If the seed still stays stubbornly in the flower head, once the herb is dry try gently rubbing the dried flowers between the palm of your hands and it should then be released. Typically, you will be able to garner seeds within two to four weeks. Remember that some plants, such as true peppermint, are sterile and do not produce seed.

For herbs that have easy to see seeds—such as marshmallow, cleavers and yellow dock—you can easily pick the seeds off the plant (marshmallow and cleavers) or strip the stems (yellow dock).

For seeds that are lodged in pods—fenugreek and mustard, for example—always allow the pods to dry on the plant and harvest before they burst. You may need to watch the plant carefully to decide on the optimum time for pod harvesting. Remember that some seed pods on the same plant will mature faster than others. I like to cut the pods off individually as they are ready and toss them in a brown paper bag. Keep the bag open so that air can circulate. As the pods dry, they will pop open and release the seed. This can be quite entertaining by itself. I had a bag full of dried mustard pods which took on a life of its own one day when all the pods decided to burst within a period of hours. I may be mistaken, but I could have sworn the bag twitched and even slightly jumped a few times from the internal explosions.

PLAYING GOD IN YOUR GARDEN

One good point to remember when collecting seed is that you only want to choose seed from herbs that are healthy and are providing you with a sufficient amount of leaves, flowers, fruits and/or roots. Consider this your chance to take part in natural selection. If you choose seed from herbs that are stunted, bearing little flower or fruit and have withering roots, it doesn't take a NASA scientist to know the seeds from that particular herb will reproduce low quality offspring.

This specific selection process is termed choosing a "cultivar" seed. It allows the herb grower to not only choose the healthiest plants for next year's growth but also gives one the opportunity to reproduce certain characteristics in future strains. For example, the medicinal part of red clover is the flower. If you spot a particular red clover plant in your yard that has lovely fat, vibrant light pink flower heads with no brown discoloration, there is a very good chance that seeds from that plant will yield the same type of flowers. Obviously, you have to know which part of the herb you are going to be using for medicine before you start choosing your specific plants. In other words, if you didn't know that the flower heads are the desired medicinal part of the herb, you might see a red clover plant with enormous leaves and puny flower heads and think "Now, there's a healthy, big leaf herb. I think I'll pick it."

Cultivar seeds should never be confused with hybrid seeds. Cultivar seeds produce true to type. Hybrid seeds either do not reproduce at all or produce stunted or odd looking offspring.

STORING YOUR SEED

Seeds are best stored in sealed envelopes or in dark colored glass jars. DO NOT store seed in plastic bags. Plastic tends to "off gas" (release trace amounts of toxins) as well as conduct heat—both of which ruin the seed. Make sure you label each envelope or jar with the name of the seed, the location it came from (i.e., "yard" or "wild"), and the date it was harvested. Place the envelopes or jars in a dark, cool, dry cupboard. Typically, most herb seeds can be stored for one to four years. However, I don't like using seed that is over two years old since the germination rate tends to go down dramatically.

Now that you have gathered your harvest, discover how to store your herbs properly in Chapter Five.

Chapter Five

~

WHERE DO I STORE ALL THIS STUFF?

After taking such great care with planting and harvesting your herbal treasures, don't forget how important it is to store them properly to guarantee a long and potent life.

Herbs are always best stored in glass jars with a tight fitting lid that prevents moisture from entering. If you can find large mouthed, amber colored glass jars, all the better. Light is one factor that can greatly reduce your herb's life and amber jars are renowned for limiting light to be passed through them. You don't need to necessarily purchase amber jars specifically for your herb collection. Old vitamin jars are often well suited for this purpose if they are large enough and have a wide opening. I had trouble finding larger wide-mouthed amber glass jars until a friend brought me several empty Ovaltine containers. These are perfect for storing herbs and tall enough to hold sections of dried roots.

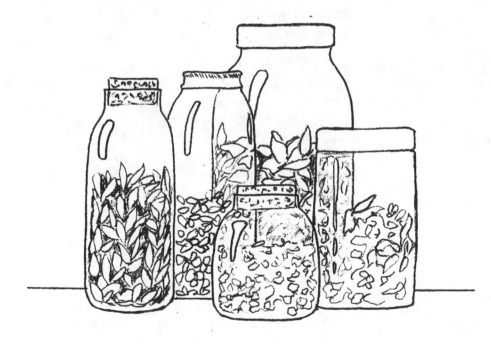

If you cannot find amber glass jars, you can always store your herbs in clear glass if you keep the bottle away from sunlight. If you are so inclined, consider covering the clear glass jar with brown paper cut from a grocery bag. Do not paint the jar since it is too easy for the paint to chip off and land inside the jar.

Heat is also a factor since heat will be transferred through the glass and dry out the herbs faster. For this reason, do not store your medicinal or culinary herbs on or near your oven or stove.

As convenient as they are, plastic containers are not recommended for storing herbs long term. After being sealed in plastic containers for several weeks or months, the herbs tend to take on the odor of the plastic. This "plastic odor" can even be tasted in the tea.

This same "no plastic" rule applies to long term storage in plastic bags. Short term use—i.e., transferring herbs into plastic bags for a few days while traveling—is okay.

Brown paper bags, while convenient, are also not recommended for storing herbs. Since there is no way to adequately seal them, the herb's aroma easily escapes and the medicinal potency can be lost within months.

HOW LONG WILL DRIED HERBS LAST?

When stored properly in airtight glass jars and kept out of heat and humidity, dried herbs can last up to two years from harvesting. Powdered herbs have a shorter shelf life—approximately one year. For this reason, do not crush your herbs into a powder until you are ready to use them in that form.

Roots can keep their healing vitality for as long as three or four years if they are stored in airtight, moisture-proof containers.

Bugs should not be a problem if your storage containers are airtight. However, one natural "insurance policy" against bugs in your herbs is to place one dried bay leaf in each jar.

Remember to always label your herb containers with the name of the herb as well as the date of storage.

~

Chapter 6

WILL THIS GREAT HERB FIT IN MY CUTE CONTAINER?

If you do not want to invest time in an outdoor garden or you live in an apartment but you would still like to reap the benefits of growing your own herbs, indoor container gardening may be for you.

Herbs outlined in-depth in this book that can be grown indoors are anise, blue violet, chickweed, fenugreek, horehound, lemon balm, mustard, rosemary, sage, spearmint and thyme. Mind you, these are herbs that *can* grow indoors. That doesn't necessarily mean it is the best place for them. For example, anise is not an herb that is typically found growing inside. However, I wanted to see if it could be successfully done. The answer was "yes." Unfortunately, it didn't look too happy and tended to be a tad on the stunted side even though I had it in a deep container.

PROPER PLANTING

There are some basic rules to container planting. First, find a pot large enough to hold the plant as well as the expected growth of that plant. Always allow space for root development. If you fail to do this, your herbs will never reach their full height and/or never blossom.

Once the proper sized container is chosen, place a layer of gravel on the bottom of the pot to prevent waterlogging. Make sure you don't seal up the container's drainage holes with the gravel.

Next, fill the container with either a sterile potting mix or a rich, non-sterile soil to within one or two inches of the rim. This allows plenty of room to water the plant. I like to mix in several handfuls of sphagnum peat moss which provides proper aeration. It also allows the roots to hold more water and nutrients. I think it's also a good idea to include a few handfuls of perlite which increases air pockets in the mix, giving the roots more "breathing" room. Both sphagnum moss and perlite can be purchased at your local nursury either separately or mixed into pre-packaged potting mixtures.

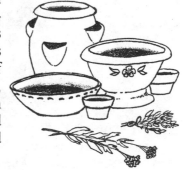

Plant your seeds directly into the pot or transplant established seed-lings/plants into it. If you are seeding directly into the container, plant sparingly, keeping in mind that you are dealing with a limited space. Water sufficiently using lukewarm water without drowning the seeds/transplants. Too much water can cause mold to form.

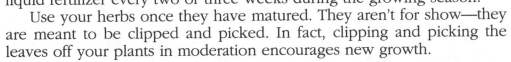

If you are starting from seed and find that some of the seedlings are too close together, thin them immediately to provide adequate room for the others.

For transplanted herbs, hold off on fertilizer until they have formed good root contact with the soil. This takes about four weeks. After that point, you can use a weak, liquid fertilizer every two or three weeks during the growing season.

Use your herbs once they have matured. They aren't for show—they are meant to be clipped and picked. In fact, clipping and picking the leaves off your plants in moderation encourages new growth.

COMMON MISTAKES

The most common mistake people make with container gardening is trying to plant too much in too small a pot. When this happens, growth is always stunted and, often, the herb never reaches maturity.

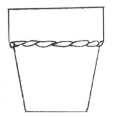

Another mistake is not giving your container herbs enough sunlight. This is not always easy since the south-facing, sunny side of your house may be the bathroom or a room where you would rather not keep your herbal treasures. Grow lights are an option. However, constantly exposing herbs to only grow lights and not giving them natural sunlight depletes them of color, taste and limits their growth.

For this reason, try to make it a point to rotate your container planting outdoors on sunny days or at least rotate your inside plants close to a sunny window for at least five hours each day. If you have larger, less portable containers, place them on roller stands for easy transport.

PLASTIC VERSUS CLAY POT

Plastic pots are less costly than their clay or ceramic counterparts. But is one better for the herb than the other? As I mentioned in earlier chapters, plastic has a tendency to "off gas." This means that when it becomes warm or hot, traces of the chemicals that were used to create the plastic could possibly seep into the soil and the herb. The question is whether the trace amount of "off-gassing" is large enough for you to be concerned.

Plastic containers which are placed in the hot sun hold and maintain more heat than clay pots. This extra warmth can be beneficial for heat-loving herbs such as thyme and sage. But for herbs such as watercress which demand a moist, cool environment, plastic containers can quickly dry out faster in direct sunlight and, thus, require more frequent watering.

Plastic containers that don't have adequate drainage holes will obviously retain more water. Even when the top layer of dirt feels dry in this type of plastic pot, there's a good chance the soil beneath it is still soaked. This can lead to root rot over time. For this reason, look for plastic containers that have good drainage holes. To save your carpeting, place heavy plastic planter trays under the containers to catch residual water. I'm not a real fan of the lighter, bendable, clear plastic trays since they have a tendency to easily crack, leak and break apart when exposed to direct sunlight.

One plus for plastic pots is the fact that they are certainly lighter to carry when you need to shift the container from one location to the other. Often times, simply carrying an oversized empty clay pot can be back breaking. When you add dirt and then water to that equation, the results can be a dead weight. One way around this "heavy" concern is to place the clay pot on a roller stand.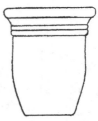

ROLL OUT THE BARREL

Another option over plastic or clay pots is to purchase wooden "whiskey barrels." They are found at most nursery and hardware stores. These are not meant for indoor use due to their size. I like using whiskey barrels for several reasons. First, they are wide enough and deep enough to accommodate most herbs that can be grown in containers. Secondly, they "breathe," meaning the wood allows water to sufficiently drain while at the same time maintaining a cool, moist environment. The only problem I can see with whiskey barrels is that their size might give the impression that you can cram more herbs into the space allotted. As with *any* of the containers mentioned, you still have to allow enough room for suitable root growth. Another consideration with wooden whiskey barrels is that over time, they tend to rot and fall apart due to water and sun. Still, for outdoor container gardening, they are my favorite choice.

GROWTH STUNTED

Your container plants will never have the same large growth characteristics as their outside garden counterparts. Because the herb's roots are confined, the plant cannot reach the same height or fullness. However, this fact can be a plus in some cases. For example, some herb gardeners purposely plant herbs in the mint family—which are known for their rapid growth via underground runners—in the ground within containers. If this idea appeals to you, use clay pots or smaller sized whiskey barrels over plastic containers since wood and clay absorb and release water and heat whereas plastic pots hold it in—especially when the pot is buried and insulated under dirt. There have been cases, however, when a particularly vigorous and determined herb with strong roots has literally broken through the pot, defying the gardener's wishes.

DRAWBACKS

There are some drawbacks to exclusively using containers for your herb garden. First, unless you are using one enormous container, your herb production will be limited to whatever that container can generate. There are some herbs that you will need a lot of in order to prepare extracted oils and tinctures and still have enough left over for teas—cleavers, stinging nettle, mullein, chickweed, red clover, skullcap, fenugreek and yarrow fall into that category.

Some aren't practical. For example, I'm not saying you can't grow corn in a pot, but do you really want to? Onion is another herb that doesn't rank high on the practical meter.

Some herbs mentioned in this book are wild and require unique growing conditions. For example, herbs such as the lichen usnea often require a forest setting to support its growth. While I have grown watercress indoors simply to prove it could be done, it was a constant battle to make sure the herb had a steady supply of water. Simulating an outdoor stream in my home is not my idea of stress-free herbal gardening. I can honestly say I put more energy into keeping that watercress alive than I've put into some relationships. It goes without saying that aspen and pine and oak trees aren't exactly built for indoor or outdoor containers. Herbs that are grown specifically for their roots (burdock, marshmallow and yellow dock) really need room to develop in order to produce a useable end result.

THE PLUS SIDE TO CONTAINER GARDENING

There is a plus side to container gardening. Some herbs are best used fresh (lemon balm and chickweed are good examples). Having a year round supply of these at your fingertips is an advantage. If you live in an apartment with no access to a garden, the idea of being able to surround yourself with a few of your favorite medicinal herbs can help bring the outdoors inside and serve as an empowering tool towards your well being.

Yes, container planting has its limitations. But it still offers the indoor herb gardener an opportunity to be part of the wonderful world of herb gardening.

Wildcrafting Ethics
&
Plant Character

*The Earth does not
belong to Man.
Man belongs to the Earth.
All things are connected like the blood
which unites a family.
Man does not weave the web of life,
he is only a strand of it.
Whatever happens to the Earth,
happens to all of us.
Whatever Man does to the web of
life on Earth,
he does to himself.*

Native American Belief

Chapter 7

THE ART OF
WILDCRAFTING

~

LISTENING TO THE PLANTS

Wildcrafters (herbalists and nature lovers who traipse through fields and streams and across mountain tops and low lying deserts in search of wild plants) are an odd sort of folk.

I, of course, include myself in this group.

We can tell you what month it is by what is blooming or about to bloom. In turn, we dutifully mark our collective calendars, highlighting dates that remind us of the "peak" times in our area for picking this or that herb.

We use the term "stand" too much. As in, "Did you see that stand (grouping) of aspen over there?" Most of us are passionate about keeping our harvesting locations to ourselves so that our herbal gems won't be snatched by every picker in the county. We are often embarrassingly enthusiastic when we encounter an unexpected herbal ally in the field, effusively talking about it as though we had found the Holy Grail.

But most importantly, we wildcrafters learn after years of sloshing through mud, baking in heat, and hanging off sides of mountains that all this green stuff surrounding us has a life, a presence, a character, a soul and an odd dignity that most people never knew existed. I believe it is then, and only then, when an herbalist truly comprehends the magnitude of what they are pursuing as well as the responsibility that is attached to it.

I could try to write about what it feels like to finally spiritually connect in the wild with an herb. But the fact is that feeling is elusive and defies words. Even if I tried to describe the incredible moment when, for a split second, you suddenly unite with a plant, I'm sure it would come out sounding like some kind of New Age rambling. I think it is best to leave that wilderness encounter—which is by all accounts a private and individual experience—for you to discover on your own.

THE ENERGY OF THE "WILD ONES"

One thing is certain about herbs that grow in the wild, they have an energy about them that is different than their garden counterparts. Their appearance can even be more striking in the forests and fields, partly due to the fact that they are growing in the precise location that is needed for their development. Instead of being forced to stand next to a herb they may not care for in the tamer garden scenario, they cozy up to other plants that share their unique likes and dislikes for soil, altitude and location.

There is a definite survival of the fittest mentality that emanates from these non-pampered "wild ones" and trees when you step out of the garden and onto the back roads. The ones that make it through the wind, rain, snow and drought have a kind of rugged individuality that, when harvested and used to make medicine, tend to get delivered into the tea, tincture, oil, salve or poultice. The idea that an herb could actually transfer its energy into whatever you wish to make out of it might sound odd to some readers. But most herbalists who work with both cultivated and wildcrafted herbs, will tell you that there really is something stronger and more intense about the wild varieties. That doesn't mean they are stronger in the sense that they taste stronger or react faster on the body. Rather, wildcrafted herbs tend to have a unique personality that shifts their intensity of purpose within the body when they are used as medicine. Wildcrafted plants are not necessarily better than those you grow in your garden, but they are different.

INTENT IS EVERYTHING

This isn't to say that your carefully grown garden varieties don't have an energy worth writing home about. It all depends on one little word: intent. I don't think enough is written or discussed about the importance of intent, especially when it comes to making medicine out of what you grow or harvest in the wild.

Intent is the feeling or feelings that you consciously or unconsciously project into the herb. I believe that good intent should be present during every step of medicine making, from planting the seed in the garden to harvesting the herb and creating the finished tea, tincture, salve and so on.

One of the first things I tell students on field walks is "Don't pick angry." If you harvest plants with the intent of using them for medicine—an endeavor that holds tremendous responsibility and demands serious concentration—**you have to be in the right frame of mind**. If you are angry, preoccupied with worries, involved in heated discussions with others during the harvest, depressed, or simply "not in the mood," **do not wildcraft**. Wildcrafting demands thoughtfulness, focus, attention to detail and a clear sense of purpose. I strongly believe that what you feel at the time of harvesting is projected in an energetic way to the plant. Again and again, I have seen people harvest medicinal herbs while they are upset only to produce a finished product (i.e., a tea, tincture, salve) that lacks healing power. I know this idea might sound "off the wall" to some readers, but I know it to be true. The recipient of the medicine may not consciously feel the poor intent that was put into the plant, but their body will most likely react to it on some subtle level.

DON'T FAKE IT

So what is good intent? First, it's not about faking it. The following suggestions should not be done in jest or with the idea that if you "follow the program" all will be well. Good intent comes from the heart. The idea is to put the best part of yourself into the plant in a thankful and always respectful manner.

The first thing I do before I even set out for the hills and valleys is ask myself why I need this or that plant. Is it for a friend or family member who needs help? Will I benefit from having it? These questions help clarify your purpose before you even get into the field. I would never pick a plant just because I heard it was good but had no idea how to use it.

LISTENING TO THE PLANTS

When I get to the area for harvesting, I proceed in a meditative, contemplative way. I'm not in some sort of hypnotic daze—I'm simply quiet and focusing my attention on my surroundings. Sometimes I talk to the plants as I pass but I assure you it's nothing deep or thought provoking. I might say a simple "Hello" or "You're looking quite well today." I don't do it because I think it's funny, cute or will put me in good stead with the plant divas. I do it because it helps me form a closer bond with the herbs. If this is not something you feel comfortable doing, don't do it.

I rarely bring other people with me when I wildcraft because there have been too many occasions when they have wanted to get into intense discussions or started complaining about the heat, the rain, the mud or whatever else is making them uncomfortable at that moment. Nothing

Your Wildcrafting
Checklist For The Road

Here are some important items to bring along on the trail.

✓   A sturdy backpack that can take a beating without re-treating.

✓   A quart of drinking water and a smaller container of water for rinsing off hands, cleaning muddy roots or, in some cases, washing the dirt out of various cuts and scrapes.

✓   A sharp knife (for slicing roots and stripping bark) and garden clippers (for cutting small branches). Make sure the knife has a locking blade to prevent accidents.

✓   A small shovel. The folding type is the easiest to carry.

✓   Waterproof boots or hiking shoes with a good traction sole.

✓   Wide brimmed hat. (Preferably one that ties around your chin to keep it in place).

✓   Canvas gloves. These especially come in handy when you are working with thorny bushes or obstinate roots and barks that can cause blisters.

✓   A good receptacle for your herbs. The best are burlap and canvas bags, paper sacks and wicker picnic baskets that have hinged tops that close.

✓   A good field book with clear, illustrations *and* color photographs for proper identification. Two of my favorites are put out by Peterson Field Guides: *Eastern/Central Medicinal Plants* by Steven Foster & James A. Duke and *Edible Wild Plants* by Lee Allen Peterson.

✓   Fresh or dried fruit, jerky, carrot and celery sticks, cookies or whatever you enjoy as snack food. Try to limit the amount of packaging so that you are not hauling back a lot of trash.

✓   A light, compact poncho for those unexpected rain showers.

✓   A map of the area you are visiting if you are not sure of your surroundings. A compass wouldn't be a bad idea either.

✓   A small flashlight just in case you lose track of time and the sun goes down.

✓   Matches or a butane lighter to be used in an emergency for making a campfire.

✓   Bug repellant (for summer time harvesting).

✓   If you are new to wildcrafting, try to find an experienced herbalist or naturalist who knows the area and can accurately identify the herbs.

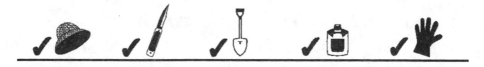

blows your good wildcrafting intent like taking someone with you who is not in the same frame of mind. I will say, however, that there have been a few people who have shared my perspective on wildcrafting and who I gladly invited on the trip. Rather than verbal sparring matches, we shared some of the most insightful, sometimes philosophical conversations that seemed to be encouraged by the green surroundings.

Another important point: I never bring portable radios, cassette players or CD players with me while I'm wildcrafting. Listening to music— even the good stuff such as Mozart—does not allow you to listen to the plant. Listening to the plants is not an easy thing to do. It takes time, patience, reverence and the ability to lose yourself in the heart of nature. No matter what anyone tells you, this cannot be taught. It is something that develops over time.

DISCOVERING "GRANDMOTHER"

When you are absolutely sure you have found the right plant you are seeking, look around the area. Hopefully there is more than one growing there. If there is only one, do not pick it. Move on and see if you can find it in more abundance somewhere else. Obviously trees and large shrubs are exempt from this "only one" rule.

If you see a grouping of the plant that you need, take a good look at each one of them. Native Americans believe that each grouping of plants has a "Grandmother" which oversees the others and gives them their medicinal power. The "Grandmother" plant was never harvested for medicine, thus allowing successful development of the plants in her care. Now the obvious question is always, "How do I identify the Grandmother plant?" No one can answer that definitively. It is at this point when listening to plants becomes important. Sometimes, if you are attuned to the rhythms of the wild and/or have visited the site many times, you will feel a sense of power, mystique or authority coming from one particular plant in the group. Whether this is the true "Grandmother" or not is completely between you and the plant.

I realize that this kind of information has not been written about in many mainstream herbal books and articles. However, spend enough time with a dedicated, thoughtful wildcrafter and you will undoubtedly learn about this "wild etiquette."

A LITTLE TOBACCO OR CORNMEAL WILL DO

Another aspect of wildnerness etiquette is bringing some kind of offering or gift to leave at the base of the plant. A typical plant offering is a pinch of tobacco, cornmeal, oats, corn or a simple prayer of thanks. Contrary to what some people believe, this is not plant "worship." It is giving something to the earth to show your gratefulness for what that plant can offer you. It is a recognition that for everything you take, you need to give something in return. The act of sprinkling a pinch of tobacco or cornmeal under a plant or tree sets up the conscious intent. The herb ceases to become a servant and is, instead, transformed into a willing partner in the healing process. If you don't feel comfortable leaving an offering under a plant, please consider a quiet "Thank you."

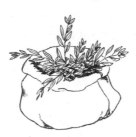

The Best Containers For Your Wild Ones

Everyone has their favorite gathering containers for wild plants. Some people like baskets or large brown paper bags, while others prefer more durable burlap or canvas sacks. Baskets are handy and a good choice if you are harvesting on flat land. I recommend picnic baskets that have secure, hinged covers over the top that help contain the harvested herb. Baskets work fine when you are collecting plants on flat land. However, they are not your best bet if you are planning to climb over hill and dale. Paper bags are plentiful and allow plenty of room for harvested plants to breathe. The only drawback is that if they get soaked in water due to wet ground or a sudden rainstorm, your precious herbal harvest can attract mold and go bad. Burlap and canvas bags are the best options since they allow a free flow of air between plant cuttings. They can be closed during transport to avoid loss of the harvest, do not absorb water easily and are easily slung over a shoulder or arm while you wander through the wild places.

Two textures you do not want next to your herbs are plastic and leather. Both hold heat which tends to make herbs wither as well as release odors into the plant matter that can alter the taste and quality of the herbs.

THE ONE DAY I'LL NEVER FORGET

When you harvest any plant, pick less than a fifth of the plant. Some herbalists say to pick less than what we *think* we need since there is a tendency to over harvest. I know from personal experience that this is absolutely true.

Greed is a powerful persuader when you are out in the wild. Obviously, greed is not part of that "good intent" I mentioned earlier. If you "rape" the plant, you might end up with what they call "bad medicine." Bad medicine is defined in a lot of different ways. I define it as a remedy that lacks the inherent healing power, does nothing at all or, in the worst case scenario, backfires on the recipient.

This idea might be controversial to some readers, but I've personally experienced the angry hand of nature. When I was younger and had not fully appreciated the power of plants, my wildcrafting approach lacked in the spiritual department. But there was one wilderness experience that opened my eyes. I set off on a beautiful, serene, cobalt blue sky day in late spring with the goal of collecting a small handful of aspen buds. After an afternoon hiking through deep snow in search of the perfect sticky buds, I finally found a small tree that offered a cornucopia. I was effortlessly able to get that single handful that I needed from the lower branches.

However, I looked up and saw two higher branches that were chock full of more buds. I had what I needed for my formula, but now I wanted more. Yes, greed had reared its ugly head. I tried shaking the tree to release the buds but they wouldn't budge. Then I hatched another plan. I would jump up, grab onto the upper branch, inch my body higher up toward the tree trunk and then shake the branch vigorously with the weight of my body. It all seemed so simple. After two attempts at the branch, I made contact. I did everything possible to shake those buds loose, but they were stubborn little creatures. "Come on! Drop!" I yelled, exasperated. And then, without so much as a warning, the entire branch gave way and split halfway apart from the trunk. I, in turn, was thrust directly into the waist deep snow.

Now I was really annoyed. I got up and grabbed the broken branch and attempted to harvest the buds. But within seconds, a strong, bitter cold gust of wind blew angrily through the forest. As I leaned over to stick my face inside my jacket to protect my skin from the freezing chill, a five foot branch about as wide as a pool cue from another aspen tree came smacking down across my back. I turned around quickly, stepped onto a soft section of snow and fell through the icy powder up to my waist. As I stood there, tangled up in the undergrowth that sliced my jeans in several spots, I stopped fighting and slowly looked around the forest. Suddenly, I could feel the whole place come to life and let me tell you, it wasn't a warm, happy place. A most unusual thing happened at that point. The words weren't audible but the message was loud and clear. "*Knock it off and get out of here!*" I wriggled out of the layers of undergrowth and looked up at the broken aspen branch. "I'm really sorry," was all I could say at that point.

I mention this story as an example of the *cooperative respect* you need to have with nature. It's not that nature is some violent, punishing entity that you should fear. You should approach the plants and trees as you would approach someone to ask an enormous favor. Demanding that they give you what you want or taking more from them than you need tends to create hostility. The great thing about nature, is that it will let you know quickly when you've gone too far. Take it from someone who went too far once and learned her lesson. It's not worth it.

Along those same lines, if you are out harvesting and find that a leaf, flower, branch, bark, bud or root is especially difficult to remove from the plant, stop what you are doing and move onto another site. For whatever reason, that particular herb or tree does not want to be picked that day. Continuing to struggle with a plant lacks dignity and means you are not listening to the plant when it is yelling, "Don't pick me today!" You also risk getting smacked in the back with a tree branch.

> To learn more about proper harvesting and drying of plants, refer back to Chapter 4, *What Do I Do With All This Stuff?* To find out how to process your wildcrafted herbs into tea, tinctures, salves, oils and more, turn to Chapter 40, *How to Make Herbal Stuff.*

A SENSE OF SELF-SUFFICIENCY

On the practical side, respectful wildcrafting gives you a sense of self-sufficiency and trust in yourself that can be very empowering. There's nothing like being in the middle of nowhere and knowing that you can rely on nature's bounty to heal any number of ailments. Suddenly the woods, meadows, creeks and deserts come alive with dimensions you never knew existed. When you don't understand plants and what they can do for you, the landscape is simply a blur of color. But when you realize the potential of what is growing out there and take the time to learn how plants work with the body, suddenly that blur of color takes on shape, texture and detail. It is a feeling like no other.

The more time you spend harvesting plants respectfully in the wild, the greater your personal responsibility. It is up to you to show others the lay of the land. Freely share your adventures and misadventures and stress the rules that go along with ethical wildcrafting.

With the proper guidance, you may soon find yourself marking the months of your calendar with your favorite "in bloom" dates and actually looking forward to the mud, dust, rain and piercing sun.

Rules of Wildcrafting

Before setting foot in the great outdoors, please remember to follow these important wildcrafting rules.

❁ Don't wildcraft any herbs if you feel you cannot complete the entire process from harvest to finished dried tea, tincture or salve.

❁ Know exactly how you plan to use the herb or herbs and, if possible, the approximate amount of the plant that will be needed.

❁ Learn which parts of the herb should be harvested and at what time of year. For example, leaves are typically picked in the spring or early summer before the plant flowers. If you were to harvest them after the plant flowers, they would be tougher and less active medicinally.

❁ Find out which medicinal plants are endangered and **do not pick them.** More than 28,000 plant species are lost worldwide annually due to over harvesting and no regard for replenishing what is taken. For example, goldenseal – a popular natural antibiotic – is extinct in 28 states. Slippery elm bark is also quickly becoming more difficult to obtain due to over enthusiastic herbalists and others. If you can grow any of the endangered varieties, please do so and help contribute to the repopulation of these wonderful medicinal friends.

❁ If the plant is going to seed when you are harvesting it, please take the time to sprinkle as much seed as you can around the area to encourage next year's growth.

❁ Whenever you are in doubt about proper identification of an herb, **don't pick it!** *If possible, I strongly encour-*

age you to grow all herbs that you have an interest in so that you can observe their many growth stages as well as have a better visual for the plants in question. Their wild counterparts may look more straggly and/or be taller or shorter, but you will still be able to properly identify the plants.

✿ **Do not** taste a wild herb as a means of identifying it. This has led to serious regrets.

❀ Invest in a good field guide that includes excellent line drawings and clear color photographs.

✿ **Do not** harvest wild plants within 75 feet of power lines, electrical boxes, near sewage drains or in stale or stagnant water. In addition, keep in mind that chemical pesticides are used in many public places which means the herbs are off limits. Such locations include any city or country road sides, public parks, shopping mall parking lots, freeway medians, train tracks, frequently traveled public trails and well established campsites.

❀ Take great care when you are collecting low lying plants in crowded growing areas that you don't mistakenly grab a little bit of other plants that might be nearby. The other plant may be harmless or it could knock you out.

✿ Be aware of poisonous look-alike herbs that may resemble the plant you are seeking.

❀ Harvest only 1/6 to 1/4 of the herb. Don't let greed get the better of you.

✿ Harvest a little less than what you think you need.

❀ Never destroy a tree or herb in the harvesting process.

✿ Don't wildcraft any plant in a hurry. This often leads to uprooting and killing herbs that you only needed for their leaves or flowers.

❀ When picking on hillsides or steep slopes, always try to pick the herbs that are downslope and leave the ones at the top of hill alone so they can re-seed and/or send roots down the slope.

❀ Gather herbs in the cool of the morning after the dew evaporates or in the early evening before the dew forms. Never harvest at high noon or when there is intense heat since the leaves have a tendency to droop and the volatile oils in the plants are not as potent.

❀ If you are digging up the roots of any plant, always fill in the empty hole with dirt, packing it down firmly **with your foot**.

❀ **Do not** destroy any wild area in the harvesting process. Make sure the area looks the same when you leave as when you arrived. That also means **leave no litter behind**.

❀ If you want to collect seed from the wild plants for later planting in your garden, pick plants that have a healthy appearance and an abundance of medicinal parts. For example, if you wish to collect wild mustard seed, choose a mustard plant that has large seed pods that are filled with well formed seeds.

❀ When you make a tincture, oil or salve out of the plant or simply dry and bottle the tea, mark the bottle with a "WC" which stands for wildcrafted. This way you can see if you notice any difference with the wild versus the garden cultivated varieties.

❀ Never underestimate the significance of what you are doing. Be grateful for the plants and they will serve you well.

When I first glimpse a long sought plant,
I sometimes seem to enter into the herb
and feel its virtues and uses.
I am one with its long history of
healing man's ills and ministering to his comfort.
And when I carry the plant home and
transmute it into some grateful remedy
it has a soul-healing power far beyond
anything it might do for my body,
and it brings a satisfaction no purchased
product could ever provide.

Euell Gibbons, *Stalking the Wild Asparagus*

~

Chapter 8

THAT HERB'S GOT CHARACTER!

Spend enough years in the outdoors rubbing elbows with wild or garden plants, and you might start to notice an unusual thing. In fact, ask any gung-ho gardener and I'm certain that he or she has made a similar discovery.

Quite simply, plants have character. Some are loners—others love to grow amongst compatible compatriots. There are those that tend to cling, either to trees, each other or a passerby in an insecure, needy way. Then there are the plants and trees that give off a superior attitude, as if to say "Of course you like me. I am the best of the bunch after all."

PLANT TALK

I am far from the only one who has picked up on this wild temperament. Native Americans, backwoods folk healers and modern day herbalists have all recognized the amazing and often quirky demeanor of plants.

For example, Native Americans had no books or field manuals to help them identify the healing plants. Instead, they gave names to healing plants based on what the herb or tree communicated to them. Sitting for hours and sometimes days in front of a particular herb, they meditated deeply, eventually moving their spirit into the plant and becoming one with it. They would emerge from this communion with a complete understanding of the herb's purpose and how to use it to heal. Sometimes the herb's use lent itself to a common name–other times an actual name would be given by the plant.

When I first heard about this tribal practice, I thought, "Well, isn't that interesting." Then I got to thinking about it one day when I was hiking through the woods. Suddenly, the whole idea became so profound. To think there's the possibility that hundreds of years ago a Native American was given healing information directly from the "plant's mouth" and that today, we are using some of those herbs based upon that esoteric guidance has to be one of the most wondrous possibilities.

DOCTRINE OF SIGNATURES

Others throughout history used a more visual approach to define a plant's character. There were those who believed that God had a hidden agenda when he created each plant and tree. Essentially, the idea was that God was giving us a hint as to the healing uses of each plant and tree by granting individual species specific signs, patterns or "signatures" that related to their ultimate purpose. This theory became known as the "doctrine of signatures." For example, the herb lungwort has leaves that are curiously marked with white blotches that resemble the lungs. This "signature" led to the belief that lungwort would be effective for respiratory complaints. Interestingly enough, they were right. Was it a lucky guess? Maybe. But there are many other plant signatures that are amazingly accurate. Take a close look at the herb self-heal (*Prunella vulgaris*). The tiny purple flowers that grow in tightly compacted tubular spikes resemble a chorus of mouths wide open, exposing the back of the throat. Is it any wonder that one of the uses for self heal is as an astringent gargle for tonsillitis?

Herbalist and author Matthew Wood believes strongly in plant signatures. In his book *The Book of Herbal Wisdom*, Wood states that the doctrine of signatures requires "two different subjective faculties, the intuition and the imagination." I would have to agree. However, I think it is important to remember that too much imagination could override your intuitive senses. You don't want to turn a forest into your own personal Fantasia, imagining the weeping willows depressed and sobbing and then proclaiming that willow must obviously be good for melancholia when accompanied by fits of crying. Discovering plant signatures is a true art that takes patience, willingness to quietly observe, the ability to trust your intuition without letting your ego get in the way and the wisdom to know the difference between what you want the plant to be and what it simply is.

PERSONALITY PLUS

There are many words that could be used to define a plant's character. One of my favorites was coined by Tom Brown, Jr., author, naturalist and wilderness expert. In his book Tom Brown's *Guide to Wild Edible and Medicinal Plants*, Brown describes the diverse "personalities" of herbs. I read that and I realized there was at least one other person in this world who acknowledged the existence of that marvelous mystique hidden within each plant and tree.

I hesitated somewhat to include my personal observations on plant character in each of the following herb chapters because I didn't want readers to think that my "take" on each herb was the definitive truth. The fact is, we are all going to look at herbs in different ways and, perhaps, see character traits that no one else notices.

If you live your life surrounded by concrete and four walls, it is difficult to fully grasp the unusual dynamic that occurs in the wilderness between humans and plants. I encourage city dwellers to either plant a garden or resolve to spend more time amidst wild plants, away from traffic noises and the steady hum of technology. It is only within these quiet, solitary moments when you can begin to hear the plants speak to you. The process takes time and a willingness to let go of preconceived belief systems from modern day society that attempt to separate mankind from the heart of nature. Plants and trees have always talked to us. We just haven't been taught how to listen.

What you perceive a certain tree or plant's character to be has a lot to do with what you are willing to believe. The magic happens when you allow that tree or plant to speak for itself.

The Herbs

**The doctor of the future
will give no medicine
but will interest his patients
in the care of the human frame, in diet,
and in the cause and prevention
of disease.**

Thomas Edison

~

Chapter 9

HOW TO USE THE HERB CHAPTERS

The following chapters cover 30 popular wild and cultivated medicinal herbs. Most are easy to grow–others need to be bought as a seedling, full grown plant or located in the wild.

Each chapter is broken down into five sections:

- **The plant's "character"**
- **Where to find the herb in the wild**
- **How to grow the herb in your garden or container**
- **When and what part of the herb to gather for making medicine**
- **How to use the herb medicinally**

If the letters "W.F." appear under the herb's name, it means the herb is both medicinal as well as a wild food. To learn how to use the herb as a wild food, look for the "Wild Food Facts" within that chapter. There you will learn which parts of the herb are edible and how to prepare them.

At the end of each herb chapter, you will find a box titled "The Dirt On..." This extensive list works as a quick reference guide, summarizing the chapter's contents as well as offering additional detailed data on that specific herb. If "N/A" follows any of the listings, it means that the information was not available for that plant.

Happy herbal gardening and hunting!

Chapter 10

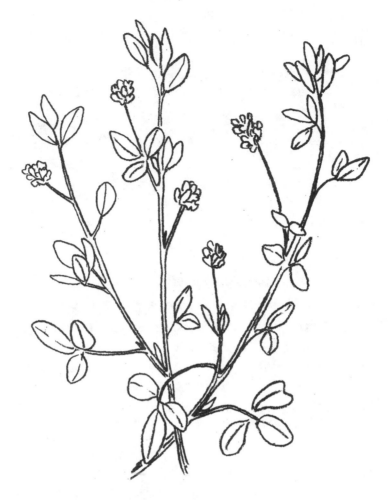

ALFALFA

WHAT'S GOOD FOR THE COW IS GREAT FOR YOU!

Medicago sativa
("W.F.")

Hardy perennial

Medicinal Uses: *Mineral tonic, fights anemia, combats fatigue, increases stamina, mild diuretic, promotes breast milk, estrogen precursor for menopause*

Medicinal parts of plant: *Leaves, flowers, seeds*

Forms: *Tea, capsules, sprouts (grown from the seeds)*

WHAT IS ITS CHARACTER?

Alfalfa is a tough, resilient, enduring herb but it gives the impression of being rather delicate on the outside. Once it likes where it lives, it digs its roots in deeply and stays around for years. Alfalfa tends to ignore those who refer to it as "just another weed." I can almost hear it saying, "Call me what you like, but I'm stronger than you and I'm planning to hang around for a long, long time."

WHERE DO I FIND IT?

Alfalfa is usually found growing along foothills and throughout mountainous regions between 3,000 and 9,000 feet. I've seen it flourishing in dry, rocky soil as well as fertile, composted fields. Whenever you see alfalfa in the wild, it is a good indicator of a high mineral content in the soil–especially iron. Additionally, the soil is normally easier to till due to alfalfa's 20 to 125 foot root system which helps break up underground deposits.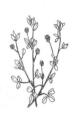

HOW DO I GROW IT?

Broadcast handfuls of seed across freshly tilled fields, in full to partial sun, pressing the seed into the soil with your foot. For small areas, consider pre-soaking seed in water that has a drop or two of liquid kelp fertilizer added to it. Try to allow eight to ten inches of space between clusters of seed. Make sure there is no hardpan or large rock formations underground since alfalfa's deep roots need plenty of room to spread. Sow alfalfa seed in the spring for a summer crop or in the fall for a spring crop. If you sow seeds in the fall early enough so that the seedlings can take hold, alfalfa can work as an excellent, vitamin/mineral enriching cover crop which can be tilled under when spring arrives. Due to alfalfa's nitrogen fixing ability (meaning it takes available nitrogen from the air and "fixes" it into the soil), this herb is great for soil that lacks nutrients or has been overworked for too many seasons. Combining it with red clover seed really increases its soil nourishing abilities. While it is not imperative, you can ensure alfalfa's nitrogen fixing ability by coating the seed with an "inoculant." Inoculants, which can be purchased at your local nursery or through mail order seed/garden companies, are covered with a specific strain of nitrogen fixing bacteria suited especially for that particular seed. When the seeds sprout and mature, the bacteria enter the root hairs, grab the nitrogen from the air and bring it down to "fix" on the nodules of the root hairs. Read and follow the instructions carefully on each package of inoculant. I've had good luck planting alfalfa using no inoculant. But other herb growers I know wouldn't be without it. As for moisture, alfalfa seed needs moderate water to establish itself. However, once it is established do not over water.

HOW DO I HARVEST IT?

Harvest alfalfa June through August. Cut the entire upper half of the plant as it begins to flower. If you harvest alfalfa immediately after the first sign of flowering, you might be able to get another cutting one or two months later. Hang the stems upside down in small bunches in a cool, dry area. Once the leaves are brittle to the touch, strip them (and any flowers) from the stem. Toss the stems away or, better yet, add them to your compost pile. Seeds can be gathered once the plant begins to fade. However, often much of the seed has already hit the ground. Personally, I've found it easier to purchase alfalfa seed in the bulk herb/seed section of health food stores and herb/seed catalogs rather than hand gather it. The seed is inexpensive and abundantly available.

HOW DO I USE IT?

If cows could talk, it would be a mighty strange world. But if they did chat with us, I'm sure they'd put in a good word for their owners who feed them alfalfa. Besides better health, an alfalfa diet produces richer milk for cows. Give alfalfa feed to chickens and they're likely to lay more eggs with the added benefit of those eggs having more nutritional value. To these creatures, alfalfa isn't so much an herb as it is a food. Herbalists

---

Can Alfalfa Turn a 90 Pound Weakling Into a Strong, Muscular Giant?

I'll never forget a story that was told to me several years ago. An herbalist I know claimed that he was able to defy all logic and give his sons the gift of height and stamina. You see, my friend wasn't exactly the tallest tree on the block. His three sons, all under the age of twelve, were all proportioned like their father—short and round. My friend had heard through the herbal grapevine that if he started giving his sons three to six alfalfa capsules every day of their life from pre-puberty through their teenage years, they might just shoot up in height as well as build a stronger more resilient body. It was worth a try, my friend thought, and so he had his sons follow the program. They resisted at first, but the promise of one day being able to look down on their "old man" was enough to convince them to dutifully take their alfalfa capsules every day. What happened in the end? Well, all I know is that by the time the boys were in their mid-teens, they were taller than any other members of their family and muscular to boot! Science may scoff at this story and claim a dozen other reasons for the boys' towering appearance. As far as my friend is concerned, he's just sorry his father hadn't heard about this miraculous remedy from nature.

consider alfalfa a tremendous all around tonic that supports your system. Don't ask what alfalfa *can* do for your body—ask what it *can't* do.

Alfalfa is *so* rich in vitamins, minerals, amino acids and digestive enzymes that it boggles the senses. The reason for this kaleidoscope of nutrients is due to the root structure of alfalfa. These babies are deep. How deep? Try up to *125* feet! Alfalfa is such a **rich vitamin source**, you could look on it as a one-stop herb shop for all your nutritional needs. Let's see, it contains major amounts of calcium and iron along with vitamins A, B_1, B_2, B_6, B_{12}, C, D, E, K (important for normal functioning of the heart and liver, alfalfa has 20,000 to 40,000 units of vitamin K for every 100 grams), P (also known as "bioflavonoids" which help to support the immune system as well as strengthen the capillaries), niacin, pantothenic acid, biotin, folic acid, saponins, phosphorous, potassium, magnesium, zinc and copper. All this healthy stuff pulsates through the root and shoots up into the plant, filling the leaves and flowers with every last drop.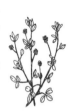

Alfalfa has numerous medicinal possibilities. Here are just a few that may surprise you.

RESISTANCE TO DISEASE

It's not exactly a stretch of the imagination to say that any herb with this many vitamins and minerals is good for **fighting off the latest cold/flu**. The next time the latest "bug" is buzzing around, try sipping two to four cups of alfalfa tea a day as a preventative measure. If you've already got that "bug", drinking up to six cups a day can help to fortify your system and quickly pour much needed minerals and vitamins into your bloodstream. If you are having a difficult time **recovering from a debilitating illness**, alfalfa tea might just be the ticket to renewed well-being. Start drinking one or two cups each day and work up to four or five.

ANEMIA/MENTAL & PHYSICAL FATIGUE

I always associate the word "endurance" with the alfalfa plant. Any herb with this much iron charging through it has got to be helpful for **battling anemia**. Try three to four capsules with each meal or as much as one quart of the tea sipped throughout the day. Along the same lines, regular use of alfalfa—either in capsules or tea form—helps **sharpen the mental faculties** as well as **supports the body against physical fatigue**.

RHEUMATOID ARTHRITIS

Arthritis (along with **bursitis**) is often caused by an over acid condition in the body. The acid settles in joints causing inflammation. Alfalfa alone won't help with this problem if you still eat sugar, white flour, processed chemical-laden foods, salt, caffeine and alcohol. However, cutting these out of your diet and adding the mild diuretic action of alfalfa to your daily regimen can, over time, gradually reduce the inflammation and alkalize the body to empty those nasty acid deposits. You can take it in either the capsule or tea form. You will need to take nine to eighteen capsules per day to benefit from the herb. If you prefer the tea, one to two cups a day is usually sufficient, taken usually first thing in the morning and again sometime during the afternoon.

BLOOD PRESSURE REGULATOR & CHOLESTEROL

There is hard, scientific proof that alfalfa **helps regulate high or low blood pressure** as well as inhibits high cholesterol by 25%! In addition, alfalfa also works to **strengthen the arteries and blood cells** throughout the body which can, in turn, provide major support to the heart. Two capsules taken with each meal or several cups of the tea sipped throughout the day are recommended. Once again, diet plays a big role.

MENOPAUSAL SUPPORT

Alfalfa contains what researchers like to call "plant hormones" These plant hormones are called "phytoestrogens" and are similar in some ways to human estrogen hormones. Phytoestrogens bind to estrogen receptor sites in the human body but know instinctively to keep the delicate balance of estrogen at an even balance. Since phytoestrogens work *with* the body and listen to what it needs at that moment, they don't produce the negative, unbalanced reactions caused by their chemical counterparts. (Other phytoestrogen herbs featured in this book include red clover and fennel). It should come as no surprise to know that alfalfa is considered one of the **natural answers for women during menopause**. Drinking one cup of alfalfa tea during menopause, two weeks out of every month, helps nourish the ovaries and adrenal glands as well as supports the pituitary gland. The tea's mild diuretic action also comes in handy when a woman feels a bit on the bloated side.

LABOR & NURSING

It might sound weird to add alfalfa ice cubes to the labor room repertoire but it's a surprising aid for the mom-to-be. Make a double strength tea–two teaspoons of the herb to eight ounces of hot distilled water–allow it to cool and then pour the liquid into an ice cube tray. **Sucking on the ice cubes during labor** not only eases tension but replenishes the body with minerals and vitamins. When it comes time for **nursing**, alfalfa works much like it does on those alfalfa-grazing cows. (This is not to compare a

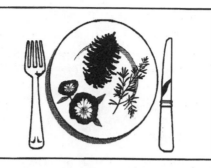

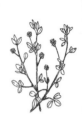

Wild Food Facts

Did you know that alfalfa sprouts contain 150% more protein than wheat or corn? Best of all, alfalfa sprouts only take five days to mature in plastic sprouting trays when exposed to an average temperature of 70⁰ F. A mere two tablespoons of seed can yield a whopping *quart* of one to two inch tall sprouts! Sprinkle the sprouts into soup right before serving, add them in abundance to salads and sandwiches or consider them a healthy, energy-giving snack during that late afternoon "sinking spell" we often encounter.

mother with a grazing cow, mind you). Alfalfa **enriches mother's milk**, filling it full of vitamins for the baby. Mothers can sip a cup of alfalfa tea before each feeding or one cup in the morning and one in mid-afternoon.

PEPTIC ULCERS

Alfalfa has long since been regarded as an A-1 herb for **peptic ulcers** since it nourishes the body and aids in digestion. Three to four capsules spread throughout the day or one cup of tea sipped slowly throughout the morning can be beneficial and soothing.

ALCOHOL, DRUG ADDICTION
& PRESCRIPTION MEDICATION

While it's not going to take away the craving for alcohol or drugs, it has been shown that alfalfa tea, capsules, sprouts and powders added to drinks, foods or taken alone help to **reduce the desire for your addiction**. The premise is that if your body is getting a hefty nutritional punch through the use of this herb (and dare I say again, a well-balanced, whole food diet), your system will not crave anything that will be destructive. The same holds true if your body is **addicted to prescription drugs**. In fact, some herbalists recommend drinking alfalfa tea while taking a course of **antibiotics**—especially **sulfa drugs**. It gives the body support, while replenishing it with the vitamins and minerals that are lost due to the drug's systemic effect.

DENTAL DECAY

While it's no excuse to stop brushing and flossing, many herbalists feel that taking two to three alfalfa capsules daily helps to **prevent cavities**. Along with proper dental care, alfalfa tends to **ward off dental decay**–especially for those people who are prone to problems no matter how well they take care of their teeth.

RADIATION DAMAGE

It's not one of the most well known attributes of this formidable weed, but alfalfa can help to **protect the body against radiation damage due to traditional cancer treatment**. Try up to six capsules each day or three cups of the tea.

THE DOSE

The taste of alfalfa tea has been compared to "drinking grass clippings"–not a particularly enticing thought. For this reason, add a pinch of lemongrass and/or peppermint to your brew and you'll perk up that "grassy taste."

TWO CAUTIONS TO CONSIDER

There are two cautions to consider. The first one is that **alfalfa has been shown to aggravate lupus and other autoimmune disorders**. If you have lupus or an autoimmune problem, do not take alfalfa. Secondly, **never eat alfalfa seeds**. They have a toxic amino acid called *canavanine* which can cause a wicked blood disorder called pancytopenia which interferes with the platelets that help the body fight infection.

Aside from those two cautions, this rich green herb can be your best friend when you want to flood your body with "liquid" vitamins. Cows may not be the brightest bulbs in the box, but when it comes to chewing their cud with alfalfa, they are truly moo-ved.

THE "DIRT" ON...ALFALFA

Botanical ~ *Medicago sativa*

Growth cycle ~ Hardy perennial.

Medicinal uses~ Mineral tonic, fights anemia, combats fatigue, increases stamina, mild diuretic, promotes breast milk, estrogen precursor for menopause.

Part(s) used for medicine ~ Leaves, flowers and seeds.

Vitamins/Minerals ~ High amounts of iron, calcium and vitamin K, along with vitamins A, B_1, B_2, B_6, B_{12}, C, E, D, trace minerals, chlorophyll, protein, potassium, chlorine, sodium, silicon and magnesium.

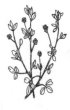

Region ~ Generally found in mountain and foothill areas between 3,000 and 9,000 feet.

Wild or Domestic ~ Both.

Poisonous look alikes in the wild ~ None that I know of.

Hardy or Delicate ~ Very hardy.

Height of mature plant ~ One to three feet.

Easy or hard to grow ~ Easy.

Cultivation ~ Seed. Directly broadcast seed in the fall for late spring crop; sow in the early spring for summer crop. One-half pound of seed covers approximately 1000 square feet.

Plant spacing ~ Eight to ten inches apart.

Pre-soak seeds ~ Yes, but not imperative.

Pre-chill seeds ~ No.

Indoor seed starting ~ No.

Light/dark seed requirements ~ Light.

Days to germinate ~ Two to three.

Days to full maturity ~ Approximately 60 days.

Soil type ~ Well drained soil with moderate fertility. Make sure it is not too acid. Okay in clay as long as it doesn't get boggy. In the wild, alfalfa enjoys moist soil in dry regions and dry soil in moist regions. Hint: Make sure there is no hardpan or rock under soil. Alfalfa's deep root system needs lots of "elbow room" to travel.

Water requirements ~ Keep moist but well drained. Needs water to establish itself. Once it is established, alfalfa is fairly drought resistant.

Sun or shade ~ Full to partial sun.

Propagation ~ Seed.

Easy/hard to transplant ~ Not an herb that is commonly transplanted. Typically, sow directly where you want it.

Pests or diseases ~ Can host the alfalfa mosaic virus which can endanger peppers growing nearby.

Landscape uses ~ Low lying filler where a sprinkle of purple flowers amidst the green is desired.

Gathering ~ Upper half of the plant, collected June through August. Hint: Harvest first flowering immediately and you may get a second harvest later in the season.

Best fresh or dried ~ Can be used either way, however some people feel the fresh plant is too strong for their taste buds.

Drying methods ~ Hang in small bunches in dry, cool area. Once dry, strip leaves and any flowers from stem, discarding the stem.

Amount needed ~ Moderate use: 5 plants. Regular use: 10 or more plants.

Seed collection ~ Since alfalfa is in the legume family, it develops hairy, spiral seed pods after flowering in mid to late summer. Instead of picking the seed pods off individually, cut the plant several inches above the ground, place it tops down into a brown paper bag, secure the top of the bag with string or a rubber band and allow it to dry in a cool, dry place. Pods will either pop open on their own or, after they are completely dry, can be broken open to expose the seeds.

Companion planting ~ Red clover, plantain, nettle.

Container planting ~ Not suited as a container plant.

Common mistakes ~ Planting alfalfa in an area that hinders its extensive root growth.

Interesting facts/tips ~ Finding alfalfa in the wild indicates that soil is high in minerals. Alfalfa's roots can be as deep as 125 feet. They help to "fix" nitrogen in the soil. Alfalfa, either alone or combined with red clover, makes an excellent cover crop (see page 14 for more info on cover crops).

Chapter 11

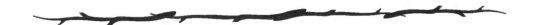

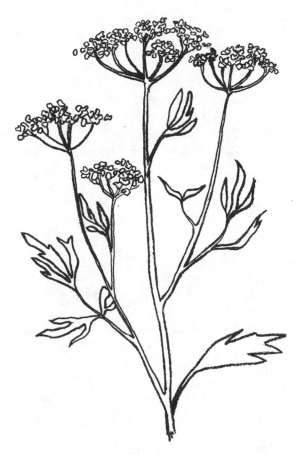

ANISE

FINALLY, AN HERB THAT TASTES GOOD

Pimpinella anisum

("W.F.")

Hardy Annual (If seed heads are completely harvested)
Perennial (If plant is allowed to go to seed)

Medicinal Uses: *Aromatic, carminative, expectorant, mild sedative, galactagogue, possible aphrodisiac, hangover relief, mouse bait.*
Medicinal parts of plant: *Seeds*
Forms: *Tea, pure essential oil*

WHAT IS ITS CHARACTER?

Anise has a bit of a perfectionist mentality, in my opinion. It takes such a long time to reach maturity that it feels a little on the insecure side, never wanting to make a mistake. When it finally does produce its umbel of tiny flowers, it again spends more time creating its perfectly shaped aromatic seed. Anise hates to be rushed and will not move any faster than absolutely necessary. The strain of being a perfectionist is evident for anise when it sometimes bends over and breaks its stalk under the weight of its seed head. For the ones that make it through the pressure and remain upright, there is a brief moment of pride as its seed head clusters wave in the breeze as if to say, "You see? Perfection sometimes pays off."

WHERE DO I FIND IT?

Anise prefers the cool corners of gardens and wild places where passing birds have dropped its seed. It can be found anywhere from sea level to 9000 feet. However, you don't usually see it growing wild in regions that have less than 130 frost-free days since it takes that amount of time to fully mature. If you think you have found anise in the wild, *examine the plant very carefully*. What looks like anise to the untrained eye could easily be either poison hemlock or water hemlock. These toxic, deadly look-alikes obviously have different leaf structures and other identifying features. However, I have seen novices on plant walks point to one of these plants and say, "Hey, look. It's 'wild anise.'"

HOW DO I GROW IT?

Direct seed anise into rich, composted soil in early to mid-spring after the threat of frost has past. Anise needs 120 to 130 frost-free days to reach full maturity. If your region does not meet that requirement, consider growing anise in a deep container with one or two seeds in a pot that measures approximately eight inches wide and one foot deep. Place the container outside when the days are warmer. The optimum temperature for germination is 70°F. This speeds germination, it will *not* make the herb reach maturity any faster. Due to anise's carrot-like tap root, it hates to be transplanted. Please go ahead and try it if you enjoy beating your head against the wall because that's exactly what you will be doing as your transplants shrivel up one by one. If any of them make it, I have found they take even longer to reach full maturity. To avoid the breakage of stalks under the weight of the seed head, consider *loosely* staking anise's stalks before the flower head matures. Don't tie it too tightly to the stake, though, or the stalk will become dented and eventually stop growing.

HOW DO I HARVEST IT?

Harvest the seeds for medicine and the fresh leaves for adding flavor to salads, ice tea or in anything where a slight licorice taste is desired. The leaves can be harvested and used fresh until the umbel flower head appears. After that, they are tough and not too tasty. Wait until the seeds are fully mature–typically one month or so after the plant flowers. However, your region's temperatures may cause anise seeds to develop faster or slower. The seeds are ready to harvest when they turn from green to a grayish brown color. I always pick a few and test them. They should be rather hard and wonderfully aromatic when you bite into them. Cut the stalk several inches from the base and hang the seed heads upside down in a brown paper bag, out of direct sunlight. Seeds that don't drop off into the bag will need to be plucked off by hand. Store the whole seeds in airtight glass jars and grind *as needed* since pre-ground seeds are nearly void of the active medicinal oils.

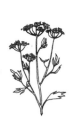

HOW DO I USE IT?

A few years ago I was asked to take a garden club on an herb walk. The location for this walk was not the hills and dales but a beautiful, rural private estate filled with acres of cultivated herbs. I arrived early so I could roam around and get the lay of the land. I noticed that the groundskeeper, a man in his mid-forties, kept following me. "You want to learn about herbs?" I asked him.

"How's that?" he yelled back, standing only about 20 feet away from me.

"You want learn how to use these herbs for their medicinal benefit?" I said a little louder.

He came closer, cupping his hand to his ear. "You'll have to excuse me," he said loudly. "Sometimes I have trouble hearing."

"How come?" I asked.

"What about the sun?" he said.

"No, I said, *how come.*"

"Oh! I think it's got something to do with the cannon."

"What cannon?" I said loudly.

"I'm in charge of setting off the town's cannon at special events. I think I might be standing too close to it." He looked down at the plant in front of us. "Hey, what's this herb?"

"Anise," I said.

"How's that?"

"*Anise,*" I said loudly.

His eyebrows furrowed. "Strange name for an herb. What can it do for me?"

"The seeds made into a tea help with digestion, gas, nausea and breaking up mucus when you've got a bad cough."

"Wow! Anything else?" he said totally enthralled.

"Well, they say anise is an aphrodisiac for some people."

"I want it!" he said.

I pulled a handful of the seeds from the plant and told him to write me and let me know how the herb worked for him.

Two months later I got a letter.

Dear Laurel,

Thank you so much for introducing me to Ann Smith. You were right. Ann Smith stops me from burping. Before Ann Smith, I had gas every night. Not anymore! And another thing, thanks to Ann Smith, my libido is back where it should be. I'm passing Ann Smith around to all my friends and family too! I'm a new man since I brought Ann Smith home.

P.S. You must admit, it's a strange name for an herb.

Whether you call it "Ann Smith" or anise, this licorice-smelling herbal favorite has been used for thousands of years to cure what ails you. One of the greatest things anise can do is **aid digestion and prevent gas**. Before there was Tums, there was anise. Before there was Gas-X, there was anise. And according to many folks who have used both anise and the brand name product, anise works better and is easier on the system.

What anise does as a digestive tea is **help prevent fermentation of food in the stomach**. Because anise is considered a "warming" herb, it **stimulates digestion by increasing heat in the digestive tract**. A great tasting tea can be made by combining four ounces of freshly crushed seeds with one pint of boiling distilled water. Simmer the seeds in the water for two to three minutes, covered. Let the mixture stand for ten minutes, strain and enjoy one sip at a time. *It is important to note that you must crush the seeds right before using them to release the active oils.* One of the compounds in the seed, *anethole*, has been found to have a certain amount of antiseptic action in the intestines.

PICK A PESTLE AND START GRINDING

Crushing (grinding) the seeds releases *anethole* as well as other helpful naturally-occurring chemicals within the seed. However, the active oils are only at their medicinal height for a short time after grinding, thus, preground seeds are practically worthless.

74

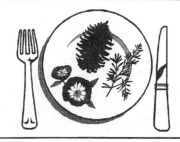

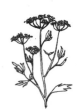

Wild Food Facts

Anise seeds perk up fruit salads, homemade breads and cookies with a slightly sweet licorice flavor. In fact, what passes for "licorice" at the candy counter is usually anise seed. Fresh anise leaves are a taste-tempting addition to salads, soups and stews. For soups and stews, it is best to add the fresh leaves as you are serving the food. This way, the delicate leaves won't lose their fragrance through cooking.

By the way, I'm not a big fan of using electric grinders with metal blades. I have found that, while these devices are quick and handy, they break the seed apart so much that there is a loss of aroma and flavor in the finished product. If you don't already own one, invest in a good mortar and pestle. I think pestles and mortars made from marble are the best with heavy duty porcelain china ranking second. I'm not much for the wooden varieties since they retain the aromas and colors of all the herbs that touch them. Purchase one that is large enough to accommodate four or more tablespoons of an herb without worrying about the various seeds, leaves and flowers flipping out of the pestle as you grind. **Always grind herbs in a clockwise direction, which increases the energy components within the plant matter**. (For that matter, stir *everything* clockwise, whether it be soups, stews or drinks). The other thing about using a mortar and pestle for grinding herbs is that you have a chance to press your energy into the plant matter and exercise that all-important *intent* that I covered in Chapter 7. As you grind the herbs, picture in your mind what you will be making with this particular plant, who it is for and what positive outcome you wish to create. Don't worry if you can't press the leaves, flowers or, in anise's case, the seeds into a fine powder. You merely want to break apart the plant matter. When grinding seeds, you just have to make a dent into the seed's hard shell to release the healing oils.

SAY "GOODBYE" TO GAS

Anise is a sweet-tasting tea to drink if you are suffering from **gas or bloating**. One classic formula worth trying is made by grinding together one ounce each of anise seeds, fennel seeds and caraway seeds. Pour 12 ounces of boiling distilled water over the seeds and cover tightly. Let the mixture steep for 10 to 20 minutes. Strain, and sip slowly.

Another *topical* way to reduce gas pains and that bloated feeling is to use anise essential oil. In one tablespoon of a base oil such as grape seed, apricot kernel or safflower, blend five drops of anise essential oil. Lie down and rub this concoction on your abdomen in a *clockwise rotation* until the oil is completely absorbed. Drinking the above mentioned tea formula in addition will also be helpful.

"NO" TO NAUSEA

Anise tea is also a godsend when you are suffering from **nausea** or an **upset stomach**. When I was in Egypt in the early 90s, I contracted what they call "The Pharaoh's Revenge" while on a cruise down the Nile. Let me tell you, this is not the place you want to get sick. I'll spare you the graphic details. Suffice to say, I was incapacitated for several days. If it weren't for the head steward on the ship, I would have missed many more days. He made an herbal tea concoction–a "secret Egyptian remedy that could cure anything," he told me. It turned out to be anise tea with a little cinnamon and honey added for flavor. Believe me, nothing tasted better than that tea. Once again, the presence of *anethole* in anise is responsible for not only soothing the stomach lining but it also acts as a **mild anti-parasitic**.

One blend I discovered for nausea that really helps is to combine a pinch each of freshly ground anise seed and cardamon seed along with a pinch of cinnamon and ginger. Pour one cup of boiling distilled water over the powders, stir and cover for 10 minutes. Strain the powders and add honey to taste. Sip this slowly whenever you feel nauseous. The combination or simply the anise seed alone is also good for those who suffer from **migraines that are accompanied by nausea**.

SOOTHE THAT COUGH

For centuries, anise seed has been used in cough teas, lozenges and syrups to **expel mucus** and **calm that tickle in the back of the throat**. Many people think anise just makes those natural cough preparations taste better. While that's true, anise is also a major ingredient on its own. You can thank two naturally-occurring chemicals in the seed, *creosol* and *alpha-pinene* for this healing benefit.

Anise seed is **especially good for hard, dry coughs when you know you've got trapped mucus in your lungs but you can't get it out**. To make the tea, pour one cup of boiling distilled water over three teaspoons of freshly crushed seeds. Cover and steep 20 minutes. Strain, add honey to taste and sip. You can drink up to three cups a day when you are fighting a dry cough. The herb works very well for children. Best of all, you don't have to force them to drink some wicked herbal brew since anise is mighty tasty. By the way, a little trick herbalists learned years ago was that **whenever you want to mask the nastiness of an herbal formula, adding a pinch of freshly crushed anise seeds to the brew will help take the edge off**. For children under the age of 12, make the above tea concoction but administer one to three teaspoons as needed. Oh, and don't be surprised when the tea starts forcing up all that trapped mucus. Remember, that's the whole point.

NURSING MOTHER'S BEST FRIEND

Another old use for anise is to **promote milk in nursing mothers**. One of the strangest herbal studies to prove this point was done at Auburn University. Researchers sprayed cows with anise oil. The fragrance alone apparently encouraged the cows to give more milk. While I can't say if simply smelling the oil or crushed seed will do the same for humans, I do know that drinking two cups of the tea daily will produce more milk for nursing mothers. And since anise relieves gas, this transfers to the mother's milk, **discouraging colic**.

MENOPAUSE AID

Anise has been found to stimulate the female glands that could help to balance estrogen levels. Its estrogenic ability is not considered top of the line. However, some herbalists feel this fragrant seed has the ability to **reduce menopausal symptoms brought on by an imbalance of estrogen**.

COULD THE SEED MAKE YOU PASSIONATE?

Due to the seed's slight estrogenic attributes, there have been many people throughout history who have considered anise a **natural aphrodisiac** for both men and women. This definitely falls more into the "folk remedy" file. Does it work? I think the herbal jury is still out. But if it doesn't trip your trigger in the passion department, at least the fragrant seeds will make your breath smell like licorice.

SWEET DREAMS ARE MADE OF ANISE SEEDS

An old remedy for **insomnia** that works quite well is made by placing one-half teaspoon of freshly ground anise seeds into six ounces of milk. Bring the mixture just to a boil (better yet, steam the milk if you have a

77

cappuccino steamer attachment), strain the seeds and sip the drink slowly. Anise seeds are warming to the stomach. The hot milk, which is easier to digest than cold milk, is a natural source of the amino acid *tryptophan* that helps to soothe the nerves. Put the two together and you have a warming, soothing blend that's a tasty alternative to counting sheep.

HANGOVER HELPER

I am not able to obtain any evidence to support their claim, but I know several herbalists who believe that the herb tea as well as the pure essential oil work to reduce the effects of a **hangover**. I would try two or three cups of the strong tea and perhaps add eight to ten drops of the pure essential oil to a lamp ring or oil diffuser which will broadcast the aroma into the air. If it doesn't make the hangover go away, at least your house will smell great.

THE SCENT THAT STIRS VERMIN AND FISH

Apparently, anise's licorice-like perfume is **an instant draw for mice and fish**. For mice, try crushing a few seeds once every day and place them on a mousetrap. Adding a few drops of the pure essential oil wouldn't hurt either. As for those fish, herbalist Jeanne Rose mentions in her book *The Aromatherapy Book* that fisherman entice their catches by rubbing anise essential oil over their hooks. If this does indeed work, I imagine it will make a lot of night crawlers very relieved.

TWO CAUTIONS

There are two cautions that come to mind. First, the tea was once thought of as a menstruation promoter. While there has never been one reported case of anise seed tea causing a miscarriage, **the conservative herbalist warns against pregnant women drinking the tea or using the essential oil**. Secondly, if you have **sensitive skin, the essential oil may be too strong and cause some burning**. So use caution and try only a small amount of the essential oil on your skin to avoid unnecessary problems.

Obviously, this is one herb you should keep on the shelf for those little emergencies. Just remember when you buy it, the name is *anise*. If you ask for Ann Smith, there's no telling what you'll get.

THE "DIRT" ON...ANISE

Botanical ~	*Pimpinella anisum*
Growth cycle ~	Hardy annual if seeds are completely harvested; perennial if left to go to seed.
Medicinal uses~	Aromatic, carminative, expectorant, mild sedative, galactagogue, possible aphrodisiac, hangover relief, mouse bait.
Part(s) used for medicine ~	Seeds.
Vitamins/Minerals ~	N/A
Region ~	Prefers cool climate from sea level to 9,000 feet.
Wild or Domestic ~	Both. Domestic species that are coddled may grow larger than their wild counterparts.
Poisonous look-alikes in the wild ~	To the untrained eye, poison hemlock and water hemlock.
Hardy or Delicate ~	Hardy if planted in cooler regions.
Height of mature plant ~	Ten inches to two feet.
Easy or hard to grow ~	Easy.
Cultivation ~	Direct seed into tilled soil in mid-spring. Cover with 1/8" of dirt and press down.
Plant spacing ~	Six to twelve inches.
Pre-soak seeds ~	No.
Pre-chill seeds ~	No.
Indoor seed starting ~	No.
Light/dark seed requirements ~	Dark, (i.e., make sure seed is fully covered with dirt).
Days to germinate ~	Six to fourteen days. However, if the soil is too cold, seedlings may germinate sporadically. Germinates best with a constant temperature of 70°F. Since anise often has a low germination rate (i.e., sometimes only 50% of the seeds planted actually germinate), you might want to plant a little more than you want. If you get lucky and a large percentage of seeds germinate, simply thin out what you don't want.
Days to full maturity ~	120 to 130 days of *frost-free* weather to mature. You might want to grow anise in a container if you reside in a region that has a short growing season.
Soil type ~	Best in rich soil with a touch of compost added. However, it will also grow in poor, sandy soil as long as it is well drained.
Water requirements ~	Likes light moisture but it must be well drained.
Sun or shade ~	Full sun.
Propagation ~	Seed. If seed umbel is not harvested, seeds should drop and germinate. Fresh anise seed tends to germinate better than dried. However, if you live in a region that gets frost or an average winter temperature that hovers around 50°F or 60°F, the soil and air temperature will not be warm enough to allow proper germination.

Easy/hard to transplant ~ Hard. Due to anise's long tap root, it doesn't take well to transplanting. Some growers feel you can transplant it in the seedling stage, but I've found that you lose more than you gain. Save yourself misery and direct seed anise.

Pests or diseases ~ Almost none. However, I had one beautiful stalk devoured by a late fall onslaught of aphids.

Landscape uses ~ Makes a nice, aromatic low hedge or worked into the garden as filler.

Gathering ~ **Seeds** ripen approximately one month after the flowering stage, typically August or September. However, your particular region may dictate a different time table. You want to wait and gather the seeds when they are hard, turn from green to grayish-brown and are blissfully aromatic when eaten. If you harvest the seeds too early, they will be soft and may not reach their true aromatic potential. Gather the **leaves** as needed before plant flowers. The younger leaves are the most flavorful and contain more aromatic oils. Older leaves are tough and not too tasty.

Best fresh or dried ~ **Seeds**: fresh or dried; **leaves**: fresh, as needed.

Drying methods ~ Cut stalk several inches above base and hang upside down in a paper bag. Seeds may need to be hand-picked off the seed head for storing once they are sufficiently dry.

Amount needed ~ If you really love anise, you may need a minimum of 10 plants.

Seed collection ~ Same method as for drying seeds. Helpful hint: you can plant the same anise seeds that you are using for medicine. However, due to possible problems with age and improper storage, the germination rate is not as high as seeds packaged especially for growing.

Companion planting ~ Anise likes coriander. Yarrow and stinging nettle may help to boost the aromatic oil content of anise.

Container planting ~ Not considered to be a typical container plant. However it can be done. Seed only one plant into a container six inches round and one foot deep to give the tap root room to grow.

Common mistakes ~ Not planting the seed early enough to accommodate the 120 to 130 day growing period; thinking you are "herbally gifted" and trying to transplant a fully grown plant...even if one of the transplants takes, it's not worth the energy.

Interesting facts/tips ~ You can lose some plants if they become top heavy with their seed heads and then fall over, breaking the stalk. To avoid this, loosely stake the stalks once they are developed but before the seed head matures.

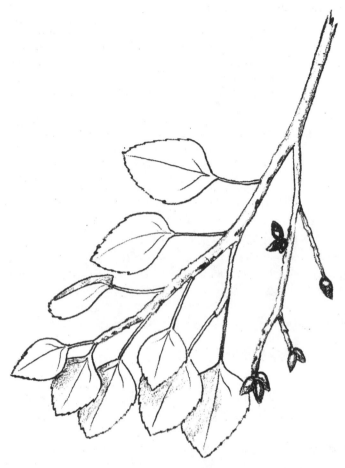

Chapter 12

ASPEN
VOTED MOST POPLAR

Populus tremuloides
(Other notable poplars species include Black cottonwood
(Populus trichocarpa), **Balsam poplar** *(P. balsamifera)* **and**
Balm of gilead *(P. x candicans)*
Perennial
Medicinal Uses: *Febrifuge, anti-inflammatory, stomachic, tonic*
Medicinal parts of plant: *Bark, fresh spring buds*
Forms: *Tea, fomentation, oil, tea wash, salve*

WHAT IS ITS CHARACTER?

Aspens can be a bit aloof in their nature. If you lie on your back with your head against the chalky white trunk and look upward, you'll notice two things. First, the aspen leaves flutter in a trembling motion, sending a soft whisper of sound through the forest that sounds like tissue paper being ruffled. This trembling of the leaves gave aspen its slang name "quakie" which stands for "quaking aspen." Some observers of aspens often say that this trembling reveals a deep seated nervous character trait. However, aspen never seems too nervous to me. With its tall, outstretched trunk arching far into the blue sky, aspen has always acted more "above it all" rather than some frightened forest tree. The second thing you'll notice as you stare up at the aspens is that the tops of each tree often softly rock to and fro, sometimes with the tiptop of one aspen bending to touch the top of another. When I see this, it always reminds me of a gossip fest, as one tree eagerly passes on its catty commentary to the surrounding members. Aspens can definitely be standoffish in character and suspicious of anyone new venturing into their domain. However, if you befriend them and they take you in, the aspen trees can help guide you on your path as they communicate with your spirit on incredible levels.

WHERE DO I FIND IT?

Aspens are found in moist areas from 5,500 feet to 9,500 feet, often in woodland settings. Some feel that the higher in altitude you go for an aspen, the better quality tree you will find. Black cottonwoods are found up to 5,000 feet, usually around shaded rivers, stream beds and creeks. Cottonwoods require a lot more water to survive than aspen trees. If you don't see any visible water source, chances are the cottonwood is being fed by an underground stream. Native Americans, trappers and mountain men used the cottonwoods to locate underground waterways. Balsam poplar and balm of gilead are also found in moist, shaded woodland areas.

HOW DO I GROW IT?

There's an old saying with aspens that if you cut down one tree, ten more will pop up. This theory is due to the deep, underground root formations that are said to interconnect each aspen in the forest. In other words, when you see a stand of aspens, they are all related to one main tree in that grouping. I think it's best to purchase a sapling from a tree nursery that has access to forest aspens. However, I don't feel that domesticated (i.e, backyard aspen trees) have the energy and power of their woodland family members. Domesticated aspens always look a bit lost, lonely and out of their element. Backyard aspens (as well as their wild counterparts) are also prone to a host of fungi diseases that range from "ink spot" on the leaves to oyster shell crawlers on the bark. These conditions along with the other assorted fungi completely destroy the tree by suffocating it. Cottonwoods can also attract the fungi but aspens tend to be more of a target. There is a paraffin-based oil application that can be sprayed on the tree in the spring which may reduce the fungi. However, I wouldn't trust the medicinal purity of the tree's bark or spring buds after a coating of paraffin had been applied. In my opinion, ethical wildcrafting of aspen is your best bet or purchase the bark and spring buds from a wildcrafter whom you trust.

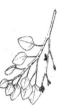

HOW DO I HARVEST IT?

Let's take the bark first. Always gather bark in the spring from *recently downed aspen trees*. They might have been downed by the wind, a lightning storm or a hungry beaver. The term "recently downed" means that the tree has fallen within the last 14 days or less and hasn't had a chance to rot or attract forest fungi. If the aspen shows an obvious formation of fungi (which might be the reason it fell down), I would leave it. I don't gather bark from standing aspens for two reasons. First, since the trunk is usually fairly small, the harvesting of bark often kills the tree. Secondly, it is so much easier to peel the inner bark off recently downed, healthy trees. When you are looking for the perfect tree, look for older, thicker-trunked trees since they yield a greater amount of inner bark. Typically, you shouldn't have to use a knife to harvest the inner bark since the outer white bark is already partially released from the heartwood. Once you lift off the outer bark, turn it over and peel away the brown inner bark. This is what you will use for medicine.

Now, onto the aspen buds. Gathering aspen buds has become a spring ritual of mine that usually ends up requiring a considerable amount of time, patience and, above all else, luck, to accomplish. You see, you don't just go out in the woods and pick aspen buds willy-nilly. They need to be as long as possible before they break open into spring catkins. They also need to be covered with a layer of sticky sap before they are considered worthy of harvest. It is that sticky sap that will eventually be medicinally beneficial. Depending upon your region, start looking for aspen buds as early as January and as late as April. They should be three-eighths to five-eighths of an inch long and a bit on the plump side, rather than narrow. I mention this because you will need a lot of them to generate enough oil and eventually salve. Picking a bunch of buds that are smaller than bee-bees will take forever and yield next to nothing in the final processing. It is vital that the buds have sufficient sap on them. When you press them between your fingers, you should feel a slight resinous quality that covers each bud. Some bud pickers who have plenty of free time and love to keep notes, require four things for optimum picking. It should be a bright, sunny day with low humidity, there should be at least a few inches of snow surrounding the trees, the nights should still be below freezing and it should be around two o'clock in the afternoon when you pick the little darlings. I'm not kidding about that two o'clock part. The sun is still hot enough at two to bring out the sap in the buds without being so hot that it dries it up. Take these four so-called "optimum requirements" for bud picking and throw in the fact that you have to find the perfect sized buds and you have an herbal spring challenge that often results in returning home empty handed.

However, there are alternatives. If you cannot find the perfect aspen buds, consider finding the perfect cottonwood buds. Cottonwood or balsam poplar spring buds are much bigger—anywhere from one-half inch to one inch long—fatter and covered with much more of that important medicinal sap. I found a recently fallen, 40-foot tall cottonwood tree on the side of the road a few years ago and was able to easily collect a little over two pounds of the fat spring buds. In comparison, the same size *aspen* tree would probably yield half the weight or less in buds. Since it takes cottonwood buds more time to grow before they pop open to reveal their strings of spring catkins, you have a longer time period to pursue them. Whereas, with aspens, the time period between the bud starting to appear and the breaking into a catkin is much shorter.

If you are lucky enough to live near a stand of balm of gilead trees, you have hit the "bud jackpot" since balm of gilead produces some of the fattest, sappiest buds I've seen. With either species of poplar trees, you will still want to follow the snow on the ground, sunny day, evening freeze, two o'clock suggestions to ensure the sappiest buds. Instead of gathering the sticky buds of either aspen or cottonwood in a paper sack or burlap bag, place them in a glass jar. This way, they can be easily removed without their sap sticking to the container.

HOW DO I USE IT?

When I was in fifth grade, I remember reading a book in school that recounted the story of a country doctor in the 1880's. In the book, the doctor spent a fair amount of time hanging out with the local Indians and learning which plants helped which ailments. As I recall, the Indians taught him about roots, barks and leaves. But when it came down to helping the townsfolk, the country "doc" always served them aspen bark tea. I couldn't understand the doc's fixation with aspen bark. Whatever condition he was treating, it was always "here's some aspen bark tea." Fevers, aching joints, malaria–even the common skin itch–and there he was with his trusty cup of aspen bark tea.

It wasn't until much later in my herbal studies that I realized the doc wasn't so crazy after all. The aspen tree has been one of the most reliable as well as effective herbal treatments for a variety of troubles throughout history. It is probably because the Indians and pioneers had to use the trees and weeds which were most plentiful around their homestead. And if the white trunked aspens happened to grow nearby, they quickly determined what the trees could do for them on the medicinal front. It didn't take them long to realize that the slender trees which turned to "gold" in the autumn were worth their weight in gold when it came to their many uses.

TAKES THE FIT OUT OF THE FEVER

One of the first uses those western folks discovered was aspen's ability to effectively **bring down a fever**. As an herb, aspen has what is called a "cooling energy" as opposed to a warm or hot, circulatory-stimulating energy. Aspen cools the fire of a fever which, in turn, brings calm and balance back to the body. When malaria was racing its way through towns during the 1800's, the suggested treatment was massive doses of quinine. Unfortunately, quinine often further upsets a weakened stomach as well as depresses the heart's ability to function. However, a person could safely take cup after cup of aspen bark tea for malaria and never experience any negative side effects. Did it always cure malaria? No. But then again, neither did quinine. The point is, aspen bark *did* help reduce the chills and fever triggered from malaria or any other common cold that came down the pike.

The stuff that gives the bark its fever-stopping bite is *populin* and *salicin*–kissing cousins to aspirin but without the chemical "middle man." In other words, instead of a laboratory extracting the active ingredients out of the bark and forming them into a little white pill, your body absorbs the whole bark and naturally converts what it needs of the *populin* and *salicin* in order to reduce the fever.

For bringing down fevers, the most effective part of the tree is the bark. However, many people complain that it's way too bitter a brew. For this, reason, the leaves are often used. However, they do not pack the same fever-killing punch as the bark. My attitude has always been that I want to use the best herb in the best form for the job at hand. If that herb happens to taste like pond scum, well, I guess that's life. After all, this *is* medicine and really strong medicine is usually never confused with "sipping tea." So, bite the bullet, hold your nose and drink the stuff down.

To make this biting brew, place a heaping teaspoon of the bark in 16 ounces of boiling distilled water. Let the bark simmer for 10 to 20 minutes. Strain the bark and then *let the mixture stand until cool*. When it is cool, sip it gradually until you have finished.

The fever-reducing aspect of aspen bark can be used as a **bath for young children and even babies**. Some scientists don't believe that your skin can absorb the healing benefits of the *populin* and *salicin*. However, experience has proven otherwise. Essentially what happens is the pores absorb the tea mixture and carry it into the blood stream which, in turn, prompt the *populin* and *salicin* into action. Obviously, this absorption method is not as effective as drinking the tea but it does work. I recommend that you drink the tea while soaking in the bath to get the most bang for your buck. You'll need to make a stronger brew for the bathtub than you would for drinking. What I do is take a big stainless steel pasta pot and fill it with tap water. Add one cup of chopped aspen bark. (Cottonwood bark will work if you can't find aspen bark). Bring the mixture to a rolling boil and simmer covered for 20 minutes. Meanwhile, pour a hot bath, making sure that the bathroom temperature is hovering around 75°F so as not to get a chill. Strain the mixture into the tub. Let the child soak in the bath anywhere from five minutes to 15 minutes, depending upon the severity of the fever and age of the child. For babies, I would err on the side of caution and keep the soak time around five minutes to start. This can be repeated up to three times a day, *changing the water each time*.

A TERRIFIC TONIC

Aspen bark tea is an excellent tonic for the system. This means that it is able to strengthen and invigorate weak organs or the entire body. The great thing about herbal tonics is that they are drawn to the exact area in the body where they are most needed. If the entire body needs a tonic effect, the herb adjusts and works on a systemic approach.

If you suffer from **chronic diarrhea that is not directly related to parasites or a bacterial infection**, aspen bark tea may help reduce the symptoms. Adding equal parts of barberry bark (*Berberis vulgaris*) to the tea will enhance its benefits.

If your **urinary organs are inherently weak** and prone to recurring problems such as **cystitis**, combine one-half teaspoon of aspen bark with one teaspoon of uva ursi leaves (*Arctostaphylos uva-ursi*) and steep the herbs in 10 ounces of boiling water for 20 minutes. Drink one-half to one cupful of the tea up to three times each day until relief is felt.

Aspen also works as a stomachic. This means it **acts on the stomach specifically to strengthen and tone the area**. For this reason, aspen bark tea is one of the oldest **digestive tonics**, especially for those who have **chronic digestive disorders or for the elderly who may have lost tone in their stomach lining**. Drink one or two cups of the bark tea per day to help build a healthier, more toned stomach.

INFLAMMATION BE GONE!

The team of *populin* and *salicin* also work wonders for any kind of **inflammatory pain** (such as a **headache, rheumatism or arthritis**) as well as for **skin rashes**, **sore throats**, **minor burns** or **inflamed wounds**. Once again, aspen's cooling energy helps to temporarily take the fire out of the inflammation. You can either drink the bark tea, try an external application in the form of a "tea wash," make a salve or employ all methods simultaneously.

The bark tea is made and consumed cool as mentioned earlier. If you are using the tea to replace aspirin for a **headache**, you will notice that the medicinal effect is quick and gives a tingly feeling to the body and head. However, the painkilling effects are mild and do not last as long as white willow bark (the herb that inspired the creation of aspirin).

The tea wash (which would work for **skin rashes**, **sore throats**, **minor burns** or **inflamed wounds**) is made as you would make the tea "fever" bath. You can either soak the affected area in a pail of the hot or cool mixture or, if that's not easy to do, saturate a clean cotton flannel cloth in the tea bath, wring it out and place it over the area to be treated. In herbal medicine, this is called making a *fomentation*. In the case of a sore throat, simply gargle with the strong tea concoction.

If you really want to "juice up" the fomentation, here's an effective little formula you can try. (This works especially well for inflamed joints or where one needs external pain relief). First, apply arnica ointment to the area you are treating. (**If there is any broken skin, do not use arnica ointment since it can cause blistering**). Dip the cotton cloth in the aspen bark tea bath. Before you place the cloth on the skin, put three drops *each* of pine pure essential oil and birch pure essential oil on the cloth. If you cannot find birch essential oil, substitute wintergreen instead. I usually secure the fomentation with plastic wrap to help seal in the essential oils.

THE SOLUTION IS IN THE SALVE

One of my favorite remedies for inflammation, however, is the oil or salve made from those sappy aspen, cottonwood, poplar or balm of gilead buds. It may be difficult to obtain "the perfect buds," but when you can find them, they hold great healing power.

The aspen/cottonwood/poplar/balm of gilead bud oil is made differently than the normal method due to the resinous coating that makes the buds so sappy. This method is easier, less of a clean-up hassle and guarantees the highest retention of "activating" ingredients. First, take your sappy buds and place them in the freezer overnight. The following day, place the buds on a food scale and determine their weight. Multiply the weight in *ounces* by four. That number is the amount of extra virgin olive oil you will need by *volume*. For example, if the buds weigh one-half pound (eight ounces), you would multiply eight by four. This gives you 32. Thus, you will need 32 ounces of extra virgin olive oil. It is important to use extra virgin olive oil since it the purest and is less processed.

Place the frozen buds into a blender and pour the olive oil over them. Hold the lid down tightly and turn the blender on the "liquefy" setting. Turn off the blender every now and again to see if any of the buds are stuck on the blade. If so, pry them off and continue to process. I must say that **I am not usually in favor of using an electric blender to make my oils and salves since I much prefer using my own elbow grease which helps to transfer my physical and emotional intent into the herb**. However, even if I pounded the buds into the olive oil, I could never get the same smooth result that the blender provides. Liquefy the buds and oil until you get a thin, runny mixture that has a beautiful, soft burgundy color. Pour the mixture into jars, place one drop of benzoin tincture for every ounce into the "bud batch," which acts as a natural preservative and keep it refrigerated. It should last up to several years if stored in this way. If you want to turn that oil into a salve, simply stir in a teaspoon of melted yellow beeswax per ounce of *heated* bud oil and allow it to set until solid. This salve is excellent for external inflammations as well as wounds and oven burns. (For more information on how to make the perfect salve, turn to Chapter 40 "How to Make Herbal Stuff" and look under the heading "Salves/Ointments").

By the way, *don't try to make this oil with unfrozen buds*. If the buds aren't frozen, their sap will cause them to adhere to the blender's metal blades. This will leave you with a blender that will be so hard to clean, you will never want to touch it again for food use. I always suggest storing your buds immediately in the freezer after harvesting, even if you don't intend to make the oil for days or even months. This way, they will always be at their height of medicinal power.

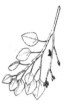

> ## *The Humorous Herbalist's*
> ### "Adiós Aches & Pains" Salve Recipe
> To give your bud salve extra pain-killing kick, try the following formula.
> For every ounce of salve, mix in two tablespoons each of St. John's wort oil and cayenne oil. Once the salve becomes semi-solid, for every ounce of salve, stir in 15 to 20 drops each of wintergreen pure essential oil and clove pure essential oil. This salve helps to "cool the fire" of inflammation while generating a gentle circulatory heat under the skin that temporarily gently numbs the area you are treating.
> It is great for arthritis, bursitis, tendinitis, pulled or over-exerted muscles, low back pain and sciatica.

A FEW THINGS YOU SHOULD KNOW...

Aspens, of course, fall under that large umbrella of "poplar trees." However, of all the other poplars mentioned in this chapter, most herbalists agree that aspen has a greater amount of those important pain-killing, inflammation-reducing ingredients, *populin* and *salicin* in its bark. That doesn't mean that other poplar trees, such as cottonwoods, are inert—you just might need an additional one or two cups of tea made from a cottonwood tree to get the medicinal effect found in one cup of aspen bark tea.

It has been found that aspen tree bark does not work as effectively on folks who have used a lot of aspirin in their life. Actually, for those who have taken aspirin every day for years at a time, aspen bark often has no medicinal effect on them whatsoever.

Whether you are treating fevers and headaches or arthritis, cystitis and inflamed wounds, it comes through like a trooper. From the bark to the buds, aspen should become one of your most "poplar" herbal remedies.

THE "DIRT" ON...ASPEN (& POPLAR)

Botanical ~	*Populus tremuloides* (Aspen) Other poplars with medicinal action include *Populus trichocarpa* (Black cottonwood), *P. balsamifera* (Balsam poplar) and *P. x candicans* (Balm of gilead) **NOTE: The yellow or tulip poplar is not a member of this medicinal family.**
Growth cycle ~	Perennial.
Medicinal uses~	Tea, fomentation, oil, salve.
Part(s) used for medicine~	Bark, fresh spring buds.
Vitamins/Minerals ~	N/A
Region ~	Aspens: in moist, woodland settings from 5,500 to 9,500 feet. Aspens can often be found growing wild in clear-cut and/or burned areas. Cottonwood trees and other poplars generally found growing near streams, rivers or over an underground water source.
Wild or Domestic ~	Generally wild, however aspens and poplars are used in landscaping.
Poisonous look alikes in the wild ~	None.
Hardy or Delicate ~	Hardy.
Height of mature plant ~	Approximately 100 feet.
Easy or hard to grow ~	Once established from a sapling, easy to maintain as long as tree does not attract fungi growth.
Cultivation ~	Buy tree from nursery.
Plant spacing ~	In the wild, aspens naturally grow anywhere from three inches apart to over 25 feet across. A good spacing would be around six to ten feet apart.
Pre-soak seeds ~	Not applicable.
Pre-chill seeds ~	Not applicable..
Indoor seed starting ~	Not applicable.
Light/dark seed requirements ~	Not applicable.
Days to germinate ~	Not applicable..
Days to full maturity ~	Not applicable.
Soil type ~	In nature, aspens grow in "quakie" soil, a rich blend of light, aerated, cool, rich earth. Try to duplicate this as much as possible when transplanting the tree into your yard.
Water requirements ~	Constant moisture is helpful without drowning the tree's roots. Cottonwoods, however, require a great deal of steady water. If you happen to have a stream running through your yard, that's a good place to plant the poplar.

90

Sun or shade ~	Partial sun.
Propagation ~	An intricate twist of underground roots.
Easy/hard to transplant ~	Nursery stock tree, easy.
Pests or diseases ~	A long list of fungi, including ink spot on the leaves and oyster shell crawlers on the bark. These affect both domestic as well as wild aspens. Cottonwoods and other trees that fall under the "poplar" umbrella, can be prone to these fungi, but not to the extent of the aspen tree.
Landscape uses ~	Wind break, dramatic electric yellow splash of color each fall.
Gathering ~	**Bark**: spring. Pick only from a recently fallen tree; **leaf buds**: late winter/early spring, sunny afternoon when buds are at their height of "stickiness."
Best fresh or dried ~	**Bark**: dried; **leaf buds**: *always* fresh
Drying methods ~	**Bark**: Peel the inner layer from the outside bark and place in air dryer or on sheets of paper towels.
Amount needed ~	One tree is sufficient for all your needs.
Seed collection ~	Not applicable.
Companion planting ~	Blue violet, cleavers, skullcap, nettle.
Container planting ~	Definitely *not* suited as an indoor container plant.
Common mistakes ~	Due to aspen's inherent fungi problems, it really doesn't make for a good backyard tree. If you choose to spray the tree with a paraffin-based oil to reduce the fungi, you shouldn't use the tree for medicine.
Interesting facts/tips ~	In the woodland setting, one aspen tree is interconnected via the underground roots to every other tree in that forest. There's a saying that goes "Cut down one aspen and 10 more will grow."

Chapter 13

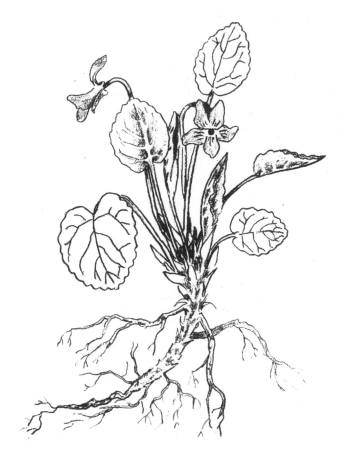

BLUE VIOLET

PICK THIS POSEY FOR PLEASANT RELIEF

Viola odorata

("W.F.")

Perennial

Medicinal Uses: *Alterative, soothing expectorant, sedative, anti-neo-plastic, febrifuge, antiseptic, anti-spasmodic, demulcent, vulnerary. Large doses of violet can produce an emetic effect (vomiting)*

Medicinal parts of plant: *Flowers, leaves*

Forms: *Tea, tincture, tea wash, fresh plant poultice, syrup*

WHAT IS ITS CHARACTER?

At first glance, you could easily mistake blue violet for a weak, tender perennial. But if you take a closer look you might see the young, eager spirit within the plant that can hardly wait to emerge from frozen lawns and snowy hillsides. No matter how old or deeply rooted a particular stand of violets may be, they seem to exude a child-like exuberance as their blue and purple flowers heads burst open, signaling the first sweet days of spring. The tender, delectable petals last only a few weeks before disappearing and giving way to the hardy, heart-shaped green leaves which give off a far more reserved energy than their petaled predecessors. To me, spring violets radiate a beautiful vitality that teaches us we all have the potential to begin again and see the future with renewed hope.

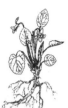

WHERE DO I FIND IT?

Blue violets can be found growing in a cool, shady, wet corner of your backyard lawn or anywhere in the wild where there is a constant source of water and partial shade. They love woodland type soil and settings. I have seen a few stands of violets in sunny locations. However, they don't last long since the heat wilts both the flower heads and leaves. They thrive in a heavy, rich, composted soil that falls somewhere on the acid to neutral pH scale.

HOW DO I GROW IT?

Blue violets can be tricky to cultivate, but it *can* be done if you follow certain specifications. Violets require a temperature of 32°F or lower to germinate. Germination is erratic so I always suggest planting a few more seeds than you desire to increase your success rate. Direct seeding is always best over cells and/or growing flats. However, your particular region will dictate what you need to do. For example, if you live in regions that have some periods of frost or snow, you should take advantage of this fact and directly sow the seeds outside in early autumn. Choose an area that is shady, cool and, if possible, near some source of water. Broadcast the seeds into rich, dark well tilled soil that has a good amount of compost mixed into it. Press the seeds firmly into the soil, making sure they are covered with dirt. Spread a layer of leaves over the soil as a mulch during the snowy winter months. Since germination is erratic, you may lose a third or more of what you sowed. The seedlings that eventually make it through come spring will be tough enough to weather the extreme elements needed for years of growth. If you don't live in areas that experience freezing temperatures, plant seeds in cells filled with the same kind of rich, composted soil you would use in the garden. Press seeds firmly and cover with a thin layer of dirt. For the seed trays, a burlap cover is a good idea since it helps create a slightly moist environment. You will need to imitate freezing temperatures. To do this, place the covered tray in a freezer or walk-in cooler where the temperature hovers between 35°F and 40°F. Keep them in that cold to freezing environment for two to three months before gradually reintroducing them to warmer temperatures and gently mist with water. Once the seedlings emerge and appear semi-hearty you can transplant them into the garden. You will need to handle the seed cells carefully since blue violets hate to have their young roots disturbed. **Remember, blue violets flourish in shady, moist areas**. Once established in your yard, blue violets propagate via underground root runners that are almost impossible to banish. Of course, the idea of getting rid of these sweet little things would never cross my mind.

HOW DO I HARVEST IT?

Some of blue violet's remedies, such as the cough syrup, require *fresh* handfuls of spring flowers which should be gathered in early spring just as they are opening. The *fresh* leaves are eaten as a wild green as well as used for medicinal remedies. They are best harvested in early spring and either used immediately or placed on an inside drying rack in a cool area and dried for later use. Don't bother drying the flowers since they quickly lose their sweet scent and potency. One important note: I don't usually harvest first year plants since they are always on the smaller side and I want them to develop a strong underground root network so they will have years of new growth.

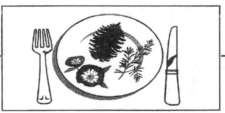

Wild Food Facts

In a world where nature often delivers some mighty bitter tasting plants, blue violet is a refreshing surprise. The fresh spring flowers add a sweet taste to salads, ice tea, lemonade and sparkling water. If you have some free time and the patience of Job, you might want to make crystallized blue violet flowers. To make this confectionery treat, gather blue violet flowers just as they are opening. Beat the white of an egg and, using a fine paintbrush and delicate strokes, coat the entire flower with the mixture. Dust the wet petals with a fine sprinkle of powdered sugar and gently rest them on waxed paper to dry. When they harden, they are ready to place on cakes, on ice cream, eaten like candy or displayed on a plate.

HOW DO I USE IT?

As a kid, I never gave blue violets much of a second glance. To me, they always seemed kind of puny and weak with their dainty heart-shaped leaves and delicate, sweetly scented blue and purple petals drooping downward in a sort of "Don't-bother-me-I'm-having-a-bad-day" kind of display. If there was a garden brawl between violets and daisies, I would have given eight to five odds on the daisy to win with a technical knock-out.

But as I became more interested in plants and their medicinal benefits, I kept hearing herbalists speak volumes about violets. Could this flower that looked to me as if it had the lowest self esteem in the forest actually rank as an incredible–and even life saving–herbal remedy? Decide for yourself.

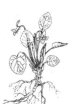

A SWEET "SPRING TONIC"

In many parts of the country, blue violets—which are also referred to as "sweet violets" because of their sweet, delicious scent—are the sign that spring has finally arrived. Back when folks turned to their backyards for medicine, blue violets were one of the first plants they eagerly grabbed as part of their "spring tonic." Spring tonics have fallen out of favor in the modern world. That's too bad because they can build a bridge between seasons and help shrug off whatever winter crud you haven't been able to shake. What a spring tonic does, in essence, is flood the body with much needed vitamins and minerals via the fresh, young, supple green leaves of spring plants. Other plants that fall into this category are spinach, lightly steamed nettle leaves, alfalfa, watercress and dandelion greens. These are all mighty fine plants and ones that you should combine as part of your spring cleaning. But few people realize that the common blue violet *beats* each one of these plants when it comes to the amount of vitamin A and C it packs in its petals and leaves. **Both flowers and leaves are high in vitamin C while the leaves rank at the top of the vitamin A list.** This means that a mere half-cup of *fresh* violet greens will give you above and beyond your daily dose of beta carotene and is equal to eating four oranges.

As a "spring tonic" of violet flowers and leaves courses through your body, you should expect some…well…movement in various areas. First and foremost, **violet leaves and flowers are an A-1 blood purifier.** This means that whatever has been "stuck" in your system over the winter has the ability to break free and find its way out of your body. There are three ways this can take place: through the pores of your skin, through urine and through the bowels. Blue violet has been known to work on all three and sometimes all at once. Thus, as with any "spring tonic" please don't overuse the remedy or you will spend a great deal of spring just trying to stop the various leaks.

VIOLETS CONQUER "THE COUGH"

One of the most common hanger-oners from winter is "the cough." And it just so happens that blue violet has the ability to **soothe, sedate and expectorate that cough** in the sweetest of ways. I'm talking about the taste. Yes, instead of recommending an herb that tastes like wet asphalt, here's a medicinal that can make you actually look forward to its tasty tingle on your tongue. And best yet, it's safe to give to children.

The tea is made by pouring eight ounces of boiling distilled water over two heaping teaspoons of the fresh leaves or one heaping teaspoon of the dried leaves. Cover and let it steep for 15 minutes, then strain, add honey if you wish and enjoy.

The tea—minus the honey—also makes a great **anti-inflammatory gargle for sore throats.** But don't spit out the tea when you are finished gargling. Swallow the tea and enjoy the sweet taste.

Some herbalists feel that blue violet works better in combination with other cough-related herbs. One formula combines one-half ounce *each* of dried coltsfoot, hyssop, horehound and blue violet leaves. Pour six cups of boiling distilled water over the herbs and cover, steeping for 20 minutes. Every few minutes, uncover and rapidly stir the herbs into the water to encourage their medicinal extraction. After 20 minutes, strain the herbs, add honey if you desire and drink the tea in eight ounce doses every two hours.

While the tea works well, many old time and modern day herbalists think that the syrup beats the best tea combo. As with the tea, the syrup can be given to children. The only prerequisite is that blue violet syrup must be made from the *fresh* petals and leaves. Here's how to make it: Combine one cup of tightly-packed fresh blue violet flowers (which have been torn into small, "thumb nail" pieces) and one-half cup of finely chopped fresh blue violet leaves and place them into a wide mouthed glass jar that can hold two cups of water. *Do not use any kind of metal or plastic containers.* Pour two cups of boiling distilled water over the plant. Secure it with a tight fitting lid and allow the flowers and leaves to steep for 24 hours. I like to stir the tea every hour or so and even shake the jar vigorously to stimulate the release of the herb's healing ingredients. After 24 hours, strain the liquid through a layer of clean muslin cloth. You should have a lovely blue colored tea. Take the blue tea and pour it into a glass or stainless-steel saucepan. Warm slowly on very low heat. *Do not boil the liquid!* As you heat it, gradually add four cups of unfiltered honey, stirring constantly. Remove from the heat and, when beginning to cool, add the juice of one fresh lemon. Store in amber or blue bottles in the refrigerator. To lengthen the syrup's life span, add a tablespoon of fresh grated ginger to the blend. It should keep for up to two months. The dose is one to two tablespoons as needed. Blue violet syrup has been used for centuries in the treatment of **sore throats, whooping cough, chronic dry coughs, dryness of the upper respiratory chest and asthma.** As always, if your cough persists for longer than one week or becomes worse, discontinue use of the syrup and see a doctor.

HEADACHE RELIEF

One of the major advantages of blue violet is that it is considered a **gentle sedative**. In ancient Greece, the populace used violets to "**moderate anger, comfort and bring about sleep.**" These days, this sweet little plant made into a tea can be used to **relieve severe headaches—especially when there is a congested feeling in the head.** While it is not exactly known how this herb works to allay headaches, *salicylic acid*—the ingredient they make aspirin out of—was extracted from the herb. This would account for blue violet's anti-inflammatory abilities and possible connections to headache relief. A friend of mine was given blue violet years ago when she suffered from intense **migraines** that left her incapacitated for days at a time. She told me that several cups of the fresh flower tea taken every two hours helped get her through the rough times. No, the tea didn't "fix" the migraine, but according to what she said, it didn't make it worse either. If you can't find fresh blue violet flowers, look for a tincture that is made from the fresh plant. The tincture dose is 25 to 45 drops in two ounces of warm water. Adding the tincture to warm water speeds its delivery into the bloodstream.

Another way you can use the tea for headaches is in a compress. Using the dried leaves or the fresh flowers, make a double-strength tea (i.e., steep two heaping teaspoons of the dried leaves or four heaping teaspoons of the fresh flowers in eight ounces of boiling distilled water for 20 to 30 minutes). Soak a clean, cotton cloth in the liquid, wring it out and then place the compress over your forehead. Some people like to place a compress against the nape of their neck as well. Once the cloth becomes cool, dip it into the warm tea, wring it out and repeat. As always, it is best to lie down when you're doing this. Feel free to sip a cup of blue violet tea for added relief.

FOLK CANCER REMEDY

Read any old herbal book and blue violet often comes up as an aid for **cancerous growths**. The leaf tea was typically taken often throughout the day. Handfuls of the fresh leaves were also mashed into a juicy paste and placed over areas of the body where tumors were found. *The Encyclopedia of Herbal Medicine* by Thomas Bartram mentions the successful use of blue violet in the treatment of cancer. In one entry, he notes that a 67-year-old woman was "cured of a malignant tumor in the throat (epithelioma of tonsil) with (blue) violet leaf tea (one ounce to one pint boiling water) taken freely." He goes on to say that the woman placed mashed poultices of the fresh leaves against her throat and experienced "immediate relief from pain and breathing difficulties." According to Bartram, "Within seven days the swelling disappeared; within 14 days the tonsil growth also." Obviously, cancer is a multi-dimensional disease that requires examination of the physical, mental and spiritual aspects. Herbal medicine can certainly play a role in the healing process as well as in the reduction of pain caused by the disease. It is completely up to you to decide which avenue of healing you wish to embrace.

ULCER RELIEF

The fresh or dried leaf tea has been used for many years to **soothe internal ulcers and, in some cases, provide mild pain relief**. One of the nice effects of drinking blue violet tea is that it has a lovely quieting effect on the nerves—something that proves quite useful for those who suffer from ulcers.

THE POWER'S IN THE FRESH LEAF POULTICE

The same fresh leaf poultice which was used externally for cancerous growths can be **applied over the eyes to reduce puffiness and inflammation**. If you suffer from **cracked nipples**, try the fresh leaf poultice and see if you get some relief. In addition, the fresh leaf poultice is one of the natural cures for **relieving the sting from stinging nettle**. In the wild, you will sometimes find nettle and blue violet growing within eyesight of each other. If you plant nettle in the garden—or if it happens to be there already—you might want to place blue violet near it.

A WONDERFUL TEA WASH

Blue violet tea can be used as a gentle wash for **minor skin diseases**, **mouth infections and sores**, **cooling and cleaning minor wounds** and as an **eyewash**. Make the tea as you normally would—eight ounces of boiling distilled water poured over two heaping teaspoons of the *fresh* leaves or one heaping teaspoon of the *dried* leaves—but allow the liquid to cool down completely, unless you are using it as a mouthwash. For the

eyewash, you can make the tea from the flowers at the ratio of four heaping teaspoons of flowers to eight ounces of water.

BLOOD PURIFYING BLEND

Blue violet also works as a **gentle blood purifier** to rid the body of toxins that could be contributing to **recurring skin diseases such as psoriasis and eczema**. While the fresh or dried leaf or the fresh flower tea work well on their own, adding equal parts of red clover flowers (either fresh or dried) really pumps up the herbal action. To get the most benefit from this blend, you should take three cups each day until you feel the condition is relieved.

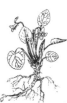

THE WILDER THE BETTER

According to herbal observation over the years, many practitioners believe that wild blue violets have more healing power than backyard cultivated ones. Also, many feel that the tea is much superior to taking the alcohol tincture. However, if you prefer the tincture, purchase a brand that is made from the *fresh plant* instead of dried. You can always make your own fresh tinctures from your herbal garden. To learn more about this, turn to Chapter 40, "How To Make Herbal Stuff" and check under the "Tincture" heading.

COMMON SENSE CAUTIONS

The cautions actually involve common sense more than anything. If you are picking the plant in someone's yard or in the wild, make sure you are picking the right plant. Once you are sure it is blue violet, you are safe. In addition, make sure the herb has not been sprayed with pesticides. If it has, stay away from it.

Eating too many fresh violet flowers and/or leaves can make you nauseous and create a nasty laxative effect. How many is too many? That's entirely up to your own body chemistry. The old adage, "You'll know when you've had enough" is my advice.

While the root is used by some herbalists, I would avoid it unless you enjoy vomiting. However, on the positive side, if you're out of Ipecac and you have a good crop of pesticide-free violets in the yard, try a mild decoction of the root in *very small doses*.

My first impression of blue violet wasn't on target. With all the vitamins it contains, it's more like a wolf in sheep's clothing. Let's just hope the common daisy isn't looking for a fight.

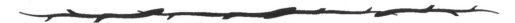

THE "DIRT" ON...BLUE VIOLET

Botanical ~ *Viola odorata*

Growth cycle ~ Perennial.

Medicinal uses~ Alterative, soothing expectorant, sedative, anti-neoplastic, febrifuge, antiseptic, anti-spasmodic, demulcent, vulnerary. Large doses of violet can produce an emetic effect (vomiting).

Part(s) used for medicine ~Flowers, leaves (either fresh or dried). Some herbalists use the root, but it is an emetic.

Vitamins/Minerals ~ Flowers and leaves have high doses of vitamin C. The leaves also have sizable amounts of vitamin A.

Region ~ Prefers cool, shady woodland environment. Found 4,000 to 13,500 feet.

Wild or Domestic ~ Both, although many wild varieties have been over harvested. If you correctly identify blue violet in the wild, make sure the stand is plentiful before harvesting a portion of it.

Poisonous look-alikes in the wild ~ Before blue violet flowers appear, the heart-shaped leaves resemble arnica (Arnica montana), a poisonous plant. To avoid confusion, always wait until the distinctive blue violet flowers appear before harvesting.

Hardy or Delicate ~ Hardy.

Height of mature plant ~ Three to six inches.

Easy or hard to grow ~ Moderately easy if you follow directions given in this chapter.

Cultivation ~ Direct seeding is best idea, however, it can be started in seed cells. For direct seeding, plant seed in loose, rich soil in early autumn. Press seed firmly into soil, covering it completely with dirt. Blue violet requires a temperature of 32°F or lower to germinate. Mulch seeded area with leaves during the winter. Seedlings should emerge in early spring. For seed cells, cover seed with dirt and place tray outside (if temperatures are below freezing) or in a cooler/freezer for two to three months. Reintroduce gradually to warmer weather and mist with water.

Plant spacing ~ Three to six inches. As blue violet reproduces each year, it tends to bunch together, so give it plenty of room to spread.

Pre-soak seeds ~ No.

Pre-chill seeds ~ Yes.

Indoor seed starting ~ Yes, but in controlled (i.e, below freezing) environment.

Light/dark seed requirements ~ Dark.

Days to germinate ~ Germination is erratic. Once seed has been exposed to freezing temperatures and is then introduced gradually to heat, germination can occur anywhere within 21 days. However, don't be surprised if seeds continue to germinate long after that.

Days to full maturity ~ 60 to 70.

Soil type ~ Rich, woodland-type soil with compost added is best, acid to neutral.

Water requirements ~ Must have adequate moisture without drowning in pools of water.

Sun or shade ~ Shade and cool.

Propagation ~ Seed, underground roots.

Easy/hard to transplant ~ Easy if transplanting already established plants. More challenging with seedlings since they dislike having their delicate roots disturbed. When transplanting established plants, make sure you bring along some soil from where they have been growing and pack it around the plants.

Pests or diseases ~ Red spider mites. One remedy for this is to use a forceful spray of the garden hose directed at the underside of the leaves.

Landscape uses ~ Makes a colorful border.

Gathering ~ Depending upon the region, blue violet is gathered anytime between early March to early May. Flowers are picked just as they are opening. Leaves should be harvested in early spring while they are still tender.

Best fresh or dried ~ **Flowers**: always fresh; **leaves**: fresh or dried.

Drying methods ~ **Leaves**: harvest tender young leaves and air dry indoors away from direct sun.

Amount needed ~ Fifty or more established plants, especially if you want to make the cough syrup which requires many flowers.

Seed collection ~ Once it is established in your garden, blue violet reproduces many more plants via underground roots. Seeds can be difficult to obtain, depending upon your region. Spring flowers are typically sterile in warm areas while fall flowers produce small "capsules" which can hold as many as 50 seeds.

Companion planting ~ Other moisture-loving plants such as skullcap, nettle and cleavers.

Container planting ~ Makes a good container plant as long as the pot is deep enough to accommodate future root growth. Regular watering is necessary, making sure there is always sufficient drainage to prevent root rot. During summer, place container in shade; during winter, place container in a cool location where temperatures hover around 45° F. If they become too warm during the winter, they may not flower come springtime.

Common mistakes ~ Not allowing the seed to pre-chill long enough to allow germination and not planting enough of the plant to satisfy your medicinal and edible needs.

Interesting facts/tips ~ A fresh leaf poultice of blue violet helps take the sting out of stinging nettle.

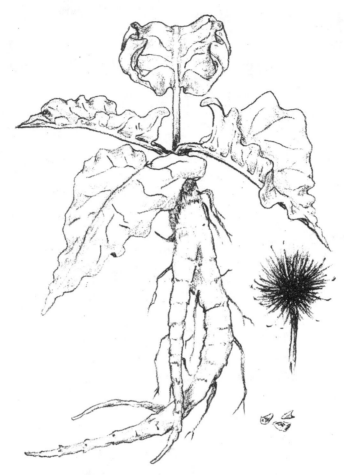

Chapter 14

BURDOCK
THE BOFFO BLOOD CLEANSER

Arctium lappa
("W.F.")
Hardy biennial

Medicinal Uses: *Alterative, aperient, depurative, diuretic, hepatic, laxative, tonic, gentle lymphatic cleanser*

Medicinal parts of plant: *Root, leaves*

Forms: *Tea, tincture, tea wash, poultice, salve*

WHAT IS ITS CHARACTER?

Many herbalists refer to burdock as one of nature's "hitchhikers" since the velcro-like burrs that develop in the second year of growth love to "hitch a ride" on clothing and shoes. However, I've never regarded burdock as a neurotic plant that felt the need to cling. Rather, I've always looked on this herb as an "old soul" that fully understands the power and importance of what it has to offer. Since it knows it only has two short years of life, it is bound and determined to reproduce itself in dozens of places so it can serve as many people as possible. Come that second and final year of growth, burdock's burrs are on a noble mission, attaching themselves to humans and animals alike and later dropping in a wide variety of areas to create the next generation of healing plants. Call it dogged, call it stubborn, it matters none to burdock. Its burrs are made for hitchin'.

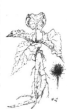

WHERE DO I FIND IT?

Everywhere and anywhere across the United States in cool, moist fields and along roadsides. You are less likely to come upon burdock as a wild plant in California and some of the southern states unless it has been planted on purpose by someone.

Proper identification of burdock is vital since the herb has been mistaken for one poisonous plant and other non-poisonous plants. The poisonous plant it slightly resembles is deadly nightshade (*Atropa belladonna*). Often, burdock grows close together in large clumps with other extraneous plants finding their way in the middle. One of those plants happens to be deadly nightshade and, while it does not have burdock's distinct shape and second year purple flowers, the leaves could be mistaken for burdock. This happened to one woman who drank a combination of burdock and deadly nightshade. While she survived the ordeal, it drives home the point that you must always be observant of what you are doing when you wildcraft herbs. On the non-poisonous front, to the untrained eye, rhubarb (*Rheum palmatum*) can be mistaken for first year burdock and vice versa. Cocklebur (*Xanthium strumarium*) could be confused with second year burdock. You also might confuse *Arctium lappa*—known as Greater burdock—from *A. minus*. *A. minus* usually grows under five feet tall, has smaller sized leaves, hollow leaf stalks and flower heads that rest on short stalks or are completely stalkless. **Greater burdock has quite distinctive tall stalks which are solid instead of hollow and leaves that can grow two feet or more in length. Overall, Greater burdock can grow as high as seven feet.** *A. minus* is sometimes called "Common burdock" although there are plenty of people who refer to

"Greater burdock" as "Common burdock." The point of this whole dissertation is that many herbalists feel that Greater burdock (*A. lappa*) is more active and the "specific" species you need to request when purchasing seed for your herb garden. When you are out in the wild, use the stalk variations mentioned above to discern between *A. lappa* and *A. minus*.

HOW DO I GROW IT?

Plant burdock from seed in the spring in a cool, moist part of the garden. Cover seed with one-half inch of dirt, setting seed two inches apart in rows six inches apart. Keeping plants close together makes for an easier root harvest since you might be able to pull up more than one at a time. Work a few shovels full of sawdust into the soil and you may have better luck getting the roots to break free come fall since it makes the soil more porous. Keep it well watered without drowning until germination which should occur within 21 days.

HOW DO I HARVEST IT?

Burdock leaves should be harvested from **first year plants** while they are still tender, usually around mid-summer. Some forest foragers have said that you can tell a first year plant from a second year plant by the fact that there is no stalk growing. However, I've seen a few first year plants with a definite stalk showing. What you are looking for in first year plants is the large rosette of huge leaves that forms at the base of burdock with *none* of the five to seven foot solid stalks and purple flowers.

For those people who want to experience the herbal joy of digging up fresh burdock root, I wish you all the luck in the world. I also hope you have a strong back, unlimited patience and aren't put off by the fact that you will work very hard to get your root. I speak from experience after spending the better part of a Saturday in early autumn digging up some of the toughest burdock roots known to Man. After three hours of shoveling, digging and pulling, I emerged with about one pound of root. I also had lower back pain and blisters. But if you're set on digging, here's the best way to approach it: Make sure the plant you're digging up actually *is* burdock. Once that's confirmed, you want to choose first year plants. The question in my mind has always been, "When does that first year end? Fall or spring?" Some herbalists swear by the roots dug in the fall from plants that were seeded six to seven months previously during spring. Others insist that if you wait until the following spring (i.e., approximately one full year from the time you planted burdock), the root is more medicinally viable. What you *don't* want to do is dig up the root from second year plants which have fully established their round-headed purple flowers.

Roots from these plants are stringy, almost inedible and lacking in medicinal energy. When you do set your shovel into the ground to dig burdock roots, realize that some of those little buggers can be three feet or longer in length. Instead of going directly in for the root, dig around the plant about one foot deep to gain better leverage and to ensure you get the whole root.

Immediately clean all dirt off the root with cool water. If you are using the root for wild food, completely pull off the inedible brown rind to reveal the creamy white inner core of the root. That inner core is quite edible and has a slight artichoke flavor. (For more ideas on how to use burdock root and leaves as wild food, check out the box on "Wild Food Facts" on page 109). If you want to use the root for medicinal purposes, DO NOT scrape off the brownish rind since it holds a vast amount of the plant's medicinal properties. To dry the roots for later use, slice the root from top to bottom and then cut them into pieces approximately two to four inches in length. Lay the pieces on a drying rack or on brown paper. DO NOT use newspaper since the ink can get into the plant matter. Make sure the roots are out of direct sunlight since extreme heat will dry up much of the volatile oils. Once they are dried, store the roots in an airtight jar and grind up portions of the roots as needed. The medicinal potency should keep for one to two years.

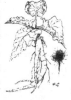

HOW DO I USE IT?

A few years ago a friend of mine offered a patch of her garden to me to "plant some great medicinal herbs." I went over to survey the area and knew exactly what would grow well in the space.

"I'm going to put in some burdock," I announced to my friend.

"Are you out of your mind?!?" was my friend's startled response. "Are you on medication? Have you recently hit your head and can't think straight? What on God's green earth would possess you to plant such a thing?"

I got the feeling that she was less than happy with my idea.

Yes, to the average onlooker, burdock is a menace that should be eradicated. But if you can convince the uninformed of burdock's blessed benefits, they might end up growing a few patches of the plant in their yard.

A BONA FIDE BLOOD PURIFIER

The root of the burdock plant is known the world over as **one of the best blood purifiers**. This herb does a mighty fine job when it comes to **toning up your system and tuning up the organs that "flush," i.e., your kidneys and your liver**.

There is nothing more important than keeping those organs that "flush" in good working order. Sluggish kidneys can create a bunch of ailments such as bladder infections and polluted blood streams. Lazy livers that don't get a chance to discharge all the crud they absorb, dump toxins into the system which can affect digestion and elimination. It can also create bouts of acne, eczema, psoriasis and my personal favorite, boils. Not a pretty picture. However, before any herb can work effectively to cleanse the body and tone the organs, there are three things you need to improve.

1. Your Diet
2. Your Diet
3. Your Diet

You can pour the best blood purifying herbs into your body but if you *also* pour in equal or greater amounts of fried foods, tons of dairy, loads of soft drinks, pitchers of booze and buckets of white sugar, you're not going to accomplish diddly-squat. No herb can combat that much garbage. In order to get the body working in sync again, you have to increase your intake of fresh fruits, lightly steamed vegetables and of course, plenty of water. Believe it or not, you should be drinking one ounce of water for every pound of body weight. That means that a 128 pound person should be enjoying one gallon of water per day. That might sound as if it is a lot of liquid but I assure you, it really works to cleanse your system of the daily accumulations of toxic waste. Once your body is flowing more naturally, it will be more receptive to what burdock can offer.

ARTHRITIS, RHEUMATISM AND GOUT RELIEF

Because burdock root acts as the ultimate "flusher," it has been considered a possible aid for those suffering from **arthritis, rheumatism and gout**. These conditions usually signal an overload of uric acid in the system which collects in the weakest part of the body—namely the joints. Once this acid collects, it sets up camp and creates more pain and stiffness. Burdock's "flushing" action helps to eliminate the uric acid via the kidneys which can, in some people, greatly reduce the pain. Diet, once again, plays a golden role. Moderating your intake of such foods as bread, dairy, red meat, salt, sugar, coffee and alcohol can help reduce the pain since these only serve to increase toxicity in the joints.

ATTACKING SKIN DISEASES FROM THE INSIDE OUT

Burdock root tea is considered a "classic" for treating skin diseases such as **acne**, **psoriasis**, **eczema** and **impetigo**. You must watch your diet for this remedy to be effective. In other words, for two to six weeks, cut out all deep fried foods, white sugar, white flour, processed foods and dairy. By doing this, you will see results much faster. Try drinking two to three cups of the tea each day with meals.

An *external* skin wash made from the *fresh* leaves is also helpful for **acne** and even **canker sores**. Dip a cotton ball or washcloth into a strong concoction of *fresh* burdock leaf tea (four tablespoons of the fresh plant to eight ounces of hot water, steeped for 20 minutes and allowed to cool) and place it over the affected areas for several minutes. This same brew and application can help reduce the pain of **minor skin abrasions**, **burns** and even **sprains** because it **reduces inflammation while drawing out the pain**.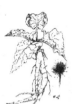

The tea made from the *fresh* root has been successful in treating **measles**. Essentially what the herb does is purge the impurities that are causing the virus from the bloodstream. The typical dose is one ounce by weight of the *fresh*, clean root boiled in two cups of water for 20 minutes. Repeat the same dose each day until relief of symptoms.

To get relief from the **external itching of measles**, herbalist Dr. John R. Christopher has a great formula made from *fresh* burdock root. Slowly simmer one pound of *fresh* burdock root in one cup of extra virgin olive oil for two hours, stirring every 10 to 15 minutes. Don't allow the oil to become so hot that it burns the plant matter. After two hours, strain the burdock root. Place a pint sized mason jar filled with one ounce of yellow beeswax in a hot water bath over low heat. Slowly melt the beeswax. Once it melts, add the hot burdock oil and stir the mixture with a wooden stick or spoon (don't use plastic since it will dissolve!) Continue to stir until you are sure both the beeswax and oil are thoroughly combined. Set it aside to harden. Once it is ready, the salve can be applied to measles morning and night or whenever they become itchy.

German researchers have discovered that the fresh root of burdock contains chemicals that kill disease-causing bacteria and fungi that could lead to such conditions as **ringworm**. The tea or tincture can be taken internally as well as applied externally to the ringworm.

ROOT FOR THIS PMS RELIEF

When your liver is congested with too much backed up estrogen, it can cause emotional fits of anger, rage and depression — all symptoms of **PMS**. Drinking two cups a day of burdock root tea from the onset of ovulation until your period arrives can help reduce these emotional reactions.

A CANCER CURE?

The famous "cancer tea" called Essiac includes burdock as one of its ingredients. That should give you an idea of the kind of healing power that is associated with this root. The Essiac formula also includes the herbs turkey rhubarb, sheep sorrel and slippery elm in specific amounts. As with any formula, this quartet of herbs work synergistically to cleanse, nourish and heal the body. There are "folk remedy" stories of burdock being used alone for treating cancer. However, whether alone or in formula, herbs should be one part of the puzzle when you are dealing with cancer. The balance of healing modalities may include other alternative therapies and/or traditional drug cancer treatment.

REGENERATE LIVER CELLS

For those who have suffered from degenerative liver conditions due to alcohol or drug abuse, one to two cups of burdock root tea each day **can help regenerate liver cells**. To increase burdock's liver protection/regeneration ability, I would combine it with the herb milk thistle. In a case like this, taking each of these herbs in tincture form is the best idea. A good dose to start off with is 25 drops of each herbal tincture in several ounces of warm water taken twice a day. As with cancer, natural liver regeneration needs a combination of healing methods to be effective. This means that proper nutrition, moderate exercise, stress reduction techniques and even deep breathing may play a role in the process.

GLANDULAR SWELLINGS

If you are feeling **fullness or swelling of glands** (such as in your neck, groin or armpits), fresh burdock leaf poultices may help reduce the puffiness. Take the large fresh leaves from either first or second year plants and "bruise" them. Bruising means that you crumple the leaves up and press them together until the juice is released. Roll the crushed leaves into a small, disc-shaped ball and hold it against the area for 10 or 20 minutes. Drinking the leaf or root tea would not be a bad idea either.

STAPHYLOCOCCUS INFECTION

Another classic formula that includes burdock root has been very successful in combatting **staphylococcus infection**. Place one tablespoon each of *fresh* burdock root, dandelion root and echinacea root in six cups of cold distilled water and bring to a boil. Simmer for 20 to 30 minutes, strain the herbs and sip the tea throughout the day.

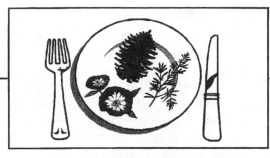

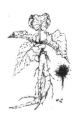

Wild Food Facts

Burdock roots (called "Gobo" in Japan) can occasionally be purchased at health food or gourmet markets. If you have space to grow the plant, however, I strongly encourage you to do so since the fresher the root the better when it comes to eating burdock root and leaf as wild food.

Unlike processing the root for medicinal purposes, you will want to pull or cut off the thick, brown rind of the root until you see the creamy white inner core. Chop the inner core into bite-sized pieces and add it to soups, stews, stir-fries or serve it in small portions as a "wild" side dish.

Collect the leaves of first year plants and cook them in two or three changes of water before serving them as a spinach-like vegetable.

One word of caution: as with *all* wild foods, take it easy when you first start eating them. Your body must gradually become accustomed to their high energy value. Too much "wild food" too fast and you'll spend a great deal of time either doubled over with stomach cramps or contemplating your herbal future in the bathroom.

DIABETES

While it is no "cure" for diabetes, burdock root has been shown to **lower blood sugar levels in diabetics**. Take two ounces by weight of *fresh* burdock root and boil it for 10 minutes in four cups of distilled water. Drink three unsweetened cups of the tea every day and keep tabs on your insulin levels.

BURDOCK FOR BALDNESS?

Burdock *root* can be used externally to **aid in stimulation of hair growth** or help stop loss of hair. It's a rather involved process but if you're going bald, what price glory? Soak four ounces of the dried root in four quarts of cold water overnight then heat the mixture slowly and strain it. Pour half of it into a basin and wet your hair with it. Using castile soap instead of shampoo, wash your hair. Rinse out the soap and then pour the remaining amount of the burdock root concoction over your hair. Do not rinse this out! I offer no guarantees that this will give you lush locks, but it's worked for some folks. Why not you?

HOW TO TAKE THE HERB

Since you are working with a root, you will want to make what is called a *decoction.* Burdock root tea is made by combining one teaspoon of the dried root to 10 ounces of distilled water. Bring the mixture to a boil, then allow the decoction to simmer for 20 minutes. Strain and drink.

Burdock leaf tea is made by combining one teaspoon of the dried leaf or two heaping teaspoons of the fresh leaf to eight ounces of hot water. Cover and steep for 20 minutes. Strain and enjoy.

For those who cannot handle drinking teas, burdock tincture is available at health food and herb stores. The tincture is effective. However, to get the most bang from your burdock, I think it's best to drink the tea.

Burdock is most effective over a long period of time which means that you can't overdo it quantity wise. Figure no more than two to three cups per day for six weeks. Burdock, slowly but surely, purifies the blood and, in doing so, rebalances and tones the kidneys and the liver.

Even if you opt for the store-bought version, I'm sure you have a new perspective on burdock. Now that you realize how much it can do, I'm certain that when you walk through a wet field next summer—feeling its hooked purple flowers taking a free ride on your pant leg and wedging its sharp needles into your socks—you'll feel somehow different toward this herb and even look forward to the experience.

Yeah, right.

THE "DIRT" ON...BURDOCK

Botanical ~	*Arctium lappa*
Growth cycle ~	Hardy biennial (if root is harvested at end of first year, treat burdock as an annual).
Medicinal uses~	Alterative, aperient, depurative, diuretic, hepatic, laxative, tonic, gentle lymphatic cleanser.
Part(s) used for medicine ~	Root, leaf.
Vitamins/Minerals ~	Rich in vitamin C, magnesium, iron, inulin (a form of starch), phosphorus, potassium, sodium and vitamin B_1.
Region ~	Found all over the United States, in cool, moist fields and roadsides. Burdock is more sparsely found in California and some of the southern states.

Wild or Domestic ~	Both. NOTE: In the wild, two burdock species co-exist, *A. lappa* (Great burdock) and the smaller sized *A. minus* (Common burdock). *A. lappa* has the greater medicinal value.
Poisonous look-alikes in the wild ~	There was an instance when wildcrafters collected handfuls of deadly nightshade leaves (*Atropa belladonna*) and mixed them in with burdock. The two plants can grow side by side and, while deadly nightshade is varied in its appearance, it could be easy to pick the leaf if it is growing in a thick patch of burdock. This deadly nightshade/burdock combination proved almost fatal for one woman. On the non-poisonous front, to the untrained eye, rhubarb (*Rheum palmatum*) can be mistaken for first year burdock and vice versa. Cocklebur (*Xanthium strumarium*) could be confused with second year burdock. There is also "Common burdock" (*Arctium minus*) which is smaller and, according to some herbalists, does not have the medicinal ability of *A. lappa*.

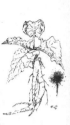

Hardy or Delicate ~	Very hardy.
Height of mature plant ~	Six to seven feet.
Easy or hard to grow ~	Easy.
Cultivation ~	Direct seed in spring, covering with one-half inch of dirt.
Plant spacing ~	Seedlings should be two inches apart in rows set six inches apart.
Pre-soak seeds ~	No.
Pre-chill seeds ~	No.
Indoor seed starting ~	No. Due to burdock's long taproot, it doesn't take well to transplanting.
Light/dark seed requirements ~	Dark.
Days to germinate ~	Varies, depending upon region. Typically 10 to 21 days.
Days to full maturity ~	Spring to fall or 120 days.
Soil type ~	Deep, loose and moist. Add a few shovels of sawdust to increase the porous quality of the dirt which will make digging roots a bit easier.
Water requirements ~	Likes light moisture but it must be well drained.
Sun or shade ~	Partial sun.
Propagation ~	Seed.
Easy/hard to transplant ~	Hard. Not recommended.
Pests or diseases ~	Virtually pest-free.
Landscape uses ~	During burdock's first year, a dramatic rosette leaf filler. The second year provides an overwhelming six to seven foot statue of a plant that could work as an interesting centerpiece.

Gathering ~	**Root**: fall of first year or spring of second year. **Leaves**: first year plants only when young and still tender.
Best fresh or dried ~	**Root**: fresh or dried, although some herbalists believe the fresh root has more medicinal power. **Leaves:** fresh or dried.
Drying methods ~	If using for medicine, DO NOT remove tough, outer rind. If using for wild food, you must remove the outer rind since it is practically inedible. Dry root by slicing it lengthwise and then cutting the root into sections two to four inches long.
Amount needed ~	Three to five plants.
Seed collection ~	Seeds are plentiful in burdock's second year. Simply pick them off the plant or off your clothes if they happen to hitch a free ride.
Companion planting ~	Stinging nettle works as a wonderful companion since it is a rich source of minerals, including calcium, which is often lacking in the soil where burdock naturally grows. Other good companion plants include dandelion, alfalfa and chickweed.
Container planting ~	No!
Common mistakes ~	Not paying attention and digging second year plants for the root. Unfortunately, second year roots are hard to eat and lack in healing energy. Another mistake is planting burdock in a shallow bed that does not accommodate its three foot plus long root.
Interesting facts/tips ~	Burdock can be used as a rotating cover crop, although it is invasive. Leftover tops from second year plants make an excellent mulch or compost ingredient. Leaves make a good emergency "toilet paper". If you have lots of burdock growing naturally on your land it often indicates soil with low pH, heavy with iron and in need of calcium. Finally, the best part of all is that once established, you can ignore burdock and it will flourish!

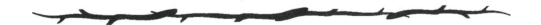

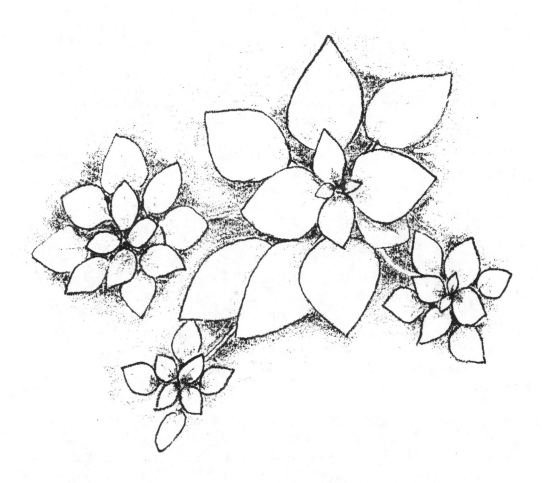

Chapter 15

AH, MY LITTLE CHICKWEED

Stellaria media

("W.F.")

Extremely hardy annual

Medicinal Uses: *Alterative, demulcent, emollient, vulnerary, anti-itch, mild laxative, refrigerant, anti-rheumatic*

Medicinal parts of plant: *Entire above ground plant*
Forms: *Tea, tincture, poultice, salve*

WHAT IS ITS CHARACTER?

Once you welcome chickweed into your garden (and even when you don't invite it), chickweed is there to stay. I've always looked on chickweed as an overly eager herb. It might be smaller than the rest of the plants, but what it lacks in size it more than makes up for in spirit. If you live in snowy climates where chickweed grows, don't be surprised if you find this ardent little plant peeking out from the frozen depths, just as green and vibrant as springtime. To say chickweed is a bit on the nervous side, is like saying Seattle gets a little rain each year. Once spring arrives, chickweed can't wait to bolt across fields and gardens, quickly forming dense mats of growth and producing thousands of tiny seed pods that burst open and start carpets of growth. It might look puny and it may get stepped on a lot, but nothing will stop this dedicated trooper. Chickweed takes a mowing and keeps on growing.

WHERE DO I FIND IT?

Chickweed can be found growing anywhere from sea level to about 9,000 feet. It loves to sprawl across shady, moist areas of fields, roadsides, lawns, ditches and creekbeds. In areas such as southern California, chickweed can grow nearly 12 months a year. In regions that get below freezing temperatures, chickweed is one of the first greens to wind its way out of the snow and lasts sometimes until after the first hard freeze.

HOW DO I GROW IT?

Chickweed is so easy to grow you could put on a blindfold, grab a handful of seeds and scatter them to the wind and this baby would emerge as healthy as ever. Direct seed in moist, rich soil in early spring, gently patting down the seed. Don't cover it with too much dirt since chickweed requires light to germinate. When you think your carpet of chickweed has died and is lost forever, gently take a trowel and stir up the soil a little bit, then add a good dose of water to saturate. Within two weeks, you should see the tiny seedlings return.

HOW DO I HARVEST IT?

Chickweed is always more medicinally potent when used fresh. For some formulas, such as the famous chickweed ointment, the tincture and the poultice, you have to use the fresh plant. Wait until chickweed reaches at least three to four inches tall before harvest. If you need to dry it for later use, harvest the plant when the tiny white flowers emerge—usually early to mid-summer. Lay the plant on a drying rack out of direct sunlight. Since chickweed naturally holds a lot of water in its leaves, you will need to turn it over each day as it dries to prevent mold from forming. The dried plant must be kept in an airtight glass bottle and placed in the dark. The healing potential is reduced with dried chickweed. I wouldn't keep the dried plant longer than six months after harvest. If you live in areas that get freezing temperatures, consider growing chickweed indoors in order to have a fresh supply.

HOW DO I USE IT?

Sixteenth century British herbalist John Gerard had this to say about chickweed: "…it comforteth, digesteth, defendeth and suppurateth very notably." Unfortunately, many modern herb books do not giveth this herb such well roundeth marks. In fact, some books omit chickweed altogether— others simply call it "too limited in use," "too mild" or plain ol' "not very valuable." This is something I simply do not understand. In some ways, chickweed can be considered mild, but in other ways, it can produce immediate and amazing results.

Perhaps chickweed is ignored by so many because of its history. It got its name because chicks and small birds feasted on the leaves and seeds. This, of course, didn't do much to create excitement when it came to healing possibilities. If that wasn't enough, it was then labeled "another green leafy food" with tons of natural vitamins A, B and C. Along with spinach and collard, chickweed was considered vitamin and mineral-rich "free food" during hard times in Europe. The "free" part comes from the fact that chickweed grows like…you guessed it, a weed. Its twisted vine-like stems grow just about anywhere, anytime in any weather. We're talking hardy.

But, alas, once you are labeled as free fodder for feathered creatures and poor folk, it is mighty tough to become respected as a quality, medicinal herb. However, I am here to tell you that this rush to judgment is unjustified! As you will soon see, chickweed has many important uses that prove it is much more than some field castaway.

SAY "GOODBYE" TO THAT ITCH!

Chickweed ointment is one of the oldest anti-itch, anti-inflammatory remedies on the herbal block. Chances are, your great, great grandmother had a jar of chickweed ointment in the medicine chest whenever **skin rashes** such as **poison ivy/oak**, **psoriasis**, or **eczema** appeared. To say this ointment is "amazing" is putting it mildly. I've seen it relieve itching in minutes, far surpassing the effectiveness of any chemical, over-the-counter lotions. In addition, chickweed ointment is an excellent topical treatment for **scrapes** and **burns** as well as a **helpful "drawing salve" to pull out thin splinters from skin**.

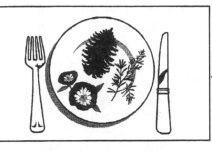

Wild Food Facts

When you harvest chickweed for wild food, be careful to trim the plant tops instead of pulling it out of the ground, roots and all. Choose only the most succulent plants—ones that show no sign of dried leaves.

Chickweed makes an excellent and tasty addition to any salad. It can be eaten sans dressing, but I prefer to perk it up with a little olive oil and lemon. Try steaming the greens for no more than three minutes and serve them as a side dish to chicken or fish or mix them in with scrambled eggs. *Never boil chickweed since it reduces its nutritional value.*

My friend, Christopher Nyerges, is an author of many wild food books as well as head of *The School of Self-Reliance* in Eagle Rock, California. In Christopher's book *Wild Greens and Salads*, he has a terrific recipe for chickweed quesadillas. With his permission, I've included it here.

Ingredients:
1 corn tortilla
About 1/3 cup of shredded cheese (jack or cheddar)
1 cup fresh chickweed
Oil for cooking
Garlic powder

Put the oil in a cast-iron skillet and heat the pan. Add the corn tortilla and cook for about two minutes. Add the cheese and let it cook at a low heat until the cheese is melted. Sprinkle the garlic powder over the cheese and remove from the skillet. Add rinsed, drained and chopped chickweed to the top of the quesadilla and serve. Serves one.

To make the ointment, you must use the *fresh* plant. Some herbalists suggest baking the plant in the oven. This might work for them. However, I have had more luck using a slower method I call the "fresh plant window extraction." It takes longer to make but I think the final ointment ends up retaining more of chickweed's healing energy.

Harvest four of five large handfuls of *fresh* chickweed. **Make sure the plant is as dry as possible** (i.e., the garden sprinklers or rain haven't dampened the plant). Water breeds bacteria and since chickweed holds a lot of water, you don't want to add to this problem. On a kitchen scale, weigh the chickweed and make a note of the weight. Place the fresh plant matter into a large bowl and *lightly sprinkle* vodka over the herb, turning it several times so that every part of the herb is coated with the alcohol.

Do not saturate chickweed with alcohol. The plant should not be dripping with vodka. The alcohol is only used as a preservative for the final oil as well as to reduce the chance of bacteria forming on the plant. Let the chickweed sit for several hours in the bowl.

To determine the amount of olive oil needed for the salve, refer back to the weight of the fresh plant. Whatever that number is, quadruple it to give you the liquid measurement. For example, if the fresh chickweed weighs eight ounces, multiply eight by four and you get 32. This means you will need 32 ounces of olive oil. If the chickweed weighs four ounces on the scale, you will need 16 ounces of olive oil by volume. This ratio is referred to as "weight to volume," meaning that it's the *weight* of the fresh plant to the liquid *volume* of the olive oil.

Place the fresh chickweed loosely into a wide mouthed glass jar (*do not use plastic!*) and pour the required amount of olive oil over it. The best olive oil is extra virgin. Make sure all the plant matter is covered with the oil. If you have to, compress the chickweed to ensure complete coverage.

Next, take a six inch square piece of muslin and fit it over the mouth of the jar, using a rubber band to hold it securely. Label the jar with the date and the ingredients. Put the jar in a south-facing window or in direct sunlight. Make sure the jar is not where rain or garden sprinklers can touch it since you do not want water seeping through the muslin top. You will need to keep the jar in a sunny place for at least four to six weeks. I know this sounds as if it's a long time, but it takes at least that long for the sun to break down the plant matter and "cook" into the oil. I usually keep the jar in a sunny window for as long as *one year*. My motto is "the longer the better" when it comes to fresh plant window extractions. Other herbal oils that benefit from this slower process include St. John's wort flowers and stems, calendula flowers and arnica flowers. The only time I would not use this method is if I'm using roots, berries, seeds or nuts. Since they have tougher exteriors, those plant parts almost always require top of the stove boiling in order to extract their healing energy. (For more information on how to make an ointment with this top of the stove method, turn to Chapter 40, "How to Make Herbal Stuff").

During the window extraction process, occasionally remove the muslin and smell the oil. You should be able to smell a hint of the vodka, the olive oil and the chickweed. However, if the odor strikes you as rancid or downright rank, bacteria has somehow found its way into the jar and the whole thing must be discarded. The alcohol treatment coupled with the muslin "lid" is meant to prevent this from happening but sometimes the bacteria win out.

After four or six weeks (or longer, if you have the patience), strain the chickweed oil through a large muslin cloth, pressing out every last drop of the oil. Measure the amount of oil by volume and make a note of this. **For every ounce by weight of chickweed oil, you will need one teaspoon of yellow beeswax**. This ratio will give you a light, creamy ointment that is easily absorbed into the skin. Place the chickweed oil and exact amount of hard yellow beeswax into a mason jar. Put the jar into a hot water bath. Heat the oil and wax gradually, stirring constantly with a wooden stick. When the beeswax has completely melted into the chickweed oil, stir the mixture rapidly for a few more minutes before removing the jar from the water. For every ounce by volume of the salve, add one or two drops of benzoin tincture (also called benzoin compound, which is available at drug stores). This acts as a natural and very effective preservative. Let the salve sit in a cool spot until it hardens. I keep all salves in the refrigerator since this further lengthens their life.

TRY A CHICKWEED BATH

If the rash or skin ailment have really got you itching, try soaking in a chickweed tea bath for 30 to 40 minutes. Pat yourself dry and then apply the ointment to the affected parts. For severe cases, you may have to repeat this process two to three times a day. To make the bath, you will need one cup of the dried herb or four good handfuls of the fresh plant. Bring a gallon of tap water to a boil and turn off the heat. Add the herbs and let the mixture steep for 20 minutes before straining it into a hot tub.

COOLING COMFORT FOR ABRASIONS, BLISTERS & BRUISES

Fresh chickweed has the admirable quality of cooling the fire while relieving the pain of **skin abrasions**, **blisters** and **bruises**. To make the poultice, take a handful of fresh chickweed and press it between the palms of your hands until the plant's juice is released. Sometimes, adding a little cool water to the herb can help but it is not mandatory. Place the fresh plant matter against your skin, holding it in place with a piece of gauze, masking tape or handkerchief. Check the poultice after an hour and replace with a new handful of fresh chickweed if needed.

REDUCE INFLAMMATION

For centuries, chickweed has been associated with **alleviating inflammation** of all kinds. It can be used as a topical poultice or taken internally in tea form to ease **rheumatism**, **bronchitis**, **colitis**, or **gastritis**. Think of any ailment that ends with "itis" (which means "inflamed") and chickweed can help take out the "ouch." One to two cups per day of the fresh or dried tea are suggested.

WEIGHT LOSS & MAINTENANCE

Check out any "slim, trim" herbal weight loss tea and 80% of the time you'll find chickweed listed as one of the ingredients. There are three good reasons. First, chickweed has been found to **aid in the dissolving of fat deposits**. Secondly, because of its mild laxative effects, chickweed helps to **rid the body of toxins that are trapped within the small intestine and colon**. And finally, chickweed works as an **appetite suppressant**. While chickweed is included in many herbal weight loss formulas, I've always preferred to use it on its own. Since its effects are so mild, it is difficult to gain any measured benefit from the herb when it is stuck in the middle of eight or ten other herbs. So, what I suggest is drinking one cup of chickweed tea on an empty stomach 10 to 15 minutes before your mid-day and evening meal. Obviously, the tea won't do anything if you continue to consume too many fatty foods in your diet. Just because chickweed is known for dissolving fat deposits, doesn't mean you can indulge on even more fat!

LAXATIVE

Chickweed is probably one of the most **gentle natural laxatives** you can take. One or two cups taken throughout the day have been able to remove bowel obstructions without the bowel-cramping, gut-twisting turmoil that other laxative herbs can produce. However, because of chickweed's reputation of "not being that strong," there are those who believe that in order to achieve the desired effect, you have to drink a really strong brew or simply cup after cup of the tea. *Neither* of these ideas is correct. Try it sometime and you'll take out permanent residency in the bathroom for about three or four days. I am not just talking diarrhea here—I'm talking violent cramping. That bowel obstruction may be gone but you'll have a new set of troubles.

Because chickweed has this potential, it is always best when treating constipation to start with a lower dose than prescribed and work up to the recommended dose if you need it. A low dose would be one half cup twice a day. If that doesn't work, then try two cups a day. The highest dose for relieving constipation is three cups a day. *However, that is only if two cups do not work.* Another thing: Make those cups normal tea to water ratio blends (i.e., one teaspoon of the dried herb to eight ounces of hot distilled water). Stronger brews can cause the same loose bowel and cramping problems.

RESPIRATORY RESCUE

Consider one to two cups of chickweed tea a day whenever there is internal inflammation or excessive phlegm due to **bronchitis**, **asthma**, a **sore throat**, **colds** and **sinus headaches**. Chickweed helps to liquefy and then remove trapped mucus from the respiratory tract. Because chickweed is gentle, it will not dry out the nasal or trachea passages in the process. There have also been cases where chickweed has been used as an **interim remedy to temporarily stop bleeding from the lungs**. However, I would only employ the herb while en route to professional medical attention.

SWOLLEN TESTICLES

As I have said, if it's inflamed or itching, chickweed is your herb. In the cases of **swollen or itching testicles**, the best approach is to fill the bathtub to hip level and pour in the same chickweed tea bath mixture mentioned earlier under the "chickweed bath" heading. Make sure the water is not too hot. In addition, drinking one cup of the tea and applying chickweed ointment to the testicles can hasten the healing process.

BLOOD CLEANSER

While chickweed is not as well known as burdock and red clover, it still acts as an **effective blood cleanser and purifier**. It can also work if **blood poisoning** is suspected. The suggested use is drinking one to two cups of the tea while applying the strained, moistened *fresh* herb to the affected part. In a case of blood poisoning, I would also take three to six cloves of raw garlic which act as a natural antibiotic. If those telltale red streaks show up, discontinue self-treatment and seek prompt medical attention.

DOSE AMOUNTS

For the fresh plant tea, use one heaping tablespoon of the chopped herb for every eight ounces of hot water. The dried herb amount is one teaspoon. Steep the herb in the water, covering the container for 10 to 20 minutes. The fresh plant tincture dose is 25 to 30 drops in several ounces of warm water, taken one to three times a day.

To cast this herb aside as "worthless" or "not valuable" is both unfair and untrue. Sure, it may not be on Harry Herbalist's top ten list. Then again, if Harry gets stuffed up, puts on a few pounds, cuts his hand, becomes constipated, needs a blood purifier or starts to itch...anywhere, he just may wish he'd taken the time to know chickweed.

THE "DIRT" ON...CHICKWEED

Botanical ~	*Stellaria media*
Growth cycle ~	Annual.
Medicinal uses ~	Alterative, demulcent, emollient, vulnerary, anti-itch, mild laxative, refrigerant, anti-rheumatic.
Part(s) used for medicine ~	Entire above ground plant.
Vitamins/Minerals ~	Healthy amounts of vitamins A, B and C. Lots of trace minerals.
Region ~	From sea level to 9,000 feet.
Wild or Domestic ~	Both.
Poisonous look-alikes in the wild ~	None.
Hardy or Delicate ~	Very hardy.
Height of mature plant ~	From three to seven inches.
Easy or hard to grow ~	Very easy.
Cultivation ~	In spring, once frost has past, direct seed in rich, moist soil. Can be planted in rows but I think broadcasting seed is easiest and fastest. Make sure you don't clump seeds together when broadcasting.
Plant spacing ~	A few inches. Chickweed will take over eventually and form a dense carpet.
Pre-soak seeds ~	No.
Pre-chill seeds ~	No.
Indoor seed starting ~	It can be done but it's not easy to transplant young chickweed seedlings.
Light/dark seed requirements ~	Light.
Days to germinate ~	Varies, depending upon temperature. Usually within 14 days if soil is moist and warm.
Days to full maturity ~	Approximately 60 days.
Soil type ~	Cool, undemanding soil. However, for a superior green crop of chickweed, add a little compost to enrich the soil.
Water requirements ~	Needs regular watering without drowning. If left to dry out, chickweed will turn yellow and lose flavor.
Sun or shade ~	Does best in full shade, but enjoys late afternoon sun to green up.
Propagation ~	Seed from the many pods that form and burst across the soil.
Easy/hard to transplant ~	Once chickweed is established in your yard or in the wild, it is easy to transplant. Make sure you dig deep enough and bring along some of the soil from where it has been growing.

Pests or diseases ~   None.

Landscape uses ~   Makes an excellent ground cover.

Gathering ~   As needed. For those who live in frost-free regions, chickweed can be gathered nearly all year long. Wait until it reaches three or four inches. Grab hold of a good handful and then snip what you need. Once it dries out or the leaves have a brown or translucent sheen to them, chickweed is not very effective.

Best fresh or dried ~   Fresh is always best when making chickweed salves, tinctures and poultices. It can be dried and stored for later use, but it loses its medicinal potency within six months.

Drying methods ~   Gather clumps of fresh, green plant and separate into smaller bunches. Lay on a drying rack completely away from sunlight. Make sure you don't have layers on top of layers or it will inhibit the drying ability. Check frequently and once plant is completely dry, store in airtight, glass canisters. Use within six months.

Amount needed ~   A dense 4' x 4' patch.

Seed collection ~   Seeds develop in minute "pods" which hold four or more tan seeds. When collecting seed, make sure the seed pod is dry before breaking it open since immature seeds are soft and not viable. Sometimes the easiest way to collect chickweed seed is to shake the freshly harvested plant over a bowl and allow the seeds to fall.

Companion planting ~   Nettle and spearmint work well with chickweed since they have similar growing needs regarding soil and water.

Container planting ~   Yes. For those who live in regions that get below freezing weather, chickweed makes an easy to grow indoor green.

Common mistakes ~   Planting chickweed in full sun and/or in soil that does not get sufficient water.

Interesting facts/tips ~   Chickweed has the remarkable ability to still be green and edible under several inches of snow. This succulent green has saved many people from starving.

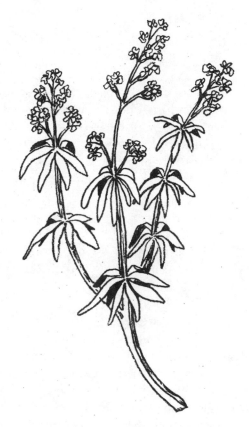

Chapter 16

LEAVE IT TO CLEAVERS

THE PLANT WITH A CAPITAL "PEE"

Galium aparine
("W.F.")
Annual

Medicinal Uses: *Diuretic, gentle lymphatic, tonic, alterative, slight laxative, vulnerary*

Medicinal parts of plant: *Entire above ground plant*

Forms: *Tea, tincture, fresh plant*

WHAT IS ITS CHARACTER?

Cleavers is one of my favorite herbs. I love discovering it in shaded gardens and dense forests. For me, it was easy to see cleavers' character emerge. I've always looked on cleavers as an herb that strives to please. It's a gentle, tender little soul that loves being loved and yearns to be needed. One of the more obvious character traits is cleavers' determination to go home with you as its tiny, velcro-like seeds latch onto shoes, socks, pants, shirt…you name it. It's a bit on the insecure side, I suppose, but it can't help it. The great thing about cleavers is that the more you love it, the more it grows. And the more it grows, the more *you* will need and want it.

WHERE DO I FIND IT?

Cleavers grows most prolifically in damp, dense, shaded forest settings and along creeks and streams. In backyards, it flourishes under shade trees as long as the planting bed is loose and well watered. It can be found growing from sea level to as high as 10,000 feet if the conditions are right. Since the square stems are weak, cleavers usually falls over once it reaches one foot in height. It continues to grow up to eight feet in length as it lays prostrate, "stuck" on its sticky self against the ground. By mid-summer, the untouched growth forms layers of soft, cool "bedding" where animals (wild and domestic) love to sleep. It also makes a nice resting place for humans to stop and take a breather after a long day hiking or wildcrafting. The sweet scent of new mown hay might come to mind as you inhale cleavers' fresh aroma.

> **NOTE:** There are other *Galium* species that can be found throughout the country. Many of them are considered perennial herbs instead of annuals. One is called sweet woodruff (*Galium odoratum*) which is smaller than cleavers and found in many gardens as a ground cover. Another is yellow bedstraw (*Galium verum*) which grows to about three feet tall and has lovely dense clusters of bright yellow flowers. All the *Galium* species are square-stemmed and share similar medicinal abilities. However, cleavers (*Galium aparine*) is the most common species and the one usually chosen for healing formulas.

HOW DO I GROW IT?

Cleavers is grown from seeds planted in late summer. Seeds need only to be firmly pressed into the ground and given no special attention. Cleavers does need to be wintered over in temperatures that fall below freezing with no special mulching or compost required. Come spring, the tiny shoots will gradually appear with their distinctive whorls of six to eight leaves appearing up and down the square stem. It's not really a plant that can be grown in seed cells since transplanting it is tenuous at best. You could start it in a flat if you need to artificially create the frozen environment. Once sprouting occurs, I would simply remove the entire flat of dirt and seedlings and lay it into a cool, moist area of the garden. Allow it plenty of room to grow and spread its vine-like mats across the soil since this will encourage further dense growth the following year.

One summer I discovered the "lazy man's way" to plant cleavers. I had gathered thick mats of the plant from the wild and, after making my formula, I had one section left over that was about one foot square. I took it out to the garden and placed it in the dirt, pressing it slightly into the soil. The following spring, seedlings happily emerged from that very spot.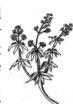

By the way, you will need a lot of cleavers to have enough to make teas, tinctures and "wild food" offerings. Keep that in mind when planning your backyard herb garden.

HOW DO I HARVEST IT?

Cleavers is ready to pick when it is anywhere from one foot to seven feet long. The younger plants are best for "wild food" use. Typically, cleavers can be harvested for medicine anywhere from April to July in most regions. Understand that cleavers will stick to itself like the strongest velcro. Thus, you will end up collecting it in interwoven "mats." Shake off any dirt or particles that may be trapped between or on the sticky stems before placing cleavers in your gathering bag.

If you want to air dry the plant, separate the herb into smaller bunches and hang the plant matter directly on hooks. It should stick with no problem. Many of the formulas, however, call for *fresh* cleavers. If that is the case, you must harvest the herb and make the formula within hours since the fresh plant tends to lose its flavor very quickly.

> **NOTE:** When you collect cleavers along with other plants, keep it separate from the other herbs since it will stick to them like glue.

HOW DO I USE IT?

Cleavers has always made me laugh. Not because of what it does but because of what it reminds me of. The first time I heard the word "cleavers" roll off someone's lips I was having a riveting conversation with a fellow about soil amendments. Between soil composition, compost mixtures and the sheer thrill of hearing the words "nitrogen-rich" spoken four times in the very same sentence, I kicked myself for not having a camera so I could preserve this Kodak moment. Just when I was thinking that one

125

doesn't have to be in a coma to be brain dead, he said the word "cleavers." You have to understand, this guy was from New England and while he looked nothing like him, he *sounded* like the elderly gentleman on those old Pepperidge Farm cookie commercials. "*CLEE-vahs*," he said, "*CLEE-vahs* is an herb I do like! Why, I can remember as a child walking through fields of *CLEE-vahs*."

I became absolutely fixated on the word *CLEE-vahs*. I had no earthly idea what the herb could do, but I knew that I'd never forget the herb's name—thanks to this guy who learned elocution from L.L. Bean himself.

AN HERB IN NEED OF PUBLIC RELATIONS

The irony is, many herbalists out there know this herb but they don't use it as much as they could. It's not one of those "Top Ten" medicinals mentioned in herb magazines nor is it widely praised in peer-reviewed herb journals. In my opinion, it needs a good public relations agent. Cleavers **(also known as "Bedstraw" or "Lady's bedstraw")** is a weed–and a somewhat bothersome one at that for some folks. The stem has backward-curving bristles that exude a stickiness. Not only do these bristles allow the plant to climb and expand across fields and gardens unchecked, the bristles also tend to catch themselves onto anything that passes by (i.e., pants, skirts, hair, dog's fur…you get the picture). Thus, the slang terms for cleavers is "catchweed," "grip grass" and my personal favorite, "sticky willie." It's also known as "goose grass" because geese tend to love the stems.

While gardeners worldwide curse the day cleavers wandered onto their property, herbalists in "the know" revel in its possibilities.

Ideally, the *fresh plant* is the most active medicinally and can be harvested from spring until late summer. Cleavers is one of the hardiest herbs on the block—often times thrusting it's little sticky stem through the snow in hopes of getting a head start on the plant competition.

When using cleavers for medicinal purposes, **it is always best to use the tea made from the fresh plan**t. If all you have is the dried plant, that is okay—I just don't think it has the same healing punch. **One alternative is to use the tincture made only from the fresh plant**. The typical dose of the fresh plant tincture is one teaspoon mixed into four ounces of hot water. This should be taken two to four times per day, depending upon the ailment you are treating. The only drawback with using the tincture is that you are not getting the additional flushing action of the tea. For this reason, I suggest that for every dose of tincture, you drink an additional 16 ounces of water.

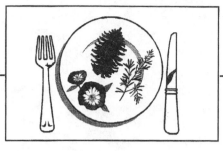

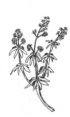

Wild Food Facts

I think fresh cleavers has a lovely taste. Don't overcook the herb since it ruins the flavor and saps much of its nutritional benefit. The early spring growth makes a nice side dish when the entire above ground plant is lightly steamed and served like spinach. Do not eat cleavers uncooked since the sticky stems may get caught in your throat. As the seeds (or fruits, as they are sometimes called) mature in mid to late summer, gather one or two cups and roast them in the oven at about 200 degrees. Watch carefully to make sure they don't burn. Once roasted, let the seeds cool and then pound them into a powder. This powder makes a pretty nice "coffee substitute" minus the caffeine.

LYMPH RELIEF

Cleavers does two basic things. First, it **activates the lymphatic system**, helping to pump toxins from the body, thereby cleansing the bloodstream. Secondly, **cleavers works like a dynamo on the kidneys**, again flushing unwanted debris from the body through the bladder. While this might not sound like something to write home about, I promise you it is. I have found that there are only a few gentle herbal lymphatic drainers that work without making the "cure" worse than the complaint. Cleavers is gentle, but be assured, it is steady and effective when used properly.

Lymph tenderness and/or swelling is usually a sign of a sluggish system. It can also be the physical trigger that says "the flu is a comin' your way." Typical lymph swelling is found on the side of your neck directly under the ear lobes, in your armpits and in your groin.

Herbal practitioner and author Matthew Wood has an interesting take on cleavers. Wood believes in using the classic "Doctrine of Signatures" as part of his healing practice. Using the Doctrine of Signatures—which says that plants reveal their healing abilities by how they look, where they grow, how they taste and how they feel—Wood has discovered a fascinating aspect of cleavers that just happens to be true. Looking at cleavers, you see a tall, angular plant that grows quickly across the ground. Wood recommends cleavers for slender, nervous, finicky, fussy and sensitive people who are occasionally bothered by stagnant lymphatic tissue in their neck. If they tend to also have a hypermobile neck and enjoy cracking their wrist as well, this could be their special little herb. Wood reports that after he gives cleavers to patients who fit this profile, "Their eyes often brighten up. Suddenly, they feel better." This doesn't mean that if you are stout, calm and nonchalant that you can't also benefit from cleavers. It just might work more effectively on those who fit the "cleavers profile."

If you feel that uncomfortable lymphatic swelling and sense that you are about to get the latest cold, there's a two step process you might try. First, place 60 drops of echinacea tincture (another excellent lymphatic cleanser) in four ounces of hot water and drink it. Secondly, add the following combination of herbs to 16 ounces of hot (but *not* boiling) distilled water.

> Cleavers (2 heaping tablespoons of the fresh plant or
> 1 teaspoon of dried)
> Red clover blossoms (1/2 teaspoon)
> Calendula flowers (1/2 teaspoon)
> Ginger root (1/4 teaspoon)

Cover the pot and steep the herbs for 15 minutes, strain and drink all 16 ounces within 30 minutes. The first day, it is best to repeat this echinacea/tea procedure three to four times a day, allowing an hour or two in between. I can almost guarantee that it will only take the first set of the echinacea and tea combo to get your kidneys flushing. Chances are, you will urinate much more than you drank. This is a good thing. This means your body is actively fighting and flushing the stuck lymphatic crud. Two words of caution here. Don't continue this process for longer than two days in a row. You can trigger too much of a discharge and become sicker than when you started. Secondly, if at any time you feel dizzy or disoriented, stop the process. This often times means that your liver is doing tailspins in an attempt to keep up with the toxic discharge. This is *not* a good thing. Learn to listen to your body and you'll soon figure out when "enough is enough."

DIURETIC SUPPORT

If your goal is to **rid your body of excess water** (such as with **edema**) or you would like to try a natural remedy for **infections of the urinary tract such as cystitis and urethritis**, you can drink cleavers tea either by itself or in combination. If you choose the herb by itself, the *fresh plant* is always better. However, the dried plant does work. The tea to water ratio is one tablespoon of the dried plant or two tablespoons of the fresh plant to eight ounces of very hot but NOT BOILING water. **Never boil**

cleavers since it will take the medicinal ability out of the plant. Drink one cup of this blend an hour before each meal.

The following formula works for those who wish to add a more antiseptic quality to the remedy. Pour 24 ounces of hot (but *not* boiling) distilled water over the combined herbs.

> Cleavers (2 teaspoons dried or 1 tablespoon fresh)
>
> Marshmallow root (1 teaspoon)
>
> Juniper berries (1 teaspoon)
>
> Buchu (1 teaspoon)

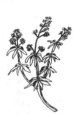

Steep the herbs covered for 15 minutes, strain and then drink one cup an hour before each meal. You can warm the tea each time if desired or drink it cold. The advantage of adding marshmallow to the blend is that this herb tends to maximize cleavers' action as well as provide soothing relief against inflammation.

As is true with any diuretic, it is best not drink the herb tea either alone or in combination for longer than two consecutive weeks. Diuretics can sap potassium from the body. While herbal diuretics tend to flood the body with vitamins and minerals, over-use of them can put a drain on the system as well. Thus, while you are taking the tea alone or in formula, up your potassium intake—especially *fresh*, green leafy vegetables.

PSORIASIS SAVIOR

Since cleavers works its little sticky bristles off to cleanse the lymph and bloodstream, the herb has been found to work very well in combination for those suffering from **psoriasis**. In holistic medicine, psoriasis has many possible physical roots. It can sometimes manifest from an impure bloodstream or sluggish lymphatic system. Poor diet often plays a role—especially where processed foods are eaten instead of the wholesome, fresh variety. Emotionally, holistic professionals consider that psoriasis is often linked with a personality that is nervous, "a loner" and unwilling to get close to other people. Minor to major stress and anxiety usually trigger the outbreaks. The point of all this is to stress that while the herbal combination has proven itself effective, the deeper more fixed personality traits are what need to be altered if psoriasis is to be completely eradicated.

The psoriasis formula is as follows:

> Cleavers (1 teaspoon dried or 1 tablespoon fresh)
>
> Red clover blossoms (1/2 teaspoon)
>
> Nettle (1/2 teaspoon)
>
> Calendula flowers (1/4 teaspoon)

Combine the herbs and pour 16 ounces of hot (but *not* boiling) water over them. Steep covered for 15 minutes, strain and sip the 16 ounces over a two to three hour period. This should be repeated twice a day for maximum effectiveness. Continue for two consecutive weeks and then take a break for one week.

CLEAVERS COOLS A FEVER

Next time you come upon a large patch of cleavers in the wild, take a moment and lie down in it. Press your face against the plant and feel the cool energy. That same cooling energy can be put to use when someone is suffering from a **high fever** that cannot be broken. It is important to note that a fever is not necessarily a bad thing—it is the body's way of naturally burning out the invading germs. However, there are times when a fever may hover two or three degrees above normal and does not want to break. At times like this, there are two things you can do. First, and most importantly, you want to clean the colon of any toxic debris. If you have been sick for three days or longer, there is a good chance that the colon has become a collection point for toxins. Those toxins create incredible heat in the colon. In turn, that heat tends to lock in the body's fever and not allow it to return to normal.

You can use herbal laxative teas such as cascara sagrada to flush the colon, but the most effective and quickest way to move out toxic poisons is with an enema. A coffee enema is a classic toxin remover. For fast fever reduction, you can't beat a catnip leaf enema. The coffee enema is best made with the ground whole bean rather than the instant stuff. The catnip enema is made as you would the tea infusion, figuring one teaspoon of the dried plant for every eight ounces of hot water. Make four cups of either and always strain the coffee/tea leaves.

The best way to give yourself an enema is to lie on your left side and insert as much of the liquid into your rectum as you can comfortably handle. I say "comfortably" and fully realize that there's nothing comfortable about an enema. The point is to try to hold as much tea or coffee as you can for 10 to 15 minutes. Stay on your left side for five minutes, roll over on your back for five minutes and then turn on your right side for five minutes. You can gently massage your abdomen during this time to move any blockages. After that point, you can release all the liquid into the toilet.

The second thing to do is drink three cups of cleavers tea each day which will release more trapped toxins from the kidneys. The *fresh* plant is preferred but the dried will work as well. If your head is still hot to the touch and you have fresh cleavers, take a handful of the plant, wad it up in a ball and pour cold water over it. Gently press it together and then place it across your forehead or wherever there is heat. It is amazing how quickly this fresh poultice often works.

WOUNDS, BLEEDING & BITES

The same poultice or tea made from the *fresh* plant works wonders at **cooling the fire from wounds and spider bites** as well as slowly **stopping the blood flow from a cut**. When using the poultice for spider bites, I always suggest that the person who has been bitten chew the plant in their mouth first before placing it over the bite. This way, the person is putting their own natural antibiotic saliva into the plant matter which I feel helps to increase the plant's healing power.

EPILEPTIC SEIZURE STOPPING

John Lust, naturopathic doctor and author of the classic reference book *The Herb Book*, suggests trying yellow bedstraw (*Galium verum*) in tea or tincture form for **reducing epileptic seizures**. While I have never heard of this before, I respect Lust's work and wanted to include the information for those who are searching for a natural way to alleviate seizures. Since all of the *Galium* species are considered interchangeable in their medicinal actions, I would think that if you can't find yellow bedstraw, cleavers will do. Try one cup of the tea each day or 15 to 20 drops of the tincture as needed.

TWO CAUTIONS WITH CLEAVERS

There are only two cautions with cleavers. First, since it can be a powerful diuretic and internal cleanser, **people with diabetes should avoid using the herb since it could alter the amount of insulin within the body**. Secondly, **cleavers is highly astringent due to its high tannin content**. It is for this reason that care needs to be taken regarding the length of time the herb is used. The best rule of thumb is two weeks on the herb (either alone or in combination) and two weeks off the herb.

Whether you call it cleavers or "*CLEE-vahs*," this is truly one herb you have to pee to believe.

THE "DIRT" ON... CLEAVERS

Botanical ~   *Galium aparine*

Growth cycle ~   Perennial.

Medicinal uses~   Diuretic, gentle lymphatic, tonic, alterative, slight laxative, vulnerary.

Part(s) used for medicine ~ Entire above ground plant.

Vitamins/Minerals ~   Rich in vitamin C.

Region ~   In woodlands and along streams and creeks where there is rich, loamy soil.

Wild or Domestic ~   Typically wild. Cleavers' cousin, sweet woodruff is more likely the Gallium species you will find growing in domesticated gardens.

Poisonous look-alikes in the wild ~   No poisonous ones that I know. However, some novices in the wild have mistaken the sometimes toxic wild lupine's (*Lupinus perennis*) whorl of leaves in its early growing stages with cleavers.

Hardy or Delicate ~   Hardy once it is established and given sufficient moisture.

Height of mature plant ~   Two to seven feet (however, once it gets to two feet tall, it has usually fallen over and is growing across the soil).

Easy or hard to grow ~   Easy if you follow growing instructions and expose cleavers' seeds to freezing temperatures.

Cultivation ~   Direct seed in autumn in shady, cool place, barely covering the seed. Allow seed to winter over in temperatures at or below freezing to spur germination.

Plant spacing ~   Since cleavers tends to grow on top of itself, this does not apply.

Pre-soak seeds ~   No.

Pre-chill seeds ~   Yes.

Indoor seed starting ~   Not the best way but it can be done. Remember to expose the seeds to freezing temperatures for two or three months before gradually introducing them to warmer temperatures and light moisture. Use trays instead of seed cells since cleavers is difficult to transplant from plugs.

Light/dark seed requirements ~   Light.

Days to germinate ~   Once the seed has had sufficient exposure to freezing temperatures, germination can occur within 21 days. However, some seed may take longer than that.

Days to full maturity ~   Approximately 60 to 70 days.

Soil type ~   Rich, aerated and mulched with leaves or compost.

Water requirements ~   Must have regular supply of moisture without drowning the plant.

Sun or shade ~	Shade.
Propagation ~	Seed and root cuttings.
Easy/hard to transplant ~	Easy once the plant is established. Difficult when it is still young and developing.
Pests or diseases ~	Virtually pest-free.
Landscape uses ~	Forms a dense "carpet" that makes an attractive and aromatic ground cover that smells of new mown hay every time it is stepped upon.
Gathering ~	Entire above ground plant should be gathered for medicine anywhere from April to July in most regions.
Best fresh or dried ~	Depends upon what you want to do with it. For "wild food" preparations, you obviously want the fresh plant. Tinctures of cleavers are best made from the fresh plant. Some herbalists believe that the fresh plant holds more nutrients and healing abilities. However, the dried herb has been successfully used for centuries and is a fine alternative.
Drying methods ~	Since cleavers will stick together in "mats," pull them apart into more manageable portions and hook them over a nail or peg to dry.
Amount needed ~	If you want to make tinctures, teas, poultices and more, you will need a minimum of a 10' x 10' square area dedicated to cleavers.
Seed collection ~	Cleavers seed can be hand-picked from the plant in mid to late summer. Once harvested, the seeds will stick to each other like velcro.
Companion planting ~	Plan to put other moisture loving herbs nearby but make sure they are not invasive since they will be difficult to extricate from cleavers' clinging stems.
Container planting ~	It can be done but you'll never have enough for what you need.
Common mistakes ~	Thinking that you can plant cleavers' seeds in spring after the frost and that they will emerge in summer even when I've told you they need a freeze to germinate. Another is placing cleavers in an area of the garden that receives direct sunlight. Extreme heat quickly kills cleavers.
Interesting facts/tips ~	The dense mat of condensed plant matter was used by farmers as a crude strainer for milk and other liquids.

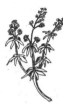

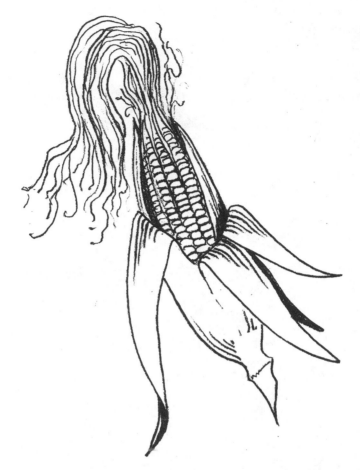

Chapter 17

Cornsilk
The Diuretic Born on the Cob

Zea mays

("W.F.")

Annual

Medicinal Uses: *Diuretic, anodyne for urinary discomfort, demulcent, alternative*

Medicinal parts of plant: *Silk that surrounds corncob, cornmeal (made from the dried, ground kernels)*

Forms: *Tea, tincture*

WHAT IS ITS CHARACTER?

It's too bad that some horror movies have taken to associating fields of corn with evil and mayhem. That's the last thing I'm feeling when I walk through rows of corn stalks. What I see is a tall, dependable personality that has the resilience to weather the strongest of storms. Even in the fall, after the harvest, the crisp stalks stand waiting for anyone who wishes to gather the dried foliage to make distinctive autumn decorations or corn husk dolls. It's an "old soul" that understands its purpose on earth and is more than willing to deliver the goods.

WHERE DO I FIND IT?

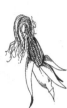

Corn can be grown in practically all regions. However, the farther north you go and the higher in altitude, the more difficult it can be.

HOW DO I GROW IT?

This hardy annual has many hybrid varieties. For some, hybrid corn has its place in that certain sizes can be created as well as "programming" the sweetness of the corn. However, hybrids of any plant cause the grower to become completely reliant on the seed company since hybrids are either sterile or do not reproduce "true to type." Another concern that is not talked about much is the long-term effects on the human body of eating hybrid (i.e., laboratory manipulated) foods. Since hybrid seeds are created with a singular purpose, what happens to the innate balance of the mature plant? In medicinal plant medicine, we are fond of talking about the synergistic interplay that happens within the herb. To reduce it down to a single component tends to erase the benefits that are found in the whole plant. And when we ingest these lab-manipulated, non-whole foods, does something happen to our bodies on a subtle level in five, ten or fifteen years? I don't know the answer. But I do know that I would much rather plant an "heirloom" seed versus a hybrid. Heirloom seeds are direct descendants from the kind of corn that was planted by our ancestors and reproduces true to type year after year. And instead of depending upon a seed company to supply you with your hybrid seed each year, each cob of dried kernels has the potential of producing rows and rows of corn.

You will want to plant that seed in a nitrogen-rich soil that has good drainage and access to plenty of water since corn needs lots of moisture to germinate and flourish. Plant each seed one foot apart at a one inch depth and cover completely with dirt. To increase the potential for successful pollination, plant corn using the "block system." In other words, instead of planting one 40 foot row of corn, plant four 10 foot rows no more than two feet apart. Pollination occurs when the top tassel (or seed head) releases pollen which falls to the waiting silk. Once that occurs, the corn begins to form on the cob.

If you have different varieties of corn, you will need to separate them from each other to avoid cross-pollination. This means you may need to place one type in the front yard and one in the backyard. Even with this system, your next door neighbor's corn can cross-pollinate with yours, thanks to the wind and hovering bees.

Make sure you have irrigation nearby since corn requires a good deal of water.

HOW DO I HARVEST IT?

The medicinal part of corn is the silky tassels that surround the cob. That's not to say you can't enjoy the corn as well. Corn is ready to harvest 18 to 24 days after the silk first appears. There is typically more silk on the corncob if you pick it before the corn is ready. However, I have a problem with discarding a perfectly good corncob simply because the silk is better before the corn is edible. You will need a lot of corn to generate enough cornsilk for medicinal purposes. This means you have to plant around 25 to 50 stalks of corn. This also means you have to eat a lot of corn or have friends and neighbors who really love corn. An easy way to harvest the silk is to remove the husks, grab hold of the brown tinged tassel and pull the strands off. Clip off the brown tassel and lay it across a well-vented drying rack. Paper towels or brown paper can also work, however, make sure you turn the sections of silk every day or so to ensure proper drying. Don't put the tassels on top of one another so that they cannot dry properly. If the cornsilk is not completely dried and stored, it can take on a purgative property (i.e., it gives you terrible stomach cramps and diarrhea). It takes about one to two weeks to dry and, once dried, the silk should be stored in an airtight, dark colored jar. It will last up to 10 months but really should be used within six months.

HOW DO I USE IT?

I distinctly remember the first time I heard the word "diuretic." I was about 10 and my mother was talking to a holistic doctor about a female friend who was retaining water faster than an old camel in a dry desert. The doctor quickly pronounced that "She needs to do a diuretic."

This doctor had a bad habit of running her words together. My young ears heard "She needs to dye her 'etic.'" This, of course, made no sense to me. But as a kid growing up within the alternative health field, many things were odd to me. So, I figured that dyeing one's "etic" was as good a treatment for urinary problems as anything else I'd heard or seen. There

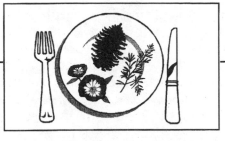

Wild Food Facts

While corn is not really a "wild food," it is still worth mentioning in this section. Corn helps to lower cholesterol as well as regulate the bowels. Cornmeal–made from the dried, kernels–can be mixed with hot water, made into a soft porridge and fed to bed-ridden folks who need a dose of nourishment.

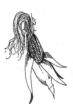

was just one little problem. I didn't know where to find the "etic" on the body and the doctor was not clear regarding what color to dye it.

Diuretic. What an odd word. When I finally figured out what it meant, I couldn't understand why someone would want or need such a thing. For myself—who as a child had a bladder the size of a pea and couldn't sit through an entire episode of *Gilligan's Island* without racing to the bathroom—it seemed like some cruel form of torture to purposely give someone an herb that triggered the "Tinkle Down" theory.

It wasn't until later in my life that I realized the value of a **diuretic**. Like the woman whose ankles were swollen four times their normal size. Or the man who wanted to urinate so badly but dreaded the idea because of the extreme pain it caused. Neither of these folks had to endure this problem when there was a safe, soothing, natural and oh-so common herb that had and still has a historical track record for solving their dilemma.

THE "MAGIC" IS IN THE SILK

It's called cornsilk. Yes, that's right, the silky strings that hug the corncob and which you probably toss in the trash. Those lovely little tassels have the incredible ability to work "magic" on the kidneys and bladder, helping to **rid the body of infection**, **uric acid build-up**, **excess water** and even **"gravel" in the urine**. And it does so in the safest manner and with absolutely *no harm* to the body.

Thank the American Indians for teaching the settlers about this most wonderful herb. Practically the entire plant is useful. Cornmeal, which is made from the dried, ground kernels, can be made into poultices by adding just enough warm milk or water until a thick paste is formed. These poultices are renowned for soothing inflammations and burns. In the Appalachian mountain region, folk healers still make a poultice out of equal parts coarse salt and cornmeal and apply it to skin problems where there is swelling.

As for cornsilk, internal use also provides pain relief when it comes to anything having to do with the kidneys, bladder and, yes, even the prostate.

Think of cornsilk whenever you experience one or more of the following:

- **Water retention**
- **Chronic or acute cystitis**
- **Excessive uric acid build-up**
- **Scalding urine**
- **Prostate enlargement**
- **Infection in the urethra, bladder, kidneys or prostate**
- **Edema**
- **High blood pressure**
- **"Gravel" in the urine (i.e., kidney stones)**

In short, cornsilk makes you "go" big time. In one study done in the Orient, it was discovered that a typical dose of cornsilk tea or tincture tripled or quadrupled urination within 24 hours. For people who measure their urine output by the drop instead of the cup, this can be an obvious godsend. The stuff that makes cornsilk do its thing is called *maizenic acid*. It acts mostly as a cardiac solution which, in turn, produces a direct diuretic action.

What I like about cornsilk is that it **cools down the "fire" in the kidneys and the bladder** and produces a lovely soothing effect on the body. I also like the fact that cornsilk has high amounts of iron, silicon and vitamin K. Synthetic diuretics only work to rid the body of excess fluid and don't add any natural vitamin or mineral content to the system. Cornsilk does not have high amounts of potassium (a nutrient that is often leeched from the body from the use of diuretics). For this reason, **I think it's a good idea to blend the herb with other kidney/bladder related plants that have natural potassium, along with other minerals and vitamins**.

For example, a good herbal formula for **cystitis** (inflammation of the bladder due to infection), is one-half teaspoon each of cornsilk, couchgrass, buchu, red clover, yarrow, uva ursi, juniper berries and parsley. The parsley is okay to use dried, but it really is more medicinally active when used fresh. If you use it fresh, you need to *double* the amount of parsley (i.e., use one heaping teaspoon of the herb) in order for it to be effective. Pour four cups of hot distilled water over the herb mixture and simmer covered for 20 minutes. If you are using fresh parsley, increase the water to five cups. Strain the herbs and drink eight ounces of the tea every three hours.

STONE SOLUTION

For "**gravel" or kidney stones**, I would highly recommend working with a holistic doctor to determine what kind of stones you have. For instance, there are certain kidney stones that are as insignificant as rock dust. There are others that could shred paper. Depending upon your overall health and/or history of kidney stones, I feel it's important not to self-treat with herbs until you have more information on the problem.

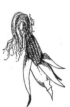

If herbs are indicated for your treatment, one formula to try is one-half teaspoon each of cornsilk, couch grass, uva ursi, goldenrod, buchu, marshmallow and one full teaspoon of gravel root. Pour four cups of hot distilled water over the herbs, cover and simmer 20 minutes. Strain the herbs and drink eight ounces of the tea every three to four hours. If you experience any discomfort or your symptoms worsen, discontinue use of the tea and seek medical attention.

PROSTATE POSSIBILITIES

Cornsilk has been used alone or in formula for **prostate complaints**. None of the research to my knowledge has dealt directly with prostate problems. However, cornsilk is considered a great help since it tends to **decrease painful swelling due to fluid build-up**.

Here's a good formula: into a bowl, combine one ounce by weight *each* of cornsilk, buchu, dried parsley and saw palmetto berries and kelp. Grind them into a fine powder. While I don't normally recommend electric grinders, you will need one for this combo since you need an extra fine powder consistency. You'll need to purchase what is called "0" capsules. Verbally, this translates to "single aught" (rhymes with the word "ought"). Fill these little capsules with the extra fine powder and take three to eight capsules for an *inflamed* prostate or two to five capsules for an *enlarged* prostate. As usual, if you feel any discomfort or pain while using this formula, discontinue use and seek medical attention.

JOINT "JUICE"

A tea made from the *fresh* strands of cornsilk has been effective in reducing the pain of **arthritis**. What researchers believe the fresh plant does is help break up uric acid in the joints. Steep four teaspoons of *fresh* cornsilk in eight ounces of warm water for 20 minutes, strain and drink. For stubborn joint pain, you can take up to four cups daily.

DOSE RECOMMENDATIONS

Many herbalists believe that fresh cornsilk is more active medicinally than the dried. However, you can't always time your urinary complaints to coincide with corn season. The tea dose for dried cornsilk is two teaspoons of the herb to eight ounces of *warm* distilled water. If you are using the fresh plant, double the amount of herb (i.e., four teaspoons) to eight ounces of warm water. Some herbal books recommend boiling the herb for five minutes. However, many herbalists feel that boiling saps much of its medicinal potential—especially when using the dried herb. I would simply pour the water over the herb, cover it and let it sit for 20 minutes. It's okay if the tea cools down—some people actually prefer it that way. It's best to drink the tea between meals, two to three times a day. Do not exceed more than one quart a day.

Cornsilk tincture, made from the *fresh* plant, is an option for those who don't like to drink teas. The suggested dose is 15 to 30 drops in several ounces of warm water, three to four times a day. To ensure a good flushing of the kidneys, I would follow each dose of the tincture with one to two cups of water.

By the way, **cornsilk is perfectly safe for children over the age of six**. However, I would adjust the dose to a quarter or half of the adult dose for children between six and twelve.

Cornsilk tea is used by some midwives to **bring contractions back when labor has stopped**. It has also been **effective during childbirth to control excessive bleeding as well as clean the urinary tract**. Even though cornsilk is used in such a way, it has been rated perfectly safe for pregnant women to use *in moderation* to alleviate occasional bouts of water retention.

You may not need what cornsilk has to offer now, but it's a good one to know. You never know when you may need to dye your "etic."

THE "DIRT" ON... CORNSILK

Botanical ~   *Zea mays*
Growth cycle ~   Annual.
Medicinal uses~   Diuretic, anodyne for urinary discomfort, demulcent, alternative.
Part(s) used for medicine ~ Silk that surrounds corncob.

Vitamins/Minerals ~	High amounts of iron, silicon and vitamin K, with moderate amounts of magnesium, phosphorus, potassium and zinc.
Region ~	All regions. Northern areas and higher altitudes may have a more difficult time due to shorter growing seasons and cooler temperatures.
Wild or Domestic ~	Domestic.
Poisonous look-alikes in the wild ~	No.
Hardy or Delicate ~	Hardy.
Height of mature plant ~	Depends upon the specific variety—anywhere from five to 10 feet.
Easy or hard to grow ~	Easy as long as you have consistently warm temperatures for proper germination.
Cultivation ~	Seed in spring. Purchase untreated seed—i.e., seed that has not been treated with fungicide protectant. Plant one inch deep in a "block system." This means that instead of planting one long 40 foot row of corn, plant four ten foot rows with two feet of space between rows. This allows for successful pollination.
Plant spacing ~	One foot.
Pre-soak seeds ~	Pre-soaking helps germination of some species. However, it is not practical for large scale planting.
Pre-chill seeds ~	No.
Indoor seed starting ~	It can be done, especially if your growing season is shorter and you don't have the consistent heat needed for outdoor germination.
Light/dark seed requirements ~	Dark. Cover seed with one inch of soil.
Days to germinate ~	Approximately seven to ten days with a prime temperature of 85°F.
Days to full maturity ~	80 to 100 days.
Soil type ~	Soil with rich nitrogen content is best. For this reason, consider cover cropping the area with alfalfa, nettle, red clover or peas the previous summer and/or fall.
Water requirements ~	Needs a lot of water with good drainage to germinate and produce an abundant crop.
Sun or shade ~	Full sun.
Propagation ~	Seed from dried cob.
Easy/hard to transplant ~	Relatively easy but not often done.
Pests or diseases ~	Earwigs (chew off the silk), earworms, corn borer. Burn off surrounding weeds or thoroughly pull them up to give corn pests less plant matter to feast upon.
Landscape uses ~	Can work as a tall hedge.

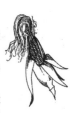

Gathering ~

There will be more silk on the cob if corn is harvested slightly before it is ready. However, you waste the actual food this way. Corn is typically ready for harvest 18 to 24 days after silk appears. Brown color of silk that protrudes out of corn husk indicates harvest time.

Best fresh or dried ~

Fresh or dried. Some herbalists feel that cornsilk is best when used fresh or somewhere between fresh and dried.

Drying methods ~

Carefully slip the tassels off the cob and place it on a plate or drying screen. Cut off any brown tassels. Make sure you don't lay the tassels on top of one another so that they cannot dry properly. The reason for this is that if the cornsilk is not completely dried and stored away, it can take on a purgative property (i.e., it gives you terrible stomach cramps and diarrhea). It takes about one to two weeks to dry and, once dried, the silk should be stored in an airtight, dark colored jar. It will last up to 10 months but really should be used within six months.

Amount needed ~

25 to 50 stalks.

Seed collection ~

Select corncobs that are healthy and relatively pest-free. Peel the husk all the way back, tie a string around the top of the husk and hang the corn from nails in a cool, dark, dry place. Basements are good as long as they are not too moist since moisture attracts mold to the corn. You don't want the area super dry either because it reduces the germination rate of the seeds. Once the corn is dry and hard— approximately after five to six weeks—seeds can be picked off or removed with a knife.

Companion planting ~

Spearmint would work since it also needs moist soil and full sun. However, you might end up trampling most of the spearmint when you are harvesting the corn.

Container planting ~

No.

Common mistakes ~

Not being aware of cross-pollination and allowing your lovely "heirloom" variety to cross-pollinate with a hybrid. Also, not providing enough water for your crop as well as not thinning the stalks if they start growing closer than one foot apart.

Interesting facts/tips ~

Some stalks of corn put out what I call "false ears." These could be the primary corn or secondary growth. These "false ears" are essentially flat husks filled with no corn and oodles of silk. Some growers believe these "false ears" might simply be unpollinated silk that never had a chance to develop. For the herbalist in search of cornsilk, coming upon a "false ear" is like striking gold.

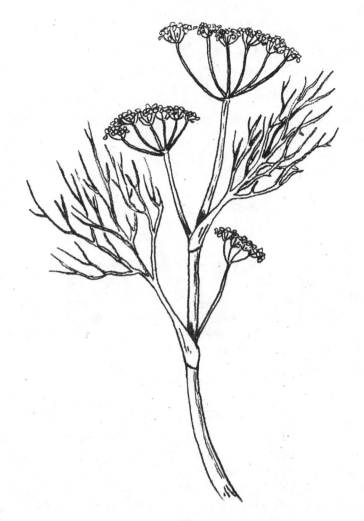

FENNEL FOR THOUGHT

Foeniculum vulgare

("W.F.")

Tender perennial (often grown as an annual)

Medicinal Uses: *Carminative, aromatic, anti-spasmodic, stimulant, galactogogue, expectorant*

Medicinal parts of plant: *Seeds*

Forms: *Tea, tincture, capsules, syrup, pure essential oil*

WHAT IS ITS CHARACTER?

Fennel always reminds me of a tall, deliberate character that is terribly preoccupied as well as proud with its appearance. During the long growing period, it develops stalk after stalk of soft fronds. Just when you think a seed head is about to develop, fennel creates yet another frond. It is in absolutely no rush. Fennel has also acquired the label of being a "loner" since it doesn't get along with other garden plants. But instead of feeling ostracized, I think fennel likes standing alone. That way, it can unfurl its regalia of fronds and showy seed heads without being overshadowed by a competing plant.

WHERE DO I FIND IT?

Fennel grows wild throughout the United States, from sea level to above 9,000 feet. It can be found along coastal areas, in vacant lots and in dense wooded areas. This showy five to six foot tall herb is hardy once established and can grow in the richest to the poorest soil.

Important note: Fennel is often confused with poison hemlock (*Conium maculatum*) which can grow near or right next to wild fennel. Poison hemlock has distinctive markings that identify it such as the red/purple spots that appear along the stem, especially at the base. Poison hemlock typically grows from 4,000 feet to 9,000 feet. From a distance, fennel and poison hemlock are hard to tell apart. If you have ANY question in your mind whether you are in the presence of fennel or poison hemlock, do not pick the plant! For novices, it is always prudent to take an experienced botanist, field guide or herbalist into the wild to help you learn proper identification techniques. Fennel can also be mistaken for the non-poisonous dill plant. They often grow next to each other and cross-pollinate which can make wild identification a tricky experience.

HOW DO I GROW IT?

Best to direct seed in April or May in 1/4 inch drills with 15 inches between rows. Space plants one foot apart. You can also plant fennel in the fall for early spring seedlings. Keep it separate from other garden plants since it can have a negative effect on them and vice versa. For example, if coriander is planted near fennel, fennel will not form a seed head. If dill is planted near fennel, they can cross-pollinate. Wormwood stunts fennel's growth as well as the development of the seed head.

HOW DO I HARVEST IT?

Harvest seed head when seeds turn from green to gray. This can be any time between August and October, depending upon your region. Clip the stem about one foot below the seed head, place it into a brown paper bag with seed heads facing down. Secure the bag with a rubber band or string and dry in a cool, dry, place. Seeds may need to be hand-picked off the seed head for storing once they are sufficiently dry. Fresh leaves are harvested as needed, while they are still vibrant. As for the fresh root, when the stalk is approximately one inch thick, push the soil around the base to form a hill. This helps create a milder flavored root which can be harvested 10 to 14 days later.

HOW DO I USE IT?

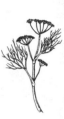

Fennel is one "old timey" herb. Back in the days of "B.C.," the Ancient Romans and Greeks prescribed this licorice-smelling plant for just about every ailment. "Take a handful of fennel seeds and call me in the morning" and "Is that your chariot?" were two common expressions.

It's hard to say which came first: fennel's folklore or the hard-core proof of its effectiveness. In the folklore department, ancient Greeks chewed fennel seeds whenever they needed courage. Many moons later, one Welsh doctor warned "He who sees fennel and gathers it not, is not a man, but a devil!"

SOLVES THE DIGESTION DILEMMA

And so, you're asking yourself "Just what has this herb done to deserve such revered treatment?" Well, for starters, it works its little seeds off when it comes to anything having to do with **digestion**. Fennel tea acts as a preventative in this arena as well as an aid. For example, one tablespoon of ground up fennel seeds sprinkled on the main meal will help *prevent* gas in the stomach as well as the bowels. Maybe you look at that main meal and think "No big deal" until after you're through and feel like a bloated, beached whale. That's when you brew up a nice hot cup of fennel tea and gently sip it until the gas pains subside.

THE COLIC KING

Fennel tea works wonders on another form of gas pain: **colic**. Ol' Hippocrates himself was prescribing fennel tea for babies back in the 3rd century B.C. It did the trick then as well as now. Today, in fact, fennel is considered the "main" herb for stopping colic in infants. Not only does the tea settle an infant's tummy, it also **sedates** them, too! That sedating part is a big selling point after hearing the constant wail of a child in pain. There are two ways to administer the herb to an infant. The first way is to make a weak tea by steeping one quarter teaspoon of *crushed* fennel seeds in 10 ounces of hot water. Cover and allow the tea to cool until warm. Strain and then give it to the infant in small mouthful doses every half hour until the pain is gone. You can also opt for the tincture. For this, simply add five to ten drops of fennel tincture to the baby's bottle of water. Small sips work best.

A classic formula for colic is made by combining equal parts of catnip (another anti-gas, digestive herb) with fennel. This can be made into a tea or used in tincture form. Some herb companies have this special combo available in tincture form so you don't have to purchase separate bottles of each herb.

There's actually a nifty way for a **nursing mother to help prevent colic**. Besides watching her own diet, if she drinks a cup of fennel tea (made from the seed or 10 to 30 drops of the tincture in eight ounces of hot distilled water) 15 to 30 minutes before nursing, there's less chance of the baby developing gas pains. What's more, the nursing mom will quickly discover that there is also an **increase in breast milk production**.

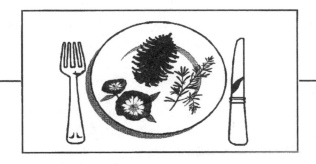

Wild Food Facts

Fennel is is a wonderfully refreshing "wild food." In spring, the tender flower stalks can be eaten raw like celery. They can also be lightly steamed for two or three minutes and served as a side vegetable. As the leaves (or fronds, as some call them) emerge, they can be clipped and added to salads, soups, stews and fish dishes. However, since heat virtually destroys the delicate licorice flavor of fennel, add the plant at the last moment before serving. The roots of the medicinal fennel can be dug up in late summer and eaten raw or slightly steamed. However, if you really love the taste of fennel root—which can best be described as licorice flavored celery—consider growing "Florence Fennel" (*Foeniculum dulce*) since you will get more root from this species. "Florence Fennel" requires a long growing period (130 + days) and plenty of moisture. Clip off the seed heads to encourage a larger root. Once the base stems are one inch in diameter, push the soil around the base to form a hill. This helps create a milder flavored root which can be harvested 10 to 14 days later. Replace all fennel plants every three to four years to ensure years of hearty crops.

UNTRAP THAT MUCUS!

So far, fennel has shown itself to be a great herb for absorbing painful poisons and expelling them. But it's not through yet. This seed made into either a tea or a tasty cough syrup can help to **bring up trapped mucus** that is stuck in the throat. The syrup is made by adding 10 to 20 drops of fennel tincture to two or three ounces of hot water. Dissolve one table-spoon of honey into the mixture (raw honey is the best) and, once cool, drink the syrup in spoonfuls. You can use this remedy once an hour for up to four hours.

POP SOME FENNEL SEEDS AND FEEL FULL

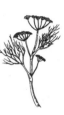

Through the ages, another popular use for fennel has been as an **appetite regulator**. Ancient Romans, in their quest to stay trim, used to pop fennel seeds like Chiclets in order to make themselves feel full. American Puritans followed suit. They nicknamed fennel "Go-to-meeting-seeds" since they were eaten to stave off hunger during marathon church meetings. Mind you, there is no substantial nourishment in fennel seeds when they are used to quell an empty tummy. They simply have the ability to make one feel temporarily full. (And **sweeten the breath** with the taste of licorice).

On its own, fennel is not the magic answer to weight loss. However, the herb can be found among other herbs in many diet/metabolism balancing herbal formulas. Basically, fennel's main purpose in the formulas is to act as a gentle stimulant and soothing herb for the digestive tract.

One old herbal book suggests a **diet tea recipe** using 1/2 ounce of fennel seeds with 1/2 ounce of dried cleavers herb or one ounce of the fresh plant. Steep the two herbs in one quart of boiling water and drink up to three cups a day before meals. Cleavers helps the body to better metabolize food; fennel aids in digestion of the food as well as catalyzes the cleavers herb. This is not a tea to take if you're looking for rapid weight loss. The average person may only see results after five to six weeks when the body has had a chance to readjust and come more into balance. Keep in mind that fennel has a tendency to **normalize the appetite**. That means that **it can suppress as well as stimulate the appetite**.

A "SEEDY" EYEWASH

Yet another favorite use for fennel is as a **gentle eyewash** for sore, tired, strained eyes. As usual, the Romans had to find something mystical in this mild eye treatment. They swore that a blind snake sucked the oil out of a fennel seed and within seconds, the snake's glazed eyes became clear. Enough people bought this snake tale and started using a mild solution of the tea to wash their eyes. Darned if the stuff didn't start to work to relieve their eyestrain. The blind did not suddenly see, but the puffy-eyed ones found an herbal wash they could depend upon. A mild solution of the tea would be approximately one half teaspoon of the crushed seed to 10 ounces of hot water. Let the herb steep in the water until it is cool to the touch, strain and then use as an eyewash.

HOW ABOUT A FENNEL BATH?

Some people swear by a **fennel bath to draw out toxins and environmental pollutants**. If anything, it will make the bathroom smell like sweet licorice candy. You'll need a good handful of the seeds. Crush them and pour six to eight cups of very hot water over them. Cover and let the seeds steep for 20 to 30 minutes while you fill the tub with hot water. Strain the seed tea into the tub. DO NOT put the seeds directly into the tub since they can cause an array of plumbing problems. I don't know about you, but I don't want to explain to the plumber why I have a cup of congealed fennel seeds stuck in my pipe. Soak in the bathtub for 20 to 45 minutes.

ANTI-GRIPING LAXATIVE SUPPORT

One of fennel's lesser known uses is **as an addition to laxative formulas to reduce extreme griping in the intestines**. If you are using a laxative that causes cramping, try adding a teaspoon of freshly crushed fennel seeds to the formula *or* enjoy a cup of fennel tea after taking the laxative product.

FENNEL ESSENTIAL OIL

The last major use for fennel comes in the form of the essential oil. The oil is found within the seeds. (Actually, the oil is what is responsible for the herb's healing abilities.) The pure essential oil on its own is much too concentrated. For this reason, you'll want to blend eight to fifteen drops of fennel pure essential oil in one ounce of sweet almond oil, peanut oil or apricot kernel oil.

This massage oil can be used two ways. First, it can be rubbed into **painful joints for soothing relief**. Secondly, when the oil is **rubbed into the breasts of nursing mothers, it can help reduce swelling and pain from "milk overload."** Even when the massage oil is used externally, milk production can still be promoted. So, take care and monitor your use. Also, since essential oils are *never* to be taken internally, make sure there is no residue of the essential oil on your breasts when the baby nurses.

DOSES & CAUTIONS

The normal tea dosage for fennel is one to two cups a day. When making the tea, it is important to always crush the seeds *as needed* with a mortar and pestle to encourage the release of the essential oils. *Do not purchase pre-ground fennel seeds since the volatile oils are lost shortly after grinding.* The herb to water ratio for tea equals one *tablespoon* of the crushed seeds to eight ounces of hot water. Steep ten minutes, strain and drink. If you prefer the capsules, take two to three a day before meals. If the tincture or extract trips your trigger, the normal dose is 10 to 30 drops in eight ounces of warm water, also taken before meals.

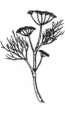

The cautions are as follows: fennel has the reputation of bringing on menstrual periods. Mind you, it takes a whole lot of fennel tea to accomplish this feat. However, there have been cases where menopausal women have had a slight return of their period after ingesting large amounts of fennel. Because it can stimulate the uterine muscles, **pregnant women— especially those with a history of miscarriage—should not drink the tea or use the tincture**. Culinary use of the herb is okay. Another study showed that, in some women, fennel had a slightly estrogenic effect. For this reason, **women who cannot take the birth control pill, have abnormal blood clotting or estrogen-dependent breast tumors should not use medicinal size quantities of fennel**. Never ingest fennel essential oil (or *any* essential oil for that matter.) It can cause nausea and seizures.

Whether fennel has the ability to "cure whatever ails you" depends upon your particular system. It could be the tea for you—especially after the "meal of the century." Consider it fennel for thought.

THE "DIRT" ON...FENNEL

Botanical ~	*Foeniculum vulgare*
Growth cycle ~	Tender perennial (often grown as an annual).
Medicinal uses~	Carminative, aromatic, anti-spasmodic, stimulant, galactogogue, expectorant.
Part(s) used for medicine ~	Seeds.
Vitamins/Minerals ~	Vitamins A, C, calcium, magnesium, phosphorus, potassium, sulphur, sodium, iron and selenium.
Region ~	Fennel grows wild throughout the United States, from sea level to above 9,000 feet. It can be found along coastal areas, in vacant lots and in dense wooded areas.

Wild or Domestic ~	Both.
Poisonous look-alikes in the wild ~	Yes. Fennel is often confused with poison hemlock (*Conium maculatum*) which can grow near or right next to wild fennel. Poison hemlock has distinctive markings that identify it such as the red/purple spots that appear along the stem, especially at the base. Poison hemlock typically grows from 4,000 feet to 9,000 feet. From a distance, fennel and poison hemlock are hard to tell apart. If you have ANY question in your mind whether you are in the presence of fennel or poison hemlock, do not pick the plant! For novices, it is always prudent to take an experienced botanist, field guide or herbalist into the wild to help you learn proper identification techniques. Fennel can also be mistaken for the non-poisonous dill plant. They often grow next to each other and cross-pollinate which can make wild identification a tricky experience.
Hardy or Delicate ~	Hardy once established.
Height of mature plant ~	Up to five to six feet.
Easy or hard to grow ~	Easy.
Cultivation ~	Direct seed in April or May in 1/4 inch drills. Figure 15 inches between rows. In areas that have temperate climates, fennel can be planted in the fall for spring arrival.
Plant spacing ~	One foot.
Pre-soak seeds ~	No.
Pre-chill seeds ~	No.
Indoor seed starting ~	No. Fennel does not transplant well.
Light/dark seed requirements ~	Dark. Cover seed with 1/4 inch of soil.
Days to germinate ~	10 to 14 days.
Days to full maturity ~	120 to 150 days for seed harvest.
Soil type ~	Rich and moist are best but fennel has been known to grow quite well in gravel or sandy soil. Do not plant fennel in heavy clay since it limits seed development.
Water requirements ~	Fennel is considered "drought hardy." However, a good, moist, well-drained soil increases the stem's succulence.
Sun or shade ~	Full sun.
Propagation ~	Seed.
Easy/hard to transplant ~	Only transplant well developed seedlings. However, it can still be a delicate proposition. Direct seeding is always your best bet.
Pests or diseases ~	Typically pest-free.
Landscape uses ~	Works as a bold, ornamental set off by itself since its development can be impeded by other garden plants. (See "Companion planting" below).

150

Gathering ~	**Seeds**: Seeds are harvested in late summer to early fall, depending upon when the seed turns from green to slightly gray. Some herbalists suggest collecting seed when it is still green. If you live in frost-free regions, plant a few of the fresh green seeds right away since their germination energy is strong and viable. **Leaves**: as needed, while still vibrant. **Root**: when stalk is approximately one inch thick, push the soil around the base to form a hill. This helps create a milder flavored root which can be harvested 10 to 14 days later.
Best fresh or dried ~	**Seeds**: fresh or dried. **Leaves & Root**: Fresh
Drying methods ~	Clip the stem about one foot below the seed head, place in a brown paper bag with seed heads facing down. Secure the bag with a rubber band or string and dry in a cool, dry, place. Seeds may need to be hand-picked off the seed head for storing once they are sufficiently dry.
Amount needed ~	Moderate use: 5 plants. Regular use: 10 or more plants.
Seed collection ~	Same method as for drying seeds. Helpful hint: you can plant the same fennel seeds that you are using for medicine. However, due to possible problems with age and improper storage, the germination rate is not as high as seeds packaged especially for growing.
Companion planting ~	Fennel needs to be a bit of a "loner" in the garden since certain other plants can affect its growth. Never plant fennel near dill since they cross-pollinate. Keep fennel away from coriander or it will not develop a seed head. In addition, never grow wormwood in the same vicinity as fennel since it also stunts its growth and seed development. Many herbalists go so far as to say that fennel is disliked by all garden plants. While I haven't seen them all dislike fennel, they certainly can grow smaller when near this aromatic herb.
Container planting ~	Yes, but it has to be a big container. Outdoor wooden whiskey barrel planters that are wide and deep enough are excellent for fennel. Since other plants have a problem with fennel, container planting is an excellent idea.
Common mistakes ~	Not paying attention to the fact that fennel needs a separate place in the garden in order to properly bloom and not disturb the development of other plants.
Interesting facts/tips ~	There are other fennel plants—some are grown for their beauty, some for their edible roots. *Foeniculum vulgare 'Purpureum'* is known as "Bronze fennel." It has distinctive purple and bronze foilage. *Foeniculum dulce* is "Florence fennel" or "Finocchio." It is grown as a vegetable crop and prized for its large roots. Removing the flower heads of Florence fennel creates a larger root. Replant every three to four years to ensure a hearty crop.

Chapter 19

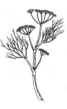

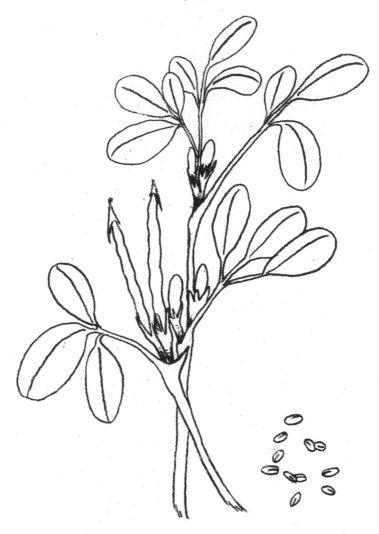

IT'S FENUGREEK TO ME!

Trigonella foenum-graecum

("W.F.")

Tender annual

Medicinal Uses: *Expectorant, mucilage, restorative*
Medicinal parts of plant: *Seeds, leaves and stems*
Forms: *Tea, capsules, poultice, sprouts (seeds)*

WHAT IS ITS CHARACTER?

I think fenugreek accepts the fact that, for most of its life, it is stepped upon and ignored. In the flurry of spring and summer growth, fenugreek tends to blend in with the rest of the meadow "weeds," fighting to stand out in the crowd. But when those three to four inch seed pods begin to mature in mid to late summer, fenugreek suddenly emerges as a seasoned veteran of fields and pastures. The other plants may begin to wither and die back, but fenugreek stands out from the rest, proud to show off its impressive little fruit pods. Sometimes I can almost hear it say, "I'm little. But don't ever underestimate me."

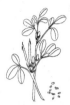

WHERE DO I FIND IT?

Fenugreek tends to blend in with other grasses and herbs ("weeds") in meadows, fertile fields and along sunny, damp roadsides. It is found from sea level to approximately 6,000 feet.

HOW DO I GROW IT?

Fenugreek grows easily from seed sown in spring once the frost danger has passed. It germinates quickly, sometimes within two or three days. It is best to directly sow the herb thickly in rows, barely covering the seed with soil since fenugreek needs light to germinate. Thin seedlings to six inches to avoid overcrowding which stunts its growth. Fenugreek can grow in sandy soil but it prefers cool, damp spring soil with an average temperature of 60°F. Avoid spring flooding or soil with poor drainage since this makes the seeds rot. Fenugreek seeds can be pre-soaked to speed germination but since they have a tremendous mucilaginous quality, they get awfully slimy once you remove them from the soaking water.

HOW DO I HARVEST IT?

Fenugreek leaves can be harvested up until the pods begin to form. The slender seed pods should be left on the plant until they become a light tan color and are dry to the touch. If you wish, you can gently pull the pod open to see if the seeds are brown and hard. The seeds should also have a lovely maple fragrance. Place the pods in partial sunshine to continue drying. Once dry, open the pods and remove the seeds, storing them in airtight, glass containers.

HOW DO I USE IT?

Leave it to those ancient Greeks to stumble upon a healing seed in the haystack.

The classic story goes that early Greek farmers, in hopes of making their moldy, rancid, insect-infested hay more palatable for their horses, spiced up the stuff with clumps of a green weed that smelled like celery. The horses and cattle went for the bait every time. What's more, the sick animals—especially those with inflamed stomachs and irritated intestines—would soon show signs of better health and an improved appetite. Word got out that this weedy concoction was the proven way to lead a cow and horse to hay and make them eat.

Soon, the herbal hay mix came to be known as "Greek hay" which later evolved into the name we know and love it by: fenugreek.

It didn't take ancient doctors long to start picking the plant apart (literally) to discover what made it so appealing. When they popped the tan seeds out of the herb's narrow pods and soaked them in water, the seeds became slick and gummy. Maybe, the doctors thought, these seeds did the same thing when they hit the stomach and maybe, just maybe, they would **soothe and heal inflamed tissues**.

No "maybe" about it. Fenugreek seeds do just that—plus a whole lot more. In fact, continuing research has discovered that this little seed has some of the most diverse uses under the sun. Keep reading and I'm sure you'll find something this seed can do for you.

CLEARING THAT "ELIMINATIVE ZONE"

One of the major uses for fenugreek is as **an effective cleanser of the "eliminative" zone. That zone includes the sinuses, lungs, kidneys and bowels.** Many acute and chronic illnesses are aggravated by a clogged up eliminative zone. Everything from **respiratory problems** (such as **chronic bronchitis**) to **diverticulitis** and **constipation** have been connected to one or more of the areas being choked with heavy, toxic mucus.

Mucus may sound like no big deal, but it is. Folks who eat lots of dairy, sugar, processed meats and white flour-filled products are unknowingly building a lovely shrine to the Mucus King. Mucus builds up over the years and is not always coughed up. Little by little, mucus trickles from the sinuses into the bronchial tubes. Next stop is the stomach, then into the kidneys before it finally builds a retirement village in the intestines and colon. There it sits until finally one or more parts in that eliminative zone become inflamed, irritated and even infected.

Antibiotics can kill the infection but they often do nothing to get rid of the mucus. That's where fenugreek steps in. Not only does this herb **work to dislodge toxic mucus, it also leaves behind a soothing layer of relief for any inflamed areas**. In addition, fenugreek cleanses all areas in the eliminative zone—especially the kidneys.

The normal dose for discharging mucus would be one fenugreek capsule three times a day or one to three cups daily of the tea made by simmering two teaspoons of the seeds in one and one-half cups of hot distilled water for 10 minutes. Feel free to add honey (*not sugar!*) to sweeten the brew. Some folks choose not to strain the seeds, opting to let them soak in the tea while sipping it and then chewing them into a pulp and swallowing. As long as the seeds have soaked until complete softness has set in, this may help in the discharge of more mucus.

One thing that's important to mention is that if you decide to use fenugreek for ridding your body of mucus, make the job easier by staying off dairy, wheat, sugar and any other mucus-inviting foods.

SOOTHING INTESTINAL RELIEF

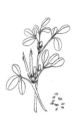

Fenugreek's natural mucilaginous ability (i.e., that slimy, slippery thing that happens when the seeds hit water) has been shown to soothe the mucosa of the intestines and stomach. For this reason, unstrained **fenugreek seed tea could help to relieve the discomfort of diverticulosis as well as Crohn's disease**. I say "unstrained" since chewing the seeds thoroughly into a pulp after finishing the tea can provide you with an added layer of relief.

CHOLESTEROL LOWERING

Research has found that fenugreek seeds are high in protein, EFA's (Essential Fatty Acids), lecithin, rich in vitamins A, B and C, minerals (especially iron and calcium) and loaded with amino acids, including lysine, tryptophan, leucine, histidine and arginine. They also have the ability to **reduce blood glucose as well as lower serum cholesterol levels**. This was discovered when mongrel dogs in the French city of Villemois-son-sur-Orge were fed their standard chow laced with fenugreek seed meal for eight weeks. Blood test showed that the fenugreek seeds contributed to the dogs' lower cholesterol readings. Scientists now knew they were barking up the right seed. They proposed that an average of two to three fenugreek capsules taken when eating meals high in fat could be beneficial in dissolving and eliminating the fat.

HELPS WITH DIABETES

Since fenugreek was shown to lower blood sugar levels, it is being looked into as a possible daily supplement for people with **late-onset, insulin-dependent diabetes**. Science has discovered that fenugreek contains six compounds that help to regulate blood sugar. The recommended dose is two to three cups of the tea a day or two to three capsules with each meal. Keep an eye on your insulin needs to see if there's any fluctuation.

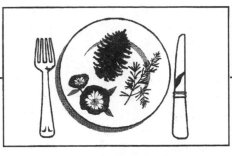

Wild Food Facts

Fenugreek leaves and stems are an excellent source of beta carotene which is thought to help slow down or prevent the progress of Alzheimer's disease. Slightly steam the greens for two to four minutes or add them at the last minute to soups and stews, since overcooking saps most of the vitamins.

Fenugreek seeds can be sprouted in plastic trays and are at their nutritional peak between the third to fifth day. If you let them sprout for seven or more days, they become awfully bitter as well as pretty slimy. When using the sprouts, add them in moderate amounts to salads and on top of stews and soups.

COULD IT PERK UP YOUR PERCOLATOR?

Another important use for fenugreek is as a **hormonal helper**. This covers a wide territory for women but men can also benefit. For example, in China, fenugreek is given to men who suffer from **impotence**. It doesn't hurt that the herb is known throughout Asia and the Middle East as an **aphrodisiac**. Whether it perks up your percolator is completely based upon one's individual chemistry. But fenugreek has been shown to "warm" the reproductive organs in both men and women, making it an interesting little seed to contemplate.

You might be interested to know that fenugreek was **fed to harem women to make them more voluptuous**. Several non-buxom women I know heard about this historical anecdote and decided to do an informal study to see if fenugreek really did give a boost to the "buxom impaired." After four straight days of taking the tea three times a day, they said they really did feel a slight lift in their chest. Of course, after they stopped drinking the tea, everything returned to normal. While I can't verify it, there are those who say that sprouted fenugreek seeds also have this bust elevating ability.

However, before women plant this seed in their mouth they should know that fenugreek might also help plant a seed in their womb. The herb contains a chemical called *diosgenin* which resembles the female sex hormone estrogen. This has varying effects on different women. **For some, fenugreek brings on a menstrual period faster than a New York minute. For others, it has turned their reproductive organs into "Camp Fertility."** Nursing women have even found that unstrained **fenugreek tea increases mother's milk, especially in small breasted women**. Obviously, more research has to be done before herbalists can make a firm judgment on fenugreek's "feminine effect." But one thing all herbalists agree upon is that because fenugreek stimulates the uterus, **PREGNANT WOMEN SHOULD ABSOLUTELY NOT TAKE THIS HERB**.

However, if you are experiencing **menopause**, fenugreek might be one of your best herbal friends. It's a natural source of calcium and iron—two important minerals women need. One to two cups of the tea each day have been known to **decrease hot flashes and curb menopausal depression**.

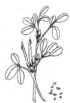

SORE THROAT AID

The tea can be used as a gargle to take the **pain out of a sore throat** by absorbing toxins and adding a soothing layer of protection from inflammation. Just mix one tablespoon of crushed seeds in eight ounces of hot distilled water and let it steep covered for 10 minutes. After straining the seeds, you can add a tablespoon of honey for added relief. Gargle with the tea up to four times a day. Don't spit out the tea once you are finished gargling! It can be extremely soothing when you are feeling ill.

I know someone who swears by fenugreek for illness the way some people depend upon echinacea when they are sick. While the two herbs are not identical in the way they work on the body, fenugreek does have the ability to pull toxic waste from the system. If I were feeling sick, I would definitely start taking my 25 drops of echinacea tincture every hour along with a cup of fenugreek tea every few hours.

If you are developing a **cough** with that cold, fenugreek can come to the rescue. One of the classic respiratory formulas is made by blending one part of thyme for every four parts of fenugreek. In other words, for every one teaspoon of thyme, add four teaspoons of fenugreek seeds. Using this measurement, make up a small batch ahead of time (perhaps one cup of the mixture) and store it in an airtight glass container. When you prepare the tea, make sure the herbs are mixed together when you add two teaspoons of the blend to eight ounces of hot distilled water.

Another good herb to add to the blend is marshmallow root. Marshmallow is suggested if you need an extra healing punch of soothing cough action. You will need three parts of marshmallow root added to the previous formula.

A POWERFUL PULLING POULTICE

Externally, these healing seeds have been used in **poultices to help draw out infection and reduce pain**. The poultice is especially good for **neuralgia**, **sciatica** and **wounds that have a hard time draining**. To make the poultice, pulverize the seeds and add just enough hot water to make a paste. Flatten the sticky mixture directly against the area to be treated, cover it with gauze and keep it warm. You can keep the poultice on the skin anywhere from 20 minutes to several hours. Keep checking underneath the poultice every hour or so to see if any drainage is taking place. An herbalist friend of mine concocted his own version of this poultice specifically for slow healing wounds. In addition to the ground up fenugreek seeds, he adds equal parts of powdered comfrey root and powdered marshmallow root. The comfrey root really works to draw flesh together. *Because of this, it is imperative that there is no infection brewing under the wound since you do not want to close a wound and trap the infection beneath it.*

LOOSENS THOSE BOWELS

I wouldn't call fenugreek a "specific" herb for constipation but two teaspoons of the seeds added to a cup of hot water have been known to **loosen the bowels**. Chewing the seeds into a fine pulp after drinking the tea is highly recommended. It is a good idea to follow the tea with two or three glasses of water to further aid in this process.

THINGS YOU SHOULD KNOW

In addition to the fact that **pregnant women should not take fenugreek**, there is another minor caution. Some people who take the herb for longer than 10 days at a time begin to smell like the herb. The odor can be compared to old celery. This may not be a problem for you, but consider this: do you really want people to associate you with an aging vegetable stalk? If your answer is "no," try to curb your fenugreek intake at eight to nine days with several days off in between. This will allow your body to throw off what it doesn't need of the herb. The tea itself smells and tastes like a strong maple flavored drink. The seeds, however, are a bit on the bitter side and it may take awhile to get used to them.

Obviously, this little seed packs a punch. Those ancient Greeks may not have understood the consequences when they tossed fenugreek into their feed. But centuries later, it's become fodder for thought.

THE "DIRT" ON...FENUGREEK

Botanical ~   *Trigonella foenum-graecum*

Growth cycle ~   Tender annual.

Medicinal uses~   Expectorant, mucilage, restorative.

Part(s) used for medicine ~ Seeds, leaves.

Vitamins/Minerals ~   Vitamin A, B, C and D, protein, EFA's (Essential Fatty Acids), lecithin, minerals (especially iron and calcium) and loaded with amino acids, including lysine, tryptophan, leucine, histidine and arginine.

Region ~   From sea level to approximately 6,000 feet, in meadows, fertile fields and along sunny, damp roadsides.

Wild or Domestic ~   Both.

Poisonous look-alikes in the wild ~   No.

Hardy or Delicate ~   Hardy.

Height of mature plant ~   One to two feet.

Easy or hard to grow ~   Very easy.

Cultivation ~   Direct seed thickly in rows two feet apart. Barely cover with soil. Thin to six inches once plant is established. Prefers cool, damp spring soil with an average temperature of 60°F. Avoid spring flooding or soil with poor drainage since this will make the seeds rot.

Plant spacing ~   Six inches.

Pre-soak seeds ~   Yes, but not necessary.

Pre-chill seeds ~   No.

Indoor seed starting ~   Yes, but only for areas that have short growing season. Use seed cells instead of dirt flats. Easier to direct sow.

Light/dark seed requirements ~   Light.

Days to germinate ~   Three to five days.

Days to full maturity ~   Approximately 60 days to seed pod harvest.

Soil type ~   Fertile, cool and well-drained.

Water requirements ~   Needs moderate water to germinate without drowning. Over watering will cause root rot and stunted plants.

Sun or shade ~   Full sun.

Propagation ~   Seed.

Easy/hard to transplant ~   Easy if the seedling is firmly established in the seed cell.

Pests or diseases ~   Watch for the occasional snail or trail of ants.

Landscape uses ~   Can be used as a soft green filler. However, make sure you can get to it easily to harvest the pods as needed.

Gathering ~	Harvest pods when they turn a tan brown color and begin to wither on the stems. Gather the clover-like leaves and stems in early summer before the pods appear.
Best fresh or dried ~	**Seeds** can be used both fresh or dried; **leaves** are used fresh.
Drying methods ~	Leave seed pods in partial sun to dry. Store in airtight container.
Amount needed ~	Each mature pod contains anywhere from 10 to 15 seeds. The amount needed is determined by how often you will be using it. If you want to use it for teas, poultices and sprouts, you will require three to four ten foot long rows.
Seed collection ~	If you live in temperate zones, replant seeds fresh from the pod that are not completely dried. If you reside in areas that get regular freezes, collect seeds for planting from the seed you dry.
Companion planting ~	Yarrow, anise, burdock.
Container planting ~	No. It takes a lot of fenugreek to provide you with a sufficient amount of seed pods.
Common mistakes ~	Not thinning seedlings enough which will stunt the growth of the mature plants. Over watering during the first week and ending up with a pile of slimy seeds that do not germinate.
Interesting facts/tips ~	Fenugreek works as an excellent fall cover crop. It breaks up heavy soil and contributes high amounts of nitrogen and organic matter to the earth. One to two pounds of fenugreek seed will cover 1000 square feet; 35 pounds will cover one acre. As with most cover crops, plant in early fall and turn plant over in spring.

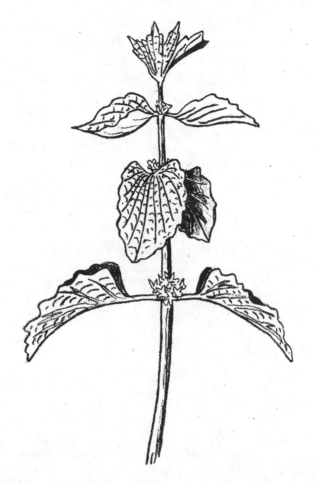

Chapter 20

THE BEST LITTLE HOREHOUND IN BRONCHUS

Marrubium vulgare

Hardy perennial

Medicinal Uses: *Expectorant, mild antispasmodic, mild sedative, mild diaphoretic, vulnerary, diuretic, stomach and bitter liver tonic*
Medicinal parts of plant: *Leaves*
 Forms: *Tea, syrup, lozenge*

WHAT IS ITS CHARACTER?

Horehound reminds me of one of the "Bowery" boys. It's a tough little herb that can be left alone in the weakest soil, given little water and still live a full life. I see horehound and I see a survivor. It doesn't really care what people think about it. When some remark on horehound's "awful musty smell" or bitter taste, I can almost hear it say, "Yeah? What's it to ya?" If you try to pamper horehound, it has absolutely no idea how to react. Horehound might like to play the tough part but it's also one of the most dependable plants. It may be bitter and some people might turn their nose up at its aroma, but when you need it, horehound always comes through for you.

WHERE DO I FIND IT?

In the wild, horehound, a member of the mint family, is often found growing in the poorest of soils. It is scattered throughout the United States from sea level to 9,000 feet. Cultivated horehound tends to grow larger and look better than the wild variety which can appear as though it has gone through its own private war with the elements.

HOW DO I GROW IT?

Horehound needs a little bit of special treatment to grow from seed. However, once it is established, you've got a perennial friend. Direct seed in the spring, covering the seed with a little bit of dirt as you press them firmly into the ground. Lightly spray with water without soaking the area. Horehound tends to like some darkness to germinate. I throw a large piece of burlap over the dirt and keep an eye on the soil every few days to check for germination. Seedlings should start appearing anywhere between seven to twenty-one days. However, germination can be erratic. Don't be surprised to see some late bloomers arrive after the rest have germinated. Once you see a few seedlings, remove the burlap and allow nature to take its course.

HOW DO I HARVEST IT?

Horehound does not typically produce a flower until its second year of growth. Some herbalists believe that you should wait until the second year to harvest horehound in order to get the most medicinal benefit from it. Harvest the late spring or early summer plants *before* the flowering stage. Clip the plant several inches above the ground, and bundle together in groups of five. Place the bundles in brown paper bags with stems poking out of the bag and leave them there to thoroughly dry. When ready, strip the leaves from the soft, woolly stems. I sometimes toss in a few chopped up stems for good measure.

HOW DO I USE IT?

When I was a kid, my parents and I would occasionally take a trip down to San Diego, California. While most youngsters begged to go to Sea World, I always wanted to visit "Old Town." Old Town—which could have easily been named "Pioneer Town," "Western Town" or "Trap & Capture the Tourists Town"—was to many, just another stop on the bus tour. But to a 10 year old who wished she had been born during the days of the covered wagons, it was a fine place to spend the day.

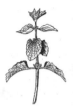

As I scuffed my feet across the sawdust-strewn streets, I looked for my favorite store. It was an old fashioned candy store, called ironically, "The Old Fashioned Candy Store." My eyes passed the thick glass canisters of lemon drops and cinnamon bears and came to rest on the one candy I loved the most: horehound. They sold the bitter, black candy in brown paper bags that said in bold lettering **"For Coughs, Sore Throats & Hoarseness, You Can't Beat Horehound!"** It didn't matter to me that my favorite candy was *also* considered to be a medicinal throat lozenge. Other kids may have loved Pez, Sweet Tarts, Milk Duds or Junior Mints. I loved horehound. Maybe I was odd, but I'll tell you right now, I would take a horehound lozenge over a pack of Pez any day—*especially* when I couldn't stop coughing.

Apparently I wasn't the only person attracted to this musty-smelling herbal helper. Valued for thousands of years, horehound—which is often referred to in herbal books as "White Horehound"—was supposedly named after "Horus," the Egyptian God. Before it was known for packing a pectoral punch, it was thought to be able to break the curse of evil magic spells. That's asking a whole lot of this humble herb. Personally, I prefer to stick with its most well known use. And that is as a **mild but highly effective anti-inflammatory herb that works directly on the bronchi to relieve coughs and bring up trapped phlegm**.

White horehound should not be confused with its sister plant Black horehound (*Ballota nigra*) which has been given the descriptive nickname "Stinking Horehound." Black (stinking) horehound smells pretty darn bad and is considered toxic in large quantities.

That stinking part has also been applied to white horehound as well. In fact, many herbal books love to remark on the "rank" odor of this herb. When I first read this, I couldn't understand what was so bad about horehound. I've always liked the herb's dusty mint aroma, which I would compare to a musty attic on a summer's day. Then again, maybe the aroma of a musty attic doesn't exactly trip your aroma trigger.

163

THE GENTLE GIANT

Horehound is the personification of gentleness. But don't let that gentleness fool you. Horehound is a giant of strength—especially when cough symptoms creep up and cause you discomfort. Horehound, taken as a tea, syrup or throat lozenge, **relaxes the bronchi while encouraging mucus to break free and be coughed up** to irritate no more.

If you drink a very hot cup of horehound tea and remain in bed under blankets, it has a tendency to **produce a mighty copious sweat**. Any herbalist worth his or her salt will look on this as a positive thing since this means the body is ridding itself of trapped toxins.

Horehound is an herb tea that can be taken freely whenever you are plagued with respiratory complaints. It may be given to children over the age of two years as well as to weakened patients who can take precious little else into their system.

Asthmatics can also benefit from horehound's congestion-clearing action, although **herbalists recommend taking the tea cold or using the syrup**.

Singers should note horehound's healing ability. Taken as a tea or throat lozenge, horehound helps **soothe vocal chords as well as relieve hoarseness and laryngitis**. To make a quick, throat-soothing remedy, pick eight to ten fresh leaves, chop them up finely and then blend with one tablespoon of raw honey. This sweet concoction helps both sore throats and dry coughs.

THE SYRUP COULD BE YOUR SAVING GRACE

Horehound syrup is a valuable home remedy. While you can buy the syrup at any health or herb store, I prefer to make it myself. Unlike most delicate leaves, it is okay to boil the horehound plant without losing the herb's healing volatile oils. The first step in making the syrup is to boil either one cup of *fresh* horehound leaves or 1/4 cup of the *dried* plant with two cups of water for 10 minutes. Turn off the heat and let the mixture sit *covered* for 20 minutes. Strain and measure how much liquid remains. Whatever this amount is, add *twice* that amount of honey. In other words, if you end up with one and one-half cups of the tea mixture, add three cups of raw honey. Stir the honey into the hot infusion until it is completely dissolved. Add a thumb-sized piece of fresh ginger to help preserve the syrup, then pour it into a bottle with a cork stopper since some cough syrups have been known to ferment and explode. Store the syrup in the refrigerator. It should keep for up to six weeks.

A LONG LASTING LOZENGE

You can also make your own horehound lozenges. Most recipes call for sugar to create the standard "hard crack" consistency. However, sugar is the last thing I want to have in my body if I am sick or trying to get over a sore throat. The following throat lozenge formula is a bit gooey due to the fact that honey is used in place of sugar. But I assure you, these lozenges are strong and effective for combatting a sore throat.

Combine two teaspoons of dried horehound, one teaspoon of dried white pine bark and one heaping teaspoon of *freshly ground* anise seed in eight ounces of distilled water. Bring to a boil and simmer for 10 to 15 minutes. Turn off the heat and allow the herbs to continue steeping in the covered pan for one to three hours. The longer the herbs steep, the stronger the lozenges will be. Strain the herbs and pour the tea back into the pan. Add one-half cup of blackstrap molasses and one cup of raw honey to the tea. Cook the mixture *uncovered* on low heat for one hour or until it reaches 300° to 310° on a candy thermometer. During this time, *do not stir the mixture.* When the scum starts to form on top, you can carefully remove it with a large spoon. The liquid is ready when a spoonful dropped into a glass of cold water forms a hard consistency. When this happens, immediately pour the thick, dark concoction on a greased cookie sheet. As it begins to harden, use a knife to score the sheet into bite-sized morsels. I have found that even though the mixture reaches a "hard crack" stage, it often returns to a rather soft, hard taffy texture. Because of this, I suggest that you keep the lozenges in a glass jar in the refrigerator so that they will retain a hard surface. Once you put a lozenge in your mouth, they will quickly dissolve and coat your throat. I must tell you that a little lozenge goes a very long way. They are strong flavored thanks to the blackstrap molasses. Start with a little chunk and work your way up to see how you like the taste.

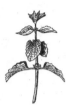

A BITTER BREW FOR DIGESTION

Another important effect of horehound tea is that its **bitter taste promotes better digestion and liver function**. This means that horehound can be used by those who need to **stimulate their digestive juices because of faulty assimilation of food in the intestinal tract.** To use horehound tea in this way, drink a strong brew 10 to 20 minutes *before* eating a large meal.

When you combine horehound's digestive benefits with its ability to soothe a cough, you get a remarkable combination. You have what herbalists refer to as **a "specific remedy" for a dry, unproductive cough** with poor appetite and sluggish digestion. Poor digestion and poor appetite are usually present when one is sick. However, this does not mean that when you are suffering from congestion and coughs that you should be dining on large meals. Most holistic practitioners will recommend a very bland, dairy-free diet when you are suffering from respiratory congestion.

APPETITE-STIMULATING

Horehound has also been known to **stimulate the appetite**. This does not necessarily mean that the herb makes you want to eat an entire smorgasbord in one sitting. Appetite-stimulating herbs get the digestive juices (bile) flowing ahead of time so that your meal is broken down more effectively when it reaches the stomach. It doesn't make you eat more, but it often makes the food taste better. Ironically, **one of horehound's secondary uses is as a treatment for obesity**. Thanks to horehound's **mild diuretic** ability, it helps rid the body of excess water weight. One doctor wrote over a hundred years ago that "Horehound should be taken in moderation for it can bring about a considerable loss of weight." You would have to drink over a quart of the tea infusion each day to see any effect. And the primary result would be water weight—not fat.

TEA DOSE

Horehound tea is made a little differently than the typical tea to water ratio. Add only *four ounces* of boiling water to one teaspoon of the dried herb. Cover and let the herb steep for 10 to 20 minutes. Sweeten with honey or blackstrap molasses to increase the soothing sensation. As I mentioned earlier, you can drink the tea freely as a remedy for respiratory ailments. This translates into four to five cups a day for up to two weeks. Remember that horehound also has diuretic capabilities so the more you drink the more you'll need to "go."

A FEW CAUTIONS....

Even though horehound is considered one of the milder medicinals, there are three things to consider. **Overdosing on the herb has been known to cause irregular heartbeats in some people as well as act as a mild laxative**.

In addition, **for some women, horehound promotes menstruation**. Thus, **pregnant women should not use horehound**. Enjoying a horehound throat lozenge now and again is fine.

Now that you know what this little plant can do, the next time someone starts coughing, toss them a homemade horehound lozenge or brew up a hot cup of tea or syrup. They may say it ain't nothin' but a hore-hound, but you'll know better.

THE "DIRT" ON...HOREHOUND

Botanical ~ *Marrubium vulgare* (White Horehound)

Growth cycle ~ Hardy perennial.

Medicinal uses~ Expectorant, mild antispasmodic, mild sedative, mild dia-phoretic, vulnerary, diuretic, stomach and bitter liver tonic.

Part(s) used for medicine ~ Leaves.

Vitamins/Minerals ~ N/A.

Region ~ From sea level to 9,000 feet.

Wild or Domestic ~ Both.

Poisonous look-alikes in the wild ~ No.

Hardy or Delicate ~ Hardy.

Height of mature plant ~ One to two feet.

Easy or hard to grow ~ Easy.

Cultivation ~ Direct seed in early spring. Cover lightly with soil and pat down firmly. Place burlap over the soil to create a dark environment. When the first seedlings appear, remove the burlap. Buying established plants is another way to get a jump on the season. Horehound can also be cultivated by root division and cuttings.

Plant spacing ~ 12 inches.

Pre-soak seeds ~ No.

Pre-chill seeds ~ No.

Indoor seed starting ~ No.

Light/dark seed requirements ~ Dark.

Days to germinate ~ Seven to 21 days.

Days to full maturity ~ 60 to 90 days.

Soil type ~ Deep, sandy, well-drained. Can tolerate poor soil. A little compost helps produce better looking plants but don't overdo it.

Water requirements ~ Needs moderate water but never the frequent soaking that other mints require. Once established, horehound needs little care.

Sun or shade ~ Partial sun.

Propagation ~ Underground roots and seeds.

Easy/hard to transplant ~ Established plants easy. Seedlings can be tricky. Direct sowing of seed is recommended.

Pests or diseases ~ Virtually none.

Landscape uses ~ Makes an attractive border or filler.

Gathering ~ Gather leaves before the flower heads appear—usually late spring to mid-summer, depending upon the region. Horehound typically does not bloom until the second year. Some herbalists believe it is best to give horehound a full year's growth before harvesting so it can achieve a higher level of medicinal potency.

Best fresh or dried ~ Both.

Drying methods ~ Gather stalks in groups of five before flowers appear. Cut stalk several inches above base and hang upside down in a paper bag. Strip the leaves off the stalks when the plant is completely dry. If you wish, you can toss in some of the dried stems as well.

Amount needed ~ A 5' x 5' patch is sufficient for those who use the herb regularly.

Seed collection ~ Leave horehound in the ground until you see the black seeds embedded in the flower heads. When you can shake the plant into your hand and see seeds appear, the herb is ready to cut and place into a white paper bag. The white bag makes it easier to see the seeds once they fall from the plant. Occasionally shaking the bag or the plant itself will help release more seeds.

Companion planting ~ Thyme and rosemary work well since they share similar soil and water requirements with horehound. Nettles and yarrow will help to increase the volatile oils within horehound. Separate horehound from other mints, such as lemon balm, spearmint and peppermint to make for an easier harvest.

Container planting ~ Yes. However, unless the container is wide and deep, horehound won't reach full maturity nor will it have room for future growth. Make sure the container is in an area that gets partial sun during the day.

Common mistakes ~ Thinking that since horehound is in the mint family, it should be treated like other mints. Horehound cannot tolerate lots of water—it stunts its development.

Interesting facts/tips ~ The fresh woolly leaves of horehound were once used to clean milk pails.

Chapter 21

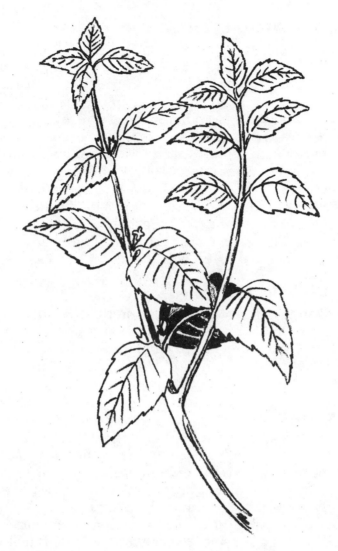

GET LEMON BALMED!

Melissa officinalis
Hardy perennial

Medicinal Uses: *Sedative, hypotensive, anti-depressant, anti-viral, anti-bacterial, antispasmodic, febrifuge, vulnerary, carminative*
Medicinal parts of plant: *Leaves*
Forms: *Tea, tincture*

WHAT IS ITS CHARACTER?

I've always looked on lemon balm as being a rather elevated member of the mint family. While other mints such as spearmint and peppermint readily take hold in the garden, lemon balm has a pickier personality. I think it senses that it is much more than "just another herb in the mint family" and it's not going to put down roots in any old place. It also has a softer, more sensitive attitude than the standard mints of the garden which often means you have to talk to it with a softer voice so as not to offend. However, once it decides it feels comfortable in your habitat, it becomes your friend for life. But as with all sensitive souls, lemon balm does not want to be ignored. If you don't give it plenty of water and thin it when it gets too dense, lemon balm can quickly fade. Never fear, though. Unlike the proverbial cat, lemon balm has many more than nine lives and will slowly return once you give it the attention it craves.

WHERE DO I FIND IT?

Lemon balm is occasionally found in the wild in some areas but it is more common to find it in the backyard garden. It flourishes at most elevations and in most regions, except for the blazing hot desert. The best plants are located in cool, moist, partially shady corners where they are given plenty of room to grow freely.

HOW DO I GROW IT?

Choose a partially shady area of the garden. Direct seed in the spring in warm, moist soil, barely covering seed with dirt. You can also cultivate lemon balm by root division and established plants. Some growers have had luck with placing flats of seeds in cool, moist environments before transferring the flats to established outdoor beds. Germination can be erratic for lemon balm, however, if the soil temperature is too cold. It germinates best at a constant temperature of 70°F. If that is possible, you could see seedlings develop within seven days. Otherwise, germination can take as long as 40 days. Average germination is usually within 21 days. Keep the soil moist but do not over water lemon balm in hopes of speeding germination. While it needs to be planted in rich, moist soil in order to ensure continued growth, the seeds cannot tolerate too much water. Do not overcrowd lemon balm either. It stunts its growth and causes a problem called "powdery mildew" on the leaves which stems from poor air circulation. With lemon balm, you have to thin, thin, *thin* those plants. This means that once you have an established stand of lemon balm, your friends will always be getting little balm plants as gifts.

HOW DO I HARVEST IT?

Lemon balm is more active medicinally when it is used *fresh*. This is due to the aromatic volatile oils found in the leaves. Yes, you can use it dried but the medicinal potential is vastly diminished. Harvest the *fresh* leaves as needed before the plant flowers while they are still vibrant green and full of natural oils. Slightly rub the leaves to check for aromatic oil content. If you decide you want to dry the plant, you must do it quickly or the leaves will turn dark and rapidly decay. Instead of placing the leafy stems in a paper bag, lay them on a drying rack with plenty of space between plants. Dry in the open air. DO NOT USE A HEATER OR ELEC-TRIC DRYER SINCE THIS SAPS MOST OF THE HEALING OILS WITHIN THE PLANT. Check the drying progress daily. Once leaves are crisp to the touch, strip from the stem and store in an airtight glass jar in a dark cupboard.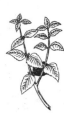

HOW DO I USE IT?

There seems to be a connection between long life and a stress-free environment. Of the 90+ year old people I have met, not one of them was hyped up. None were wringing their hands, nervously tapping their feet or riddled with worry. I get the feeling that if any of those folks discovered a lighted pipe bomb in their bed, they'd say, "Well, what *have* we got here?" and gently roll it out of the house.

Frankly, the first thing I say when I see this kind of behavior is "The medication is obviously working." But maybe, that's not necessarily so. Looking back in history, there were two men—Llewelyn, Prince of Glamorgan, Wales and John Hussey of Sydenham, England. The Prince lived to be 108 while Mr. Hussey departed at 116. They were calmer than a lazy afternoon and attributed their easygoing attitude to a light tasting herbal tea that "dispelled their melancholy and lifted their spirits."

That soothing brew was lemon balm. But the Prince and Mr. Hussey weren't the only folks who enjoyed the balm. It seems that throughout history, anyone who was feeling blue or was in need of a gentle shot of calm, reached for the balm.

FEELING GRIEF? PANIC? DESPAIR? HYSTERIA? ANGER?....

This herb which harkens from the mint family can help just about anybody and nearly any age. However, there is a certain personality profile that can *really* benefit. That profile is **people who feel grief, despair, depression, defeat, constant stress, hypochondria, panic, hysteria, anger, insomnia, nervous headaches and over-sensitivity which leads to a constant state of anxiety**. Obviously, we all fit one of these personalities at some point in our lives. But for the person who is *constantly* feeling any of the above, lemon balm can be a lifesaver.

It is important to mention that lemon balm is not some heavy duty sedative herb which works on the principle that one is simply too blitzed to care. The herb is actually very mild in its soothing properties as it **slows the respiration and pulse and lowers blood pressure**. You are eased into a state of calm without drug-like side effects *or* creating addictiveness to the herb. However, while lemon balm is considered a sedative, it also has the ability to **lift the spirits and make the emotional load a little less heavy**. This can come in very handy if you are using it as a **natural aid for mild depression**.

GET REALLY FRESH WITH LEMON BALM

The active ingredients that put the calm in the balm are the plant's volatile oils. One in particular, *citronellal* (not to be confused with the anti-mosquito oil *citronella)* has the most potent effect on the nervous system. It takes very little of *citronellal* to make the balm work its magic. However, **the volatile oils are much more potent in the freshly picked plant**. All you have to do is stroke a stalk of lemon balm and you'll instantly unleash the lemon-minty scent into the air and onto your skin. **I cannot stress it enough that fresh lemon balm leaves hold the greatest amount of healing potential**. This makes it an ideal plant to grow year-round either indoors or outside.

Because the fresh plant's oils are the active medicinal part of the plant, **you will need to take extra special care in preparing the tea so you can benefit 100% from everything it has to offer**. When brewing a tea from the *fresh* leaves, take two heaping teaspoons of the leaves and place them in a cup. Pour eight ounces of hot *but not boiling distilled water* over the leaves and immediately place a saucer over the cup. **If the water is too hot, the active oils will evaporate and you'll have a tart lemon tea which does precious little to calm**. The saucer is important because if the cup is not covered, the oily vapors escape into the air. Allow the tea to steep covered for 10 to 15 minutes. However, instead of removing the saucer from the top of the cup, tip it so the oily residue floats back into the tea. Add a little honey and you've got yourself a tranquil tea that should kick in within half an hour. If you are using dried leaves use three heaping teaspoons per eight ounces of distilled water. Always check the aroma of the dried leaves. If the lemon-minty scent is barely evident or if the leaves are over six months old, I don't think there is much healing ability left in the plant.

One can imbibe the balm up to three times each day—preferably in the morning and before bedtime. It doesn't take massive quantities of the tea for it to work. If you need an extra dose of nerve nourishment, add equal amounts of hops or chamomile to the brew. However, **omit hops if one of your symptoms is depression since hops can aggravate that condition**.

KIDS LIKE THE BREW

With its fresh, enjoyable taste, lemon balm is a great tea for children who usually turn up their nose at the idea of a "medicinal tea." It is especially **good for kids who tend to fidget before bed or can't seem to wind down**. **Nervous babies** over the age of six months can also benefit from the balm **but in small doses.** In other words, give the baby only a few mouthfuls of the prepared tea.

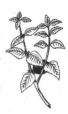

A BALMY BATH

Both children and adults can also incorporate a lemon balm bath into their evening repertoire. Nervous tension for young and old may melt away as the healing oils penetrate the skin. To make the bath, steep 12 ounces of the fresh plant or eight ounces of dried lemon balm leaves in several quarts of very hot (but not boiling) tap water. Cover the mixture and let it steep for 20 minutes. Strain the brew into the tub and soak for up to 45 minutes. For added soothing relief, you can sip a cup of the tea while you are in the tub. However, the combination of bath and tea can often make one perspire so take care not to overdo it.

EASES A NERVOUS TUMMY

There are actually many other uses for lemon balm. For those who tend to suffer from **stomach aches due to nervous tension**, lemon balm can be a lifesaver. Perhaps you have to say or do something that is turning your stomach into knots. A cup or two of lemon balm tea can help to soothe the stomach lining and put things in perspective. If that nervous tension is causing **digestive difficulties**, a cup of lemon balm tea after a meal can ease the problem as well as **relieve gas pains**. A **classic formula in this case is made by adding equal parts of peppermint leaves** to lemon balm. I have found that this simple remedy has worked wonders for folks who force themselves to eat a big meal even though they are feeling worried or anxious. Obviously, the first rule of thumb is to get the emotions under control instead of depending upon lemon balm to "fix" the problem.

SAY "NO" TO NIGHTMARES

Lemon balm tea has traditionally been used for adults and children who suffer from nightmares. It has been said that the tea helps put the mind at ease while strengthening it against those things that go bump in the night. In the same vein, this lovely little tea has the admirable gift of enhancing the brain's ability to resist shock and stress. In a case such as this, lemon balm works best when combined in equal parts with peppermint.

VANQUISHES PAIN

Lemon balm tea with just a pinch of nutmeg added to the brew is a popular remedy in Europe for **migraines** and **neuralgia**. To get the most from the tea, you will want to drink the tea or take the fresh leaf tincture —at 25 to 35 drops—at the first sign of symptoms.

AN AMAZING ANTI-VIRAL & ANTI-BACTERIAL ALLY

This lemony leaf also has tremendous **anti-viral properties that can knock out a cold**, provided you drink the herb tea at the first sign of illness. It really goes to town if one of your symptoms includes an **upset stomach**. One of the ways lemon balm works is that it forces the body to eliminate toxins through excessive perspiration. When you combine the balm bath with the tea, you increase the "sweat factor" even more. Just be careful if you try both at the same time that you don't overdo it to the point of lightheadedness.

Lemon balm also has the ability to work as a pretty impressive **anti-bacterial**. I don't think enough people realize this fact. Perhaps they think that this delicate little lemony leaf couldn't possibly have that kind of power. But consider these facts: lemon balm has been especially effective against **staphylococcus aureus**, **bacillus subtilis**, **salmonella enteritidis**, **mycobacterium phlei**, **streptococcus (various strains)** and **klebsiella (various strains)**. If you use lemon balm for any of these bacteria, it would be imperative to use either the *fresh* leaf tea or a tincture made only from the *fresh* plant.

HERPES DEFENSE

Perhaps one of the most promising possibilities with lemon balm is its use against the **herpes simplex virus**, **type 1 (cold sores)** and **type 2 (genital lesions)**. In his book *The Green Pharmacy*, Dr. James A. Duke explains that lemon balm's anti-herpes properties stem from compounds and tannins in the herb that are called "polyphenols." Duke says that "the body's cells have receptors that viruses latch on to when they're trying to

174

take over the cells. The polyphenol compounds have the ability to latch on to the cell's viral receptor sites. They take up those spaces and prevent the viruses from attaching to the cell, thus preventing the spread of infection." Duke suggests not only drinking the tea but applying it topically to the lesions in a compress to hasten the healing process.

Shingles, known as **herpes zoster**, also responds very well to lemon balm tea, used both internally and externally. For external use, try either compresses or a lukewarm lemon balm bath. To increase the anti-inflammatory ability of the tea, add equal parts of both peppermint and licorice root. Once again, in order to gain any significant benefit from the tea, you must use the *fresh* leaves.

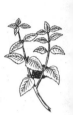

FEMALE FRIEND

Lemon balm has been found to work wonders for women, helping to **regulate as well as promote a late menstrual cycle**. It is one of the specific herbs used to aid **amenorrhea** (complete absence of a menstrual cycle). As it works with the body to regulate the cycle, women often feel a sense of calm as well as a dose of energy from the balm. In addition, lemon balm may also **ease PMS symptoms**.

WOUND BE GONE!

Still on that anti-viral front, the crushed *fresh* leaves are a **great topical first aid treatment for wounds**. In addition to being a good anesthetic, the leaves contain a number of naturally occurring chemicals which starve infection-causing bacteria of oxygen. (Two of the more "famous" bacteria balm can destroy are *Streptococci* and *mycobacteria)*. To treat a wound, simply layer four or five fresh lemon balm leaves on top of each other and then lightly chew them to release the healing oils. Place the moist fresh leaf poultice over the wound, keeping it in place for half an hour before checking it again. This same fresh leaf poultice works great on **wasp and bee stings**, too, providing a cooling and numbing sensation at the same time.

HYPERTHYROID HELP

In some studies, lemon balm has been found to decrease the levels of thyroid stimulating hormone (TSH) which reduces the amount of thyroid hormone production. This can be a welcome relief for those suffering from **hyperthyroidism (an over-active thyroid)**. On the extreme of hyperthyroidism is **Graves' disease**. Lemon balm can help here, too. The addition of the herb bugleweed—which inhibits iodine metabolism and reduces the amount of hormones released by the thyroid—is an excellent idea. Since bugleweed is most effective when used in liquid extract form, a good formula would be to add 15 to 25 drops of the extract to a cup of lemon balm tea. This tea combination can be taken up to three times a day. *One important note here:* in Europe, bugleweed—either alone or in combination with lemon balm—is used to combat Graves' disease *in the early stages.* My advice is to *only* consider this formula at the onset of hyperthyroidism or Graves' disease and only if you are working with a holistic practitioner. Hyperthyroidism and Graves' disease are nothing to take lightly. If you want to use alternative medicine in these cases, it is always best to seek the advice and perspective of a practitioner who can offer a complete treatment program that fits your individual needs.

CAUTIONS YOU SHOULD KNOW

There are two important cautions to lemon balm. First, since lemon balm can be used to promote a period, **pregnant women or women trying to become pregnant should not use the tea**.

The second caution relates to those who suffer from **low thyroid function or full blown hypothyroidism (under active thyroid)**. Since lemon balm has been shown in some people to depress the release of thyroid hormones, drinking the tea or using the tincture could negatively exacerbate an already low-functioning thyroid gland.

For everyone else who does not fit into either of those categories, lemon balm can be a wonderful herb. If people realized the potential of this herb, there's no telling how long we would live or how stress-free we could feel. It could even give a new meaning to the term "getting balmed."

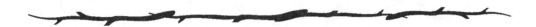

THE "DIRT" ON...LEMON BALM

Botanical ~ *Melissa officinalis*

Growth cycle ~ Hardy perennial.

Medicinal uses~ Sedative, hypotensive, anti-depressant, antiviral, antispasmodic, febrifuge, vulnerary, carminative.

Part(s) used for medicine ~ Leaves.

Vitamins/Minerals ~ N/A.

Region ~ From sea level to approximately 9,000 feet.

Wild or Domestic ~ Both, although more common as a domestic plant.

Poisonous look-alikes in the wild ~ No.

Hardy or Delicate ~ Hardy once established.

Height of mature plant ~ One to three feet.

Easy or hard to grow ~ Easy.

Cultivation ~ Direct seed in the spring in warm, moist soil, barely covering seed with dirt. Can also be cultivated by root division and established plants.

Plant spacing ~ Six to twelve inches. Understand that lemon balm will spread if planted in rich, moist soil so don't initially overcrowd.

Pre-soak seeds ~ No.

Pre-chill seeds ~ Yes, can help. Two weeks of cold moist conditioning can sometimes work.

Indoor seed starting ~ Yes. Flats are preferred over seed cells. Don't over water. Mist every three to four days until germination. Keep room temperature between 65°—70°F to ensure faster germination.

Light/dark seed requirements ~ Light.

Days to germinate ~ On average, 21 to 28 days. In warmer regions where the mean temperature is 70°F., seed can germinate in as little as seven days. In cooler regions, germination can be as long as 40 days. Be patient. Do not over water in hopes of speeding germination since you will lose a lot of what you planted.

Days to full maturity ~ Depends entirely upon your particular region. Lemon balm can be a slow grower in some areas. I've seen it take anywhere from 60 to 100 days to mature.

Soil type ~ If you want to have plenty of lemon balm for years to come, you must plant it in rich, moist soil. It can tolerate dry, sandy, rocky conditions but you won't get much of a crop.

Water requirements ~ Regular, constant moisture without flooding. Same as for most other plants in the mint family.

Sun or shade ~ Partial shade.

Propagation ~ Seed and underground roots.

Easy/hard to transplant ~ Easy, once established.

Pests or diseases ~ Whiteflies are a problem for indoor container plants if soil is poor. Scale is not natural to lemon balm but it can attack it from a host plant such as bay laurel. If this happens, separate the plants and pull up all infected plants. Lemon balm can also attract a white powdery mildew on the leaves if it is planted too close together. To avoid this, thin the patch to provide better air circulation between plants.

Landscape uses ~ Shady borders.

Gathering ~ Harvest the leaves as needed before the plant flowers while they are still vibrant green and full of natural oils. Slightly rub the leaves to check for aromatic oil content. If they feel dry, have a white, powdery film (mildew — see pests and diseases above) or have no aromatic odor, discard them.

Best fresh or dried ~ Lemon balm is always best when used fresh since much of the medicinal action comes from the natural volatile oils within the leaves. The dried plant is okay, but medicinal action can be compromised.

Drying methods ~ Lemon balm must be dried quickly or the leaves will turn dark and rapidly decay. Instead of placing the leafy stems in a paper bag, lay them on a drying rack with plenty of space between plants. Dry in open air. DO NOT USE A HEATER OR ELECTRIC DRYER SINCE THIS SAPS MOST OF THE HEALING OILS WITHIN THE PLANT. Check the drying progress daily. Once leaves are crisp to the touch, strip from the stem and store in an airtight glass jar in a dark cupboard.

Amount needed ~ Four to five medium-sized containers or a 4' x 4' backyard patch.

Seed collection ~ Wait until plant is in full flower—usually around mid to late summer. Sometimes seed production is best when the leaves are a little on the dry side. Cut the entire stem several inches above the ground and place it top down into a white paper bag. Store the bag in a cool, dry place. Shake the stems every few days to release seed. You can use a brown paper bag but it makes it more difficult to spot the seed.

Companion planting ~ Plant with other water-loving herbs such as cleavers and blue violet. However, do not plant near other mints since they will eventually all grow together and make harvesting a tedious process.

Container planting ~ Yes. Lemon balm works exceptionally well as a container plant as long as you give it enough room to grow. If you cram it into a container, it will never fully mature and can develop powdery mildew on the leaves due to lack of air circulation. The container must be deep and wide to accommodate future root growth. Once you see new plant development, pull up those sections and replant in another container. Because lemon balm should be used fresh, container planting is a great option for those who live in regions that experience freezing temperatures. Just put that container on rollers and bring it into the house during the winter months.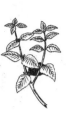

Common mistakes ~ Not keeping the patch thinned and allowing opportunistic diseases—such as powdery mildew—to attack. Also, thinking that you have killed lemon balm simply because it turns black and looks dead. If it is well established, this herb can be resuscitated with several good soakings of water. Adding a teaspoon of powdered kelp to the water will also encourage new growth.

Interesting facts/tips ~ Place lemon balm near a natural water source in your yard, such as a pond, stream, creek, or leaky hose. In late fall, cut down all the old stalks to make room for next season's growth.

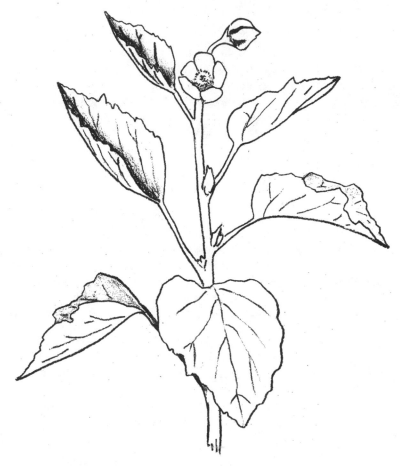

Chapter 22

MARSHMALLOW

Don't Float This Root In Your Cocoa

Althea officinalis

Also *Malva neglecta* (Known as "common" or "low mallow")

("W.F.")

Hardy perennial

Medicinal Uses: *Demulcent, emollient, mucilage, diuretic, nutritive*
Medicinal parts of plant: *Root, leaves*
Forms: *Tea, capsules, poultice*

WHAT IS ITS CHARACTER?

Some people look at marshmallow and see a weed. When I look at marshmallow growing in a moist field or vacant lot, I see a plant that exudes softness, grace and dignity. It is aloof in some ways, perfectly content to be left alone and add a touch of refinement to its living quarters. Consider it the "Miss Manners" of the wild. On the other hand, it tends to draw a person into its domain, willing to offer them whatever healing power they need.

WHERE DO I FIND IT?

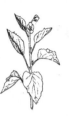

As the name marshmallow implies, this four to five foot tall herb is typically found in damp, boggy areas—especially along the eastern seaboard. It has long since been naturalized across the United States in gardens and escaping into the fields, along road sides and even in parking lots. The one requirement for marshmallow is the need for a constant water source. It doesn't have to be next to a river. But it does have to be exposed to moisture through rain or underground stream beds.

One important note: Don't confuse marshmallow with plain ol' "mallow" (a.k.a. "Common" or "low mallow.") Common mallow (*Malva neglecta*) has some mucilaginous properties but nowhere near the high percentage given to marshmallow. Common mallow only reaches 12 to 16 inches in height, grows in moist soil and always close to the ground. It is prolific all across the United States, found anywhere from sea level to 8,000 feet. Common mallow is one of the first plants to come out in spring and one of the last to die after the first hard frost. The fresh, young leaves can be eaten in moderation in salads or added to soups as a thickening agent.

HOW DO I GROW IT?

Marshmallow is grown from seed, root cuttings or root division. Plant seed in damp soil around late spring. I have found that a few days of cold temperatures help speed the germination of seed, which can take anywhere from eight to twenty-eight days. Space plants two feet apart to allow for future root development. Make sure the soil is fertile and kept constantly moist but well-drained. Most growers say that marshmallow needs full sun, however, I've had better luck keeping the soil moist when I allow the herb partial shade during the day. Indoor seed starting is fine as long as you transplant the seedlings once they reach two inches tall.

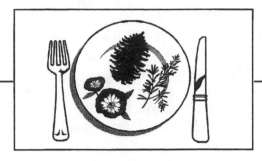

Wild Food Facts

Both marshmallow and common mallow (*Malva neglecta*) can be used as a wild edible.

Euell Gibbons was fond of boiling 1/4" pieces of marshmallow root in water for 20 minutes and then frying the boiled root with butter and chopped onions. When the marshmallow is lightly brown and the onions are clear, the dish is ready to serve.

The young, tender leaves and shoots of common mallow can be added in small amounts to salad, boiled or steamed for several minutes and served with butter or added liberally to soups and stews as a natural thickener. Don't throw out the water! It makes a highly nutritional beverage.

HOW DO I HARVEST IT?

Leaves can be gathered in early to mid-summer, before the pretty pink flowers emerge. Choose only the ones that are soft, supple and full of life. Roots should only be gathered from plants that are *two years old or older*. That's not to say that the roots gathered from one year old marshmallow lack in the mucilage department—it is just far more medicinally potent after the plant reaches two years old. Roots are easy to dig up, thanks to the amount of moisture in the soil. Scrape off the tiny rootlets and peel away the outside layer on the root to reveal the inner white core. Dry in a shaded area as is or cut it into two inch pieces.

HOW DO I USE IT?

The first time I heard about the herb marshmallow, I was thrilled to find out that those little puffy, white things that float on the top of hot cocoa were part of the herb family. Then one day, someone gently pulled me aside and informed me that while those little puffy, white things were once made from the root of marshmallow, they are in no way shape or form an herbal treatment. Well, color me embarrassed.

It turned out this pretty pale pink flowered herb with the funny name can do amazing stuff. First and foremost, it's what the herb community likes to call a "mucilage" which means that it has a tendency to become thick and form a gummy paste when water is added to it. It's no wonder candy chemists of long ago used it for making those puffy, cocoa-floating confections. That heavy duty mucilage also means that marshmallow is **great for coating and soothing inflamed parts of the body—especially the stomach lining and the small intestine**.

In the late 700's, King Charlemagne must have suffered from many stomach ailments and ulcers because he ordered his servants to plant marshmallow in every spot around the kingdom. Even back then, this herb was highly regarded as being the one plant people could count on to bring fast, soothing, healing relief. In fact, marshmallow's latin name "*Althea*" means "to heal."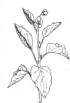

A CALMING COUGH AID

Because it soothes and coats inflammation, marshmallow is a specific herb for **upper respiratory catarrh**, **whooping cough**, **bronchitis** or coughs **that are considered "tight and harsh."** It's also a good herb tea **for people who spend much of their day talking and end the day with a rusty-feeling voice box**. To make an effective cough-fighting, throat-soothing tea, combine one-half teaspoon of marshmallow root powder in eight ounces of hot water. To kick in an additional cough suppressant action, add one-quarter teaspoon of licorice root to the blend. Cover and let the herb(s) steep in the hot water for 20 minutes. Strain and add honey to taste. It's best not to gulp this tea down quickly in the hopes of getting the job done faster. Instead, keep it warm and sip it slowly. This will ensure that the coating action takes place slowly and evenly.

THE KIDNEY CLEANSER

Marshmallow does it's herbal job on **inflamed kidneys and urinary tracts** as a **gentle diuretic** and lets you "go" without that awful burning sensation. Here's one good formula to try:

Marshmallow root (1 teaspoon)
Cornsilk (1 teaspoon)
Uva Ursi (1 teaspoon)
Juniper berries (1 teaspoon)

Place the herbs in a teapot and pour four cups of boiling distilled water over them. Cover and let steep for 20 to 30 minutes. Instead of straining, leave the herbs in the bottom of the pot as you drink one cup every two hours or so. If the condition does not clear up within three days or if it worsens, seek medical attention.

CALMS AN INFLAMED BOWEL & GUT

Anyone who has experienced ailments such as **colitis** or **gastritis** knows that the pain can be sharp, constant and debilitating. Marshmallow root tea can help take the edge off the inflammation as it coats the area with a soothing layer of its mucilaginous properties. I would definitely use the root for this condition since it contains up to 35 percent of pure mucilage. The tea to water ratio is eight ounces of hot water to one teaspoon of dried root or two teaspoons of the fresh root. This same tea helps to ease **chronic diarrhea** and even **dysentery**. However, as I learned the hard way, if you have either of these ailments, always find what the root of the problem is and treat it directly instead of addressing only the symptoms. In other words, the root of dysentery could very well be bacterial in nature. For that reason, moderate use of *fresh* garlic—*not* the tablets or oil capsules—could help kill the infection, thereby reducing the loose stool.

Marshmallow root, combined in equal parts with slippery elm powder, can be an effective palliative for those suffering from **Crohn's disease**. In a 1993 study done by researchers in England, food allergies were found to be "the most common cause of the disease." According to the study, corn, wheat, cow's milk, yeast, egg, potato, rye, tea, coffee, apples, mushrooms, oats and chocolate were the most common allergens. In addition, broccoli, tomatoes, lima beans, soybeans, Brussels sprouts, pinto beans, peas, onions, turnips, radishes and peanuts were also found to exacerbate Crohn's disease. The study claims that a "bland food diet" with little fiber and increased water intake would help the condition. One formula that might aid in relieving the pain combines one teaspoon *each* of marshmallow root *powder*, fenugreek seeds and slippery elm *powder*. Pour 24 ounces of warm water over the herbs and cover, allowing the tea to steep for up to one hour. Do not strain the herbs. Rather, stir the herbal powders and fenugreek seeds briskly as you sip the tea so that you take the herbs into your body. Chew the fenugreek seeds thoroughly before swallowing. This formula can be repeated as often as needed to bring relief.

"PASS ME SOME OF THAT 'MORTIFICATION ROOT'"

The roots of marshmallow are considered to be the most powerful part of the plant. However, the leaves are also effective. Marshmallow can grow like a weed and its root system delves deep into the soil, enriching each layer with a heavy dose of minerals and nutrients. A slang term for marshmallow is "Mortification root." This might sound as though it *causes* mortification rather than treats it. But, in truth, **the root actually arrests and reverses infected or decaying skin problems**. When you apply a marshmallow poultice, you'll notice how it immediately absorbs all the moisture around the area. You might even feel a slight tugging action which is the herb pulling out the congestion.

It really goes to town as an "A-1" **drawing poultice**. A **classic combination remedy is equal parts dried marshmallow root powder and dried slippery elm powder**. Some herbalists suggest moistening the mixture with warm milk—others simply use warm water to make the paste. Place this poultice over any **skin wound**, **bite**, **sting** or **infected cut that needs a soothing covering and an added dose of drawing power**. You can also try this poultice combo the next time you get a **splinter or piece of glass stuck under your skin**. Not only will it cool any heat caused by the inflammation, this marvelous marshmallow poultice will also help reduce the pain associated with the problem.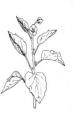

Check underneath the poultice every few hours. Don't be surprised if you see pus or liquid draining from the area. This is the drawing action of the poultice pulling the infected material out of the body. There are stories of people who have used the marshmallow/slippery elm combo to arrest **blood poisoning**, even after the tell-tale red streaks appeared. Typically, the stories involve using the poultice consistently over a period of 24 to 36 hours, replacing it as pus or toxic material is released from the wound. Whether you choose to use this natural blood poisoning remedy is entirely up to you. My advice is that if you want to "go natural" and try the poultice, do so for only up to 36 hours. If the red streaks worsen or if you experience extreme pain, a high fever or increased inflammation in the area during that 36 hour period, please discontinue use of the poultice and seek medical attention. Sometimes, depending upon individual body chemistry, antibiotics are needed in a life-threatening situation.

If the wound or bite is not critical, you can always try fresh marshmallow leaves. Take as many leaves as needed to cover the area, chew them into a moist ball and place it over the area you are treating. Cover the sticky poultice with a piece of gauze tape or masking tape. If the poultice dries out, make up a fresh one and discard the other.

AN AMAZING MARSHMALLOW COMBO

Combining equal parts of marshmallow root with astragalus root has proven to be an amazing formula to combat **auto-immune disorders**, **allergies**, and an **all around preventative remedy to strengthen and calm the immune system**.

In regard to **auto-immune disorders such as diabetes**, **multiple sclerosis** and **lupus**, the body's immune system is turning on itself. The marshmallow/astragalus combo, which was discovered by herbalist Dr. John R. Christopher, tends to make the immune system "less sensitive to itself." The easiest way to take the formula is in capsule form. Purchase eight ounces of each herb in fine powder form and a large bag of "00" sized capsules—pronounced "double aught." These are available at large herb stores such as *Herb Products Company* in North Hollywood, California. (See the Herbal Resources directory at the back of the book for their address and phone number). Thoroughly mix the two herbal powders together with a spoon and then scoop the mixture into the empty capsules. Dr. Christopher recommended taking as many as 20 of these capsules per day, spaced out every few hours, for an indefinite period of time.

The marshmallow/astragalus capsules can also work for **allergy sufferers** as well if they start taking the herbs at least six weeks before allergy season begins. The recommended dose is 15 to 20 capsules spread out throughout the day. For those who rely on this formula, it has become a "godsend" when nothing else worked.

ENCOURAGES MOTHER'S MILK

Another age-old way to use marshmallow is **to increase and enrich the flow of mother's milk**. Using either the fresh or dried leaves or the dried powdered root, make a tea and drink up to two cups a day. The ratio is two heaping teaspoons of the fresh leaves, one heaping teaspoon of the dried leaves or one tablespoon of the dried, powdered root to eight ounces of hot distilled water.

And when that little tyke starts teething, give him or her one of the oldest remedies in the herbal books: a **marshmallow root teething ring**. Choose a small root and slightly cut into it to release the mucilage. Dip it in some water to further encourage the slimy consistency and give it to the infant. The mucilage acts to soothe inflamed gums and, in my opinion, is one hundred times better than a piece of plastic.

A MARVELOUS EYEWASH

Marshmallow is also known to be a **soothing eyewash for people who do a lot of reading and computer work** or for those suffering from **sore, inflamed eyes**. Soak the *fresh* leaves or one-half teaspoon of the dried or fresh root in warm water for 20 minutes, strain and, when cool enough, bathe your eyes with the clear tea. For a soothing eye poultice, collect the warm leaves from the tea mixture and press them together. Place them over your eyelids for 15 minutes while you rest. You may be pleasantly surprised when you open your eyes.

FOR BEST RESULTS...

For best results, marshmallow root should not be boiled. You can either pour eight ounces of hot water over one teaspoon of the herb or make a cold infusion of the root or leaves. If you opt for the cold water infusion, allow the herb to steep in a covered container overnight.

Research has shown that **if you ingest marshmallow with drugs, the absorption of the drugs may be delayed**.

Other than that, marshmallow comes through like a trooper for so many of life's ills. I can honestly say that I'm always amazed by what this mellow mallow can do. I do have one complaint, though. It tastes simply dreadful when you pulverize the root and try to float it on top of your cocoa.

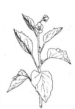

THE "DIRT" ON...MARSHMALLOW

Botanical ~	*Althea officinalis*
	A related species with similar but less active mucilaginous activity is known as "Common mallow" or "Low mallow" (*Malva neglecta*)
Growth cycle ~	Hardy perennial.
Medicinal uses~	Demulcent, emollient, mucilage, diuretic, nutritive.
Part(s) used for medicine ~	Root, leaves.
Vitamins/Minerals ~	Vitamin A, C, magnesium, iron, selenium, protein, calcium, phosphorus, potassium and manganese.
Region ~	Grows wild across the eastern seaboard. Naturalized across the United States and Canada from sea level to 7,000 feet. Prefers cooler climates.
Wild or Domestic ~	Both.
Poisonous look-alikes in the wild ~	No.
Hardy or Delicate ~	Hardy.
Height of mature plant ~	Four to five feet.
Easy or hard to grow ~	Easy.
Cultivation ~	From seed, root cuttings or root division. Plant in damp soil in late spring.
Plant spacing ~	Two feet.
Pre-soak seeds ~	No.
Pre-chill seeds ~	Yes, but it is not required for germination.

Indoor seed starting ~	Yes. Use cells to make transplanting more efficient.
Light/dark seed requirements ~	Light.
Days to germinate ~	Eight to 28 days.
Days to full maturity ~	90 to120 days.
Soil type ~	Constantly moist, fertile and well-drained.
Water requirements ~	Needs regular watering without drowning.
Sun or shade ~	Full or partial sun.
Propagation ~	Underground roots and seeds.
Easy/hard to transplant ~	Easy as long as you transplant seedlings when they are approximately two inches tall.
Pests or diseases ~	Virtually none.
Landscape uses ~	Makes a lovely, striking centerpiece or, if planted close together, a low hedge.
Gathering ~	**Root**: Collect roots that are two years old or older. After digging them up, cut away the smaller rootlets. **Leaves:** Collect the soft leaves when the plant is in flower— usually early to mid-summer. Choose only leaves that are still tender and full of life.
Best fresh or dried ~	**Root:** fresh or dried; **Leaves**: fresh or dried.
Drying methods ~	**Root:** Immediately peel the outside of the root to reveal the white core. Leave whole or cut into two inch pieces. Place in air dryer away from direct sunlight. **Leaves:** Place individually in air dryer and dry until slightly crisp.
Amount needed ~	Moderate use: 10 plants; Regular use: 10 to 25.
Seed collection ~	I like to wait until I can see the seeds appear within the flower. This can be anytime between mid-summer to late fall, depending upon your region. Either pick the seeds off individually or, if the plant is dry enough, shake several flower heads into a bag and allow the seeds to fall freely.
Companion planting ~	Fenugreek, red clover.
Container planting ~	Yes. However, unless the container is the size of a whiskey barrel, you will not be able to grow enough marshmallow for the most minimal medicinal needs.
Common mistakes ~	Many people confuse marshmallow with "common mallow" (*Malva neglecta*). This occurs since we herbalists often get lazy and refer to marshmallow as simply "mallow."
Interesting facts/tips ~	If you plan to use a lot of marshmallow, plant one or more rows every year since you will be digging up the root, thereby eliminating much of your crop.

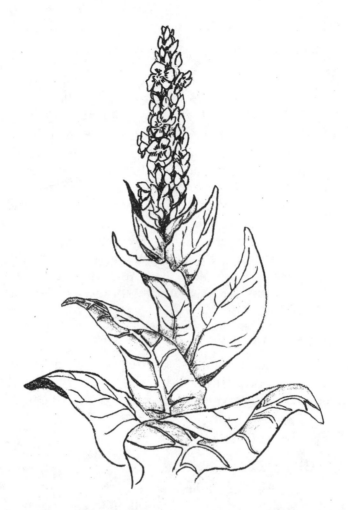

Chapter 23

A MULLEIN TO ONE

Verbascum thapsus
&
Verbascum olympicum ("Greek mullein")
Hardy biennial

Medicinal Uses: *Pectoral, demulcent, anti-tussive, lymphatic, astrin-gent, vulnerary, anodyne, antibacterial, mild laxative (in large doses)*
Medicinal parts of plant: *Leaves, flowers*
Forms: *Tea, extracted oil, syrup, fomentation*

WHAT IS ITS CHARACTER?

It's difficult to see mullein's character until its second year when it develops that distinctive, six to eight foot flower stalk. In the time it takes for the stalk to develop, mullein seems to go through a process of maturing. When the stalk is about three feet tall, mullein tends to exude a youthful, sweet, soft quality. Its leaves are like velvet and beg to be touched. But as mullein continues to grow taller and taller, it suddenly becomes an old, wise warrior, standing guard over the other plant life. Sometimes, I've come across stands of mature mullein that are so crowded together, they appear to be forming an impenetrable fence against intruders. Unlike other plants that fall to the ground during winter, mullein remains upright, albeit without its soft, velvet leaves and vibrant yellow flowers. Instead, the stalk turns a burnt shade of dark brown making mullein look as if it is a mere shadow of its former self. However, as you pass this rugged herbal veteran during the colder months of winter, it still exudes an energy that demands respect. It may be nearing the end of its life, but it will meet it head on like a soldier.

WHERE DO I FIND IT?

Mullein (pronounced "mullin," as in "I'm mullin' it over") is widespread in the Rockies and cultivated in the southern United States and on the east coast. Generally, you will find mullein above 4,500 feet but this extremely hardy herb is often found sporadically below that altitude throughout the western states.

HOW DO I GROW IT?

There are two medicinal mullein species that I like: *Verbascum thapsus* and *Verbascum olympicum* ("Greek mullein"). I discovered "Greek mullein" through the *Horizon Herbs* catalog. Owner and grower Richo Cech who resides in the tiny town of Williams, Oregon, knows that we herbalists who have spent many hours painstakingly gathering those little yellow flowers from the mullein stalks are slowly going blind. To appease us, he offers "Greek mullein," a species grown specifically for the multiple abundant flower stalks which can be *stripped* of flowers instead of enduring that one-flower-at-a-time method. Cech says that handfuls of yellow flowers can be garnered within seconds. I know all you mullein flower pickers out there are raising your hands to heaven at this news.

Both mullein species are easily planted from seed, either directly sowed in early spring or started indoors. Do not cover seed. Instead, press the tiny seed into the soil with your foot or the palm of your hand. According to Cech, "Greek mullein" is best started indoors in flats. If you start either species indoors, two or three days of exposure to cold (i.e., placing the flat in the refrigerator) can sometimes speed germination. Transplant out to a permanent location, spacing plants one to two feet apart, when the seedlings are two to three inches tall. Mullein loves poor, rocky soil with lots of sun and occasional water. It simply will not tolerate overly rich, wet soil. Take it from someone who tried and failed, pampering this plant is *not* the way to win its heart.

By the way, mullein is a good plant to have around if you decide to plant stinging nettle in your yard since *fresh* mullein leaves, crushed up and applied to the nettle sting, help to neutralize and eliminate the poison. Another good use for mullein is as a natural, wilderness "toilet paper." Learn to properly identify mullein in the wild and make a point to set up your next campsite near it.

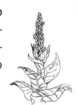

HOW DO I HARVEST IT?

Harvest of leaves, flowers and roots takes place in the second year.

Leaves should be gathered when they are, tender and vibrant, before the flowers begin to appear on the stalk. Dry the leaves separately on a sheltered drying rack or weave a thread through the stems with a fine needle (ala stringing popcorn) and hang to thoroughly dry in a cool, dark spot. Leaves can take as long as two weeks to fully dry.

Flowers are harvested as they appear, mid to late summer of the second year. *Choose only the flowers that are moist and have no sign of brown edges.* Purists prefer to go to the site where mullein grows and remove each flower from the stalk without destroying the plant. This allows the flower stalk to continue producing flowers. Those same purists will return to that same plant like a homing pigeon and continue harvesting the flowers until they all emerge. This is a wonderful idea if you have unlimited free time and are deeply infatuated with the mullein plant. The rest of us prefer to seek out a flower stalk that exhibits a large percentage of fully developed flowers, thank it for its glorious life and cut the stalk several feet above the ground. We then return home to harvest the flowers that same day so that we don't lose any medicinal quality within the flowers. The only exception to this rule is if you happen upon "Greek mullein" in the wild and are able to quickly strip the flower stalk in the field, thereby never having to remove your knife from your pocket. If you are not lucky enough to find this Greek gift from God species, you will get to experience the wonderful world of traditional mullein flower picking...one by one by one by one by one. Being that I had some spare time one day, I decided to see how long it took me to gather one ounce by weight of fresh flowers. It took over one hour of steady mullein flower picking! This might be your idea of herbal meditation, but when you need a whole lot of flowers, it is one of the most time consuming ventures. My advice: if at all possible, grow the "Greek mullein" species that promises easy pickin'. Flowers should be dried carefully, out of the sun and excessive heat and humidity since these sap much of the medicinal value.

Mullein root is dug in the fall of the second year, cleaned of dirt and dried in two to three inch pieces out of direct sunlight.

HOW DO I USE IT?

If there were commercials 300 years ago, one might sound like this:

"Hey, Bartholomew, that's a nasty cough thou hast there!"

"Yeah (cough, cough) it sure is, Nathaniel. It's so dry and unproductive. Tight, too."

"You needeth some 'cough weed.'"

"'Cough weed?'"

"Sure! A few cups of tea made from this stuff and thou shalt be back on thine horse in no time!"

(THREE DAYS LATER)

"Nathaniel, I feel great! No more dry, unproductive cough! That 'cough weed' really doth worketh!'"

That "cough weed" is better known as mullein and, through the ages, its leaves and flowers have been the **#1 herb for coating and soothing a cough**.

THAT TIGHT, DRY, UNPRODUCTIVE COUGH

You've seen the plant even though you may not recognized it. Some people mistakenly refer to mullein as "lamb's ears." ("Lamb's ears" is the entirely different two foot tall, strictly ornamental plant *Stachys lanata*). The six to eight foot mullein stalks boast velvet leaves and yellow flowers.

Mullein is one of my first choices for hacking coughs. **It works best when the cough is tight, dry and "unproductive" (i.e., not producing a lot of mucus)**. Once the infection and tightness have lessened, you should cut back on mullein and choose another tea which can bring up the mucus (such as licorice, fenugreek, ginger or yarrow).

Mullein can also be a handy herb to try when **bronchitis**, **croup** or **asthma** creep up since it has an uncanny ability to calm and quiet most respiratory problems without any narcotic side effects. Besides the flower or leaf infusion being good for coughs, it's also a **mild laxative, antispasmodic**, **pain reliever** and **gentle sedative** which can be a blessing if the cough is keeping you up all night. Of the two, I think the flowers have a better sedative and pain-killing ability. I usually combine leaves and flowers in equal parts to gain the most benefit.

I won't lie to you—the tea is not exactly a tasty treat. I strongly suggest adding honey and lemon (which also helps to soothe a **sore throat**). To make the tea, pour eight ounces of hot distilled water over two heaping teaspoons of either the dried leaves or flowers. Cover and allow the tea to steep for 20 minutes. Strain and enjoy. If you are using fresh leaves mixed with the flowers you will want to double the amount of herb. **In addition, it's a good idea to strain the tea through a muslin cloth since the fine "velvety hairs" on the fresh leaves can sometimes irritate your throat**. You can drink up to six cups a day for two weeks with no fear of overdosing on the herb. **The only "side effect" you may notice from drinking large amounts of mullein is a mild laxative effect**.

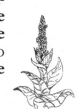

"THE HUMOROUS HERBALIST'S" ALL-NATURAL, HIGHLY-EFFECTIVE, HERBAL COUGH SYRUP

This herbal cough syrup has helped so many people get through some of the worst respiratory ailments. Best of all, you can't overdose on the stuff and kids as young as two years old can take it.

Ingredients:
- **One heaping teaspoon *each* of dried mullein leaves, dried horehound leaves, dried licorice root, dried white pine bark and *freshly ground* anise seeds**
- **Two cups of distilled water**
- **Two cups of raw honey**
- **A two inch section of *fresh* ginger root**
- **One or two peeled cloves of *fresh* garlic**

Stir the herbs into the cold distilled water. Bring the mixture to a boil and then simmer the liquid until it boils down to eight ounces. This can take anywhere from 20 to 30 minutes. When you have eight ounces, strain the herbs. Add the honey to the liquid and stir for a few minutes until completely dissolved. Remove from the heat and pour into dark glass amber bottles. (Beer and soft drink bottles are excellent for this purpose). *Use only a cork stopper instead of a screw top since syrups have been known to explode due to possible fermentation*. Add fresh ginger (a natural preservative) and fresh garlic (a natural antibiotic). Slicing the fresh garlic lengthwise before dropping it into the syrup will release the *allicin* within the garlic which is thought to be responsible for the antibiotic action.

Store the syrup in the refrigerator. It should keep for as long as six months. Dose: up to six tablespoons each hour.

Makes 24 ounces.

If you are really suffering from chest pain due to constant coughing, here is a great fomentation (compress) that gives much needed relief. The formula was created by herbalist Dr. John R. Christopher. Combine two ounces of dried mullein leaves, one-half ounce of dried lobelia and one teaspoon of cayenne powder in two quarts of apple cider vinegar. Slowly heat and allow the mixture to simmer for 15 minutes. Remove from the heat and steep for an additional 10 to 15 minutes. Cut a piece of cotton flannel that is large enough to cover the chest. Dip the cotton flannel into the vinegar tea, wring out the excess liquid and place it over the chest as hot as tolerable. Tightly cover the flannel with a piece of plastic wrap to hold in the heat and place a towel over that to further insulate. The fomentation should only be removed when it becomes cold against the skin. When this happens, simply dip the flannel back into the hot vinegar and repeat the procedure.

This **cider vinegar fomentation also works to temporarily relieve spinal tenderness and sciatica when it is placed directly on the spinal column**. The relief is temporary, but it can often help get one's mind off the discomfort and go to sleep.

PUT MULLEIN IN YOUR PIPE AND SMOKE IT!

I realize it sounds preposterous to suggest smoking an herb to alleviate respiratory congestion, but if it is done correctly and not abused, this ancient healing remedy can be extremely effective.

The smoke from mullein helps to sedate respiratory spasms after only two or three deep puffs. Within 10 to 15 minutes, you might even experience a loosening of trapped mucus. I like to combine mullein with lobelia and a little bit of yerba santa to create a formula that soothes a cough, dilates the bronchi and makes it much easier to breathe if you are suffocating with excess fluid on the lungs. To make the smoking blend, for every three parts of mullein, add two parts of yerba santa and one part of lobelia. This exact blend got me through the night when I was suffering from a terrible case of pneumonia. I couldn't lie down flat because of all the fluid in my lungs and I couldn't take a deep breath without going into a 10 minute coughing spasm. Every hour on the hour, I took two or three very deep puffs of this smoking blend. By the second puff, I could feel my lungs opening up and I could easily take a deep breath. Within minutes, I was coughing up some of the mucus that was causing my breathing to be labored.

By the next morning, I felt about a 20 percent improvement in my lung capacity and didn't feel the need to continue with the smoking mixture. Instead, I kept flooding my body with mullein and lobelia tea and taking frequent doses of the cough syrup (mentioned on page 193).

While mullein and the other herbs mentioned are non-addictive and non-narcotic, it is important to moderate their use when it comes to smoking them. Overuse can cause a very unpleasant, permanent drying out of the nasal passages. Only use mullein or the smoking blend when it is needed and keep it to two or three puffs every hour or so.

LOVE THAT LYMPHATIC RELIEF

Mullein makes an **effective tea and anti-inflammatory compress for painful glandular swelling**s. Along with its **pain-killing effects**, it has the proven ability to help **drain painful congestion from the lymph glands**. The compress can come in handy when a **sore throat is accompanied by swollen tonsils or inflammation and/or pain in the lymph nodes at the base of the ears**. The tea and compress can also be extremely helpful for **all glandular swellings**, especially when it comes to **alleviating the pain and shortening the duration of the mumps**.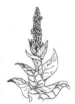

The compress formula comes courtesy of herbalist Dr. Christopher and includes three parts mullein to one part lobelia. According to Dr. Christopher, mullein cuts the pain and reduces the swelling while lobelia acts as "the thinking herb" or herbal traffic cop, directing the mullein to where it is most needed in the body. The formula ratio is three parts mullein and one part lobelia. Simmer three ounces of dried mullein leaves and one ounce of dried lobelia in two quarts of water. Remove from the heat and allow to steep covered for 15 minutes. Dip a piece of cotton flannel into the tea, wring out the excess liquid and apply to the skin as hot as tolerable. Cover with a layer of plastic wrap to secure it. Place a towel over that to hold in the heat. When the compress becomes cool against the skin, remove it and dip it back into the hot tea, repeating the process. For serious glandular swelling, you could continue using the compress for several hours. The trick to not making this a tiring venture is to figure out how to retain the heat in the compress for as long as possible so you don't have to get up and change it every 10 minutes. To encourage further drainage of the lymphatic channels, it is an excellent idea to drink mullein tea, either straight or following the mullein/lobelia formula.

After reading about this mullein/lobelia formula years ago, I wondered if I could possibly get the same kind of relief from using a salve made with the exact three to one ratio of mullein to lobelia. I made the salve the way I make every salve (i.e., combining specific proportions of olive oil to herb and cooking it on top of the stove). I quickly discovered that dried mullein leaves soak up tremendous amounts of olive oil, leaving very little in the pot. I had to adjust the amount of oil to compensate for this fact and ended up with a very good oil and salve when I added beeswax to the mixture. However, the processing of this particular home-made salve required great attention on my part to prevent the plant from burning due to the absorption of oil. While I am always in favor of making your own remedies as opposed to purchasing them, in this case I would suggest purchasing this extremely effective mullein/lobelia salve from the company that originated it, *Dr. Christopher's Herb Shop* in Springville, Utah. (Please refer to the Herbal Resource directory under the heading "Schools/Education" at the back of the book for this address and phone number). I have used Dr. Christopher's mullein/lobelia salve to reduce glandular swelling as well as a chest rub to encourage the release of trapped congestion. I can tell you that it worked far beyond my wildest dreams. In my opinion, it is a salve that should be in every person's medicine cabinet.

THE FAMOUS MULLEIN FLOWER OIL

Mullein flower oil can come in handy as a topical treatment for **leg cramps**, **inflamed joints**, **arthritis** and **rheumatism**. The oil is also excellent during the winter for **minor cases of frostbite**. Perhaps it is best known for its ability to **dissolve hardened ear wax and prevent ear infections**. It works best in this department by combining two parts mullein flower oil with one part garlic oil.

To make mullein flower oil, carefully pick the fresh flowers from the stalk and place them in a small bowl. Discard any that are dried or turning brown at the edges. As I mentioned earlier, the mullein species known as "Greek mullein" (*Verbascum olympicum*) is grown specifically for its abundant flower production and the ability to strip the stalks of flowers rather than painstakingly pull them out individually. If you grow "Greek mullein," you will have plenty of flowers; if you grow or have access to common mullein, time and patience will dictate how much you are able to harvest.

Once you have a handful or more of fresh flowers in the bowl, sprinkle a *very light* coating of vodka over them. *Do not saturate the flowers*. This is only meant to act as a "shield" against bacterial growth since the flowers hold a fair amount of natural water. Let the flowers sit for several hours before placing them into a small glass jar. Push them down firmly into the jar and then fill the jar with enough extra virgin oil to just cover the flowers. Don't substitute another oil such as sesame or safflower because mullein's healing properties are best extracted using olive oil. Instead of screwing the top on the jar, fasten a square piece of muslin over the mouth with a rubber band. This will allow the alcohol and any natural water within the plant to evaporate into the air. Set the bottle in a very sunny window for a minimum of six weeks. I've had some mullein flower oil jars sitting on the window sill for as long as two years and they turned out very well. When you are ready to prepare the oil, strain it through a muslin cloth, squeezing every last drop from the flowers. If the oil is kept in an amber bottle and stored in a dark, cool place, it can keep up to one year without turning rancid. Adding a small piece of *fresh* garlic to the bottle will lengthen its life. However, it will also make the oil quite a strong aromatic. I don't suggest adding the garlic if you are using the flower oil as an external rub.

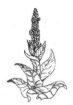

However, the garlic works well for the ear oil. The recommended amount for the ear oil is three to five drops in the ear twice a day. Sometimes, gently warming the oil is very soothing as well as massaging the ear canal afterwards. If the ear continues to hurt after two days or if there is any ringing, dizziness or a total plugged up feeling in the ear, stop using the oil and see an ear doctor immediately. You may simply have too much old, hard wax built up in the canal. A quick wash of the ear by a doctor can easily dislodge the wax in no time. **The only time you should not use the ear oil is if you have a perforated ear drum**. In fact, you should put nothing down your ears if the ear drum is damaged.

MASTITIS MIRACLE

An old folk remedy which has proven itself to be effective is lightly steaming fresh mullein leaves for several minutes and placing them on the breasts to reduce and eliminate **mastitis**. Drinking one or two cups of mullein tea in addition can further help break up the congestion and bring relief.

A FEW CAUTIONS TO KNOW

You can give mullein tea to a child under the age of two. However, instead of giving the adult dosage of one cup, administer only one tablespoon each hour. **Mullein seeds are considered highly toxic and should not be ingested**. While the herb is nearly caution-free, there is one thing to consider. Tannins are still questionable to scientists when it comes to cancer. Since mullein has a fair share of tannins, it's **best to moderately use mullein if you have cancer**.

Yes, that "cough weed" hast proved itself a winner. There's just no tullin' what the mullein will do.

THE "DIRT" ON...MULLEIN

Botanical ~	*Verbascum thapsus* and *Verbascum olympicum* ("Greek mullein")
Growth cycle ~	Hardy biennial.
Medicinal uses~	Pectoral, demulcent, anti-tussive, lymphatic, astringent, vulnerary, anodyne, antibacterial, mild laxative (in large doses).
Part(s) used for medicine ~	Leaves, flowers.
Vitamins/Minerals ~	Vitamins B_2, B_5, B_{12} and D, choline, hesperidin, PABA, sulfur, magnesium.
Region ~	Widespread in the Rockies, cultivated in the southern United States and on the east coast. Generally found above 4,500 feet but is often found sporadically below that altitude.
Wild or Domestic ~	Both.
Poisonous look-alikes in the wild ~	No.
Hardy or Delicate ~	Very hardy.
Height of mature plant ~	Six to eight feet.
Easy or hard to grow ~	Easy.
Cultivation ~	Direct seed common mullein in the early spring, gently pressing seed into soil. Be sure to spread out the tiny seeds so they don't clump on top of one another. "Greek mullein" can also be direct seeded, however, it is best started in flats and then transplanted once seedlings are two to three inches tall.
Plant spacing ~	One to two feet.
Pre-soak seeds ~	No.
Pre-chill seeds ~	Yes, but can also germinate without pre-chilling.
Indoor seed starting ~	Yes, especially for "Greek mullein."
Light/dark seed requirements ~	Light.
Days to germinate ~	Eight to 15 days. "Greek mullein" has a better germination rate than common mullein.
Days to full maturity ~	Fully mature in second year.
Soil type ~	Poor, well-drained. Cannot be too rich or mullein will not fully develop.
Water requirements ~	Needs occasional water, enough to keep it from dying. Do not over water since it tends to make the leaves turn under and stunts growth.
Sun or shade ~	Full sun.
Propagation ~	Seed.

Easy/hard to transplant ~	Easy if transplanted when seedlings are two to three inches tall.
Pests or diseases ~	If soil is poor, aphids and whiteflies can be attracted to it. Susceptible to root and leaf rot if exposed to too much moisture.
Landscape uses ~	Makes a bold centerpiece or dramatic tall hedge in the second year of growth.
Gathering ~	**Leaves:** Harvest tender, vibrant leaves before flowers appear on stalk during the second year.

Flowers: Harvest as they appear, mid to late summer of the second year. Choose only the flowers that are moist and have no sign of brown edges. Traditional herbalists recommend picking the flowers before noon, after the morning dew has evaporated. This allows for a more lively, less droopy flower. The typical mullein species that grow in the wild require that you pick each flower individually. However, the species known as "Greek mullein" (*Verbascum olympicum*) grows in such a way that the flower stalks needs only to be stripped so that in seconds you have handfuls of tiny flowers.

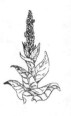

Best fresh or dried ~	**Leaves:** Fresh or dried. **Flowers:** Fresh or dried.
Drying methods ~	**Leaves:** Dry separately on sheltered drying rack or weave a thread through the stems with a fine needle (ala stringing popcorn) and hang to thoroughly dry in a cool, dark spot. Leaves can take as long as two weeks to fully dry.

Flowers: Place on a rack in the shade in a very dry area and allow to dry slowly until crisp. If flowers are exposed to humidity during the drying process, they can lose much of their medicinal ability. Store immediately in an airtight glass container.

Amount needed ~	If you just want the leaves, you will only need about five mature two-year-old plants for moderate use. For regular use, 10 to 15 plants are sufficient. As for the flowers, the amount of plants needed depends on how packed each flower stalk is and whether you are growing common mullein (*Verbascum thapsus*) or "Greek mullein" (*Verbascum olympicum*). It takes about one hour to individually pick less than one ounce by weight of flowers from the common mullein variety. On average, you will require 10 to 30 stalks of common mullein for moderate use and up to 60 plants for regular use. If you are growing the easier to harvest "Greek mullein," you will only need approximately five plants for moderate use and 10 or 15 for regular use.
Seed collection ~	This is one of the most prolific seed producers. Each dried stalk literally has thousands of tiny black seeds eager to pop out and grow. You will only need to cut a single

flower stalk approximately two to three feet in length in early fall once the plant begins to die. Place the stalk in a large supermarket brown bag and store in a dark, cool, dry closet. Occasionally shake the stalk to help release the tiny seeds.

Companion planting ~ Thyme, rosemary and yarrow.

Container planting ~ For heaven's sake, no!

Common mistakes ~ Collecting flowers that are brown and past their medicinal prime.

Interesting facts/tips ~ If the flower stalk still has a good percentage of buds that have yet to open, place it in a deep vase filled with water. Within a week or so, the remaining buds can be harvested as they open. The fresh leaves are favorably known as "nature's toilet paper" by backwoods enthusiasts. The fresh leaves are also good makeshift "pot holders" to protect your hands when gathering stinging nettle. If you do get stung from the nettle, place a bruised mullein leaf over the sting and it should quickly neutralize the acid. The dried, dead stalks that cover hillsides and roads during the winter make an excellent emergency tinder and fire starter. Centuries ago, those same dried stalks were dipped in tallow and made a suitable outdoor torch. When collecting mullein in the wild, I always look for stalks that are producing seed and give them a little shake to release the seeds. Since I often have to pick a lot of mullein in order to have enough for winter storage, I think it is important to re-seed the area to ensure many more years of continued growth.

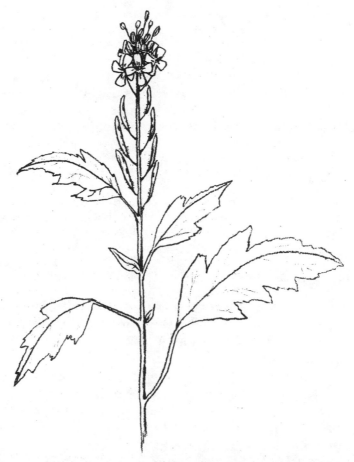

Chapter 24

GET HOT, HOT, HOT WITH MUSTARD SEED!

Brassica hirta (White mustard)
Brassica nigra (Black mustard)
("W.F.")

Hardy annual

Medicinal Uses: *Irritant, rubefacient, diaphoretic, appetizer, digestive, emetic (in large tea doses)*
Medicinal parts of plant: *Seeds*
Forms: *Tea, poultice, fomentation, sprouts*

WHAT IS ITS CHARACTER?

The mustard plant radiates a certain independence that sort of says, "Give me some dirt, a little bit of water and leave me alone to grow the way I want." It is certainly not picky about its surroundings and couldn't care less what other kind of plants crowd around it. If I had to give it a human dimension, I'd say that the mustard plant would make a fairly agreeable houseguest. It wouldn't mind sleeping on the floor, would gladly cook for itself and would never use up all the hot water.

WHERE DO I FIND IT?

The question should be, "Where do you *not* find it?" Mustard is one of the most common weeds that graces roadsides, vacant lots, meadows, hillsides, parking lots...you name the place, and mustard can probably grow there.

HOW DO I GROW IT?

You want to know how easy it is to grow mustard? It has been said that seedlings can sprout from the droppings left behind from migratory birds. Now, *that's* easy! No pre-chilling or pre-soaking of seed. No extra fertilizers. No low germination rates. And best of all, no problems. This is the herb of choice for the "gardening dysfunctional" who can finally feel successful in the yard. Mustard looks healthier when it is planted in rich, moist, slightly composted soil, but it can thrive in poor, dry, rocky soil as well. In early spring, plant the seed in one-half inch drills and barely cover with dirt. Give the seeds moderate water and germination can take place within seven days—sometimes as soon as two days. Aside from the occasional watering, care is minimal.

HOW DO I HARVEST IT?

Harvest the leaves in early spring before the flowers appear. After that, they are far too strong flavored and tough. The leaves are used *fresh* as a wild edible and have a high mineral and vitamin content. Gather the seed pods when the plant begins to die back and after one or more pods have broken open. Remove seed pods from the plant and scatter on a clean cloth. Place the cloth in the sun and air dry for one to two weeks. Most of the pods should burst open by then to reveal the seeds. The few pods that remain intact can easily be opened by hand. Black mustard seed pods hold many more seeds than white mustard. Either way, you will need to grow a minimum of 25 plants each year to obtain enough seed.

HOW DO I USE IT?

At the age of 10, I considered myself to be a junior herbalist. So when my friend Stephanie who lived down the block couldn't stop coughing, I said I could "fix it" with a mustard plaster. Taking mustard powder and a bowl in hand, I told Stephanie to lie down and unbutton her shirt. Oddly enough, she didn't ask questions. With a very serious look on my face, I plunked *four cups* of mustard powder into the bowl and added just enough water to make a paste that resembled yellow plumber's spackle. I glopped the paste on Stephanie's throat and upper chest, covered it with a towel and told her to be quiet.

In less than five minutes, she said it was getting hot.

"That's *good!*" I exclaimed, "It'll make your cough go away."

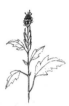

"But, it's *really* getting hot. Like *burning hot*," she insisted.

"That's what it's supposed to do," I insisted with an "I-know-what-I'm-doing-so-stop-arguing-with-me" tone.

Fifteen minutes later, Stephanie didn't look so good, but I think she was too scared to tell me. Forty-five minutes after we started, I announced it was time to take off the plaster. As I pulled the mess off her throat and chest, I noticed that her skin had turned redder than a ruby.

The next morning, Stephanie's mom came knocking at the door with Stephanie in tow. "Did you do this to my daughter?!?" she yelled. With that, she uncovered Stephanie's throat and chest. There before me was the most wicked cherry red water blister. It stretched from her throat to her chest and seemed to pulse in unison with my rapidly beating heart. "Well?" her mother said angrily, "What have you got to say for yourself?!"

I looked at her mom, then at Stephanie and said the only thing I could think of. "Well...she stopped *coughing*."

Needless to say, that was the last unsupervised visit I had with Stephanie for a long time.

The point of this biographical walk down the herbal memory lane is to drive home the most important fact about medicinal mustard: **IT GETS HOT. IT BURNS. IT WILL HURT. IT CAN BLISTER. IF YOU USE IT THE WRONG WAY, YOU WILL WISH YOU NEVER HEARD OF MUSTARD**.

This burning reputation is found in the old French term for mustard "*moult ardre*" which means "much burning" or the colloquial "Geez, that's hot." The active stuff in the mustard seed that gives it that "hell-fire" reaction is a natural chemical called "*allyl-isothiocyanate,*" found in the seed's volatile oil.

When I talk about medicinal mustard, I'm not referring to the yellow stuff people spread on their hot dogs and burgers. Mustard for healing purposes is purchased in the whole or powdered seed form. There's black mustard *(Brassica nigra)* and white mustard *(Brassica hirta)* for medicinal use, and they can be interchanged. However, black mustard is considered the best—although it is also the stronger of the two. To reduce its effect, mix equal parts of white and black together or stick with only the white. Either way, you can get a nasty blister unless you are careful.

Mustard seed can be used in a bath, a foot bath and that now-famous "plaster." Let's take them one at a time.

THE BATH

A mustard powder bath can be used medicinally or as a stimulating "tonic sweat" when you are feeling healthy. **In either case, you should soak in a mustard bath for no longer than 10 minutes**. On the medicinal front, a mustard bath works for **joint pain, sciatica, reducing fevers** and **colds and flu.** For the latter, the bath should be taken at the onset of symptoms, when you get that chilled, tired and aching feeling. If you take the bath at the early stage, you can often nip the cold or flu in the bud. A mustard bath works on the age-old principle that when the body is able to heat up and perspire freely, it can release the trapped toxins and start the healing process faster. Of course, there is also an age-old warning when you start expelling toxins through vigorous perspiration: *always stay warm and never get a chill or you will only compound the problem.*

A mustard bath can be made two ways. The first way is to mix one cup of the seed powder into a pot filled with one gallon of tap water. Heat the mixture on the stove until boiling and turn it off. Steep covered for 20 minutes. While it is steeping, bring your pajamas into the bathroom and turn on the heat so that the temperature is between 70° and 75°F. The bathroom must stay at this temperature while you are in the tub so that there is no chance of getting a chill. Pour a hot bath—as hot as you can stand it without burning your skin. After the mixture has steeped, strain it into the bath water through a fine sieve that is lined with a layer of muslin. You don't want to get the powder in the tub because that could escalate the burning and/or blistering of skin. Soak in the water for no more than 10 minutes. When you dry off, make sure you brush any mustard powder residue from your skin since it can burn. Put on your pajamas and get into bed.

The second way to make the bath is to fill a drawstring muslin bag with one cup of mustard powder and soak the bag in the hot bath water for 15 minutes before getting in. This version usually creates less heat and is a better choice for those with sensitive skin. However, you still shouldn't soak for longer than 10 minutes.

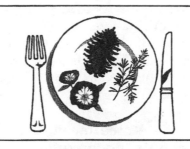

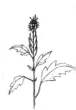

Wild Food Facts

The mustard plant offers a bevy of nature's bounty.

Let's start off with the young, spring leaves. Picked in early spring, they lend a hot, pepper flavor to salads, egg dishes and fish recipes. Use sparingly so as not to overpower the palate with their pungent taste. They also work as a nice, cooked side dish. Cook the greens in hot, not boiling, water so as to retain as much of their vitamin content as possible. Average cooking time is anywhere from 20 to 30 minutes. You will need to pick about a half more leaves than you'll need since they have a habit of shrinking when you cook them. In *The Green Pharmacy*, Dr. James Duke reports that mustard greens have a high content of the amino acid *tyrosine*. This amino acid has been shown to help increase production of the thyroid hormone "thyroxine." This means that if you suffer from low thyroid function or full blown hypothyroidism, the simple mustard leaf could be added to your diet in moderate amounts to boost thyroid hormone production.

The tiny yellow flowers are called "wild broccoli" by some wild food lovers. Higher in protein and vitamins than the leaves, the flowers should be picked just as they are opening. Wild food lover and forest forager Euell Gibbons shared a simple recipe for these flowers in his classic book, *Stalking the Wild Asparagus*. Euell boiled several handfuls of the tiny flowers in salted water for three minutes. Any longer than that and they become an awful mush. Strain the flowers and add a dash of melted butter, chopped onions, lemon and vinegar. The flowers can also be eaten raw in salads.

Mustard seeds can be easily sprouted and added to salads, soups and stews to give a peppery, hot flavor. With mustard sprouts, the hotter the environment, the faster the sprouts will develop. They are typically ready around eight to ten days. However, if you cover the seed sprouter with a plastic dome, you will be able to generate much more heat and you could have sprouts ready to eat in four days.

THE FOOT BATH

A mustard foot bath quickly draws the blood from the head and directs it to the lower part of the body. Because of this, **a mustard foot bath is great when you have a headache since it tends to literally pull blood congestion out of the head**. The foot bath also works at **the onset of colds**, **flu**, **fever** and **respiratory congestion** as well as when you simply need to **warm your feet (and body) in a hurry**. To make the foot bath, place one level tablespoon of mustard powder in a draw-string muslin bag and place the bag in a bucket of hot water that holds at least three gallons of water. Soak your feet for five to ten minutes, making sure to rinse off any of the herb powder residue from your feet.

THE "PLASTER"

A mustard plaster can be used for more than just coughs. The list includes **asthma, bronchitis, pneumonia, fever, colds & flu** (which would all require the plaster to be placed on the chest) and **sciatica, joint pain, tendinitis**, and **bursitis** (which would require the plaster to be placed on the specific area being treated). However, the way I made the plaster when I was 10 years old is the *wrong* way to make it!

The right method to make a mustard plaster is as follows: First, cover the area to be treated with castor oil or olive oil. This is the first step in protecting your skin against possible blistering. Next, mix one part mustard powder with four parts whole wheat or rye flour. (For a plaster that really pulls inflammation from joints, add an additional part of slippery elm powder). Add enough *lukewarm* water to form a paste that is the consistency of thick paint. Do not use hot water as this accentuates the heating potential. *If you have very fair and/or sensitive skin, use egg whites in place of the water. They have been shown to drastically reduce the risk of skin irritation or blistering.*

Spread the mustard paste onto a piece of cotton flannel. Place a piece of cheesecloth over the paste and lay the plaster *cheesecloth side down* against the area to be treated. Cover this with a towel and set the timer for 15 minutes. If burning becomes too much to bear before the 15 minutes is up, REMOVE THE PLASTER! When removing the plaster, make sure there is no residue on the skin from the mustard. If there is, wash it off immediately using a mild soap. Some people sprinkle flour over the area that has been treated to reduce any skin irritation that may develop. Do not re-use the plaster.

A plaster can be applied up to three times a day for chronic ailments and once a day for minor complaints.

THE "IPECAC" OF THE SPICE RACK

Mustard powder is an "old timey" remedy **when one needs to vomit due to food poisoning**. To make this retching mixture, steep a teaspoon of mustard powder in 10 ounces of boiling water. Stir the tea until it cools to lukewarm and drink it quickly. One herbal book remarks that if this does not produce the desired effect, simply "tickle the back of the throat with your finger." Personally, I only recommend performing this ritual if you really need to vomit. Other than that, let nature take its course.

THE "HOTTEST" CAUTIONS

The cautions for mustard are as follows: for internal use (i.e., **to induce vomiting), do not attempt if you are anemic, suffer from an acid stomach, ulcers or gas with distension of the abdomen**. In addition, **if you are pregnant, do not ingest large doses of mustard seed**. For example, the emetic (vomiting) tea should not be consumed by a pregnant woman.

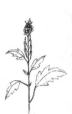

The external cautions are simple: follow the directions so that you don't end up looking like my poor neighbor, Stephanie.

Fortunately, I've become more herbally responsible since that day over two decades ago. I'm almost positive that if I met Stephanie today, she'd let me give that plaster another try.

I'm just not so sure about her mother.

THE "DIRT" ON...MUSTARD

Botanical ~   *Brassica hirta* (White mustard), *Brassica nigra* (Black mustard)

Growth cycle ~   Hardy annual.

Medicinal uses~   Irritant, rubefacient, diaphoretic, appetizer, digestive, emetic (in large tea doses).

Part(s) used for medicine ~ Seeds.

Vitamins/Minerals ~   Vitamin A, B, C and D, protein, EFA's (Essential Fatty Acids), lecithin, minerals (especially iron and calcium) and loaded with amino acids, including lysine, tryptophan, leucine, histidine and arginine.

Region ~   Everywhere from sea level to 8,000 feet. Found in fields, yards, disturbed sites, vacant lots and assorted other locations.

Wild or Domestic ~   Both.

Poisonous look-alikes in the wild ~   No. As for non-poisonous plants, some people confuse wintercress for mustard even though the leaves are completely different.

Hardy or Delicate ~   Very hardy.

Height of mature plant ~   One to three feet.

Easy or hard to grow ~   Very easy.

Cultivation ~   Direct sow in one-half inch drills in early spring. Barely cover with soil. If you live in mild, temperate regions, mustard can be sown throughout the year.

Plant spacing ~   Six inches.

Pre-soak seeds ~   No.

Pre-chill seeds ~   No.

Indoor seed starting ~   Yes. However, since mustard grows very fast, you will need to transplant it outside within weeks. If you want to speed indoor germination, place a plastic dome over the seed tray. If the tray is allowed to maintain a temperature of approximately 70°F—80°F, you can easily have four inch mustard seedlings within one week.

Light/dark seed requirements ~   Light

Days to germinate ~   Two to four days.

Days to full maturity ~   Young leaves are ready to harvest around 45 to 60 days. Seeds are well formed in the pods around 60 to 95 days.

Soil type ~   Will do fine in sandy, dry soil. However, a rich, moist soil with a little compost added produces a better plant.

208

Water requirements ~	Needs several waterings each week, but never to excess.
Sun or shade ~	Full sun.
Propagation ~	Seed.
Easy/hard to transplant ~	Easy.
Pests or diseases ~	The flea beetle can eat away at the leaves. One herbalist I know suggests growing mustard closely together to avoid this.
Landscape uses ~	Most people will probably wonder why you want to feature mustard in your herbal garden. However, if you don't mind having to constantly answer the question "Why on earth did you plant mustard in your garden?" consider using the plant as filler for areas where nothing else wants to grow.
Gathering ~	Harvest the leaves in very early spring before the flowers appear. After that, they are far too strong flavored and tough. Gather the seed pods once the plant begins to die back and after one or more pods have broken open.
Best fresh or dried ~	**Leaves**: fresh; **Seeds**: dried.
Drying methods ~	Remove seed pods from the plant and scatter on a clean cloth. Place the cloth in the sun and air dry for one to two weeks. Most of the pods should burst open by then to reveal the seeds.
Amount needed ~	Black mustard seed pods hold many more seeds than white mustard. Either way, you will need to grow a minimum of 25 plants each year to obtain enough seed.
Seed collection ~	Same as for drying. By the way, I have planted the whole mustard seeds that I bought in the bulk herb section and had very good luck with the results. Purchasing seed this way is often easier and far less expensive.
Companion planting ~	Yarrow, mullein.
Container planting ~	It can be done but you will not get enough seeds to make it worth your while.
Common mistakes ~	Waiting too long to harvest the seed pods and discovering that they have already burst open on their own.
Interesting facts/tips ~	If you live in areas that enjoy 12 continuous months of a growing season, use the fresh seeds from one crop to start the next. Fresh seeds have greater vitality and often produce a stronger plant. Black mustard makes a good cover crop, planted in the fall and turned over in the spring. However, realize that it can become invasive.

Chapter 25

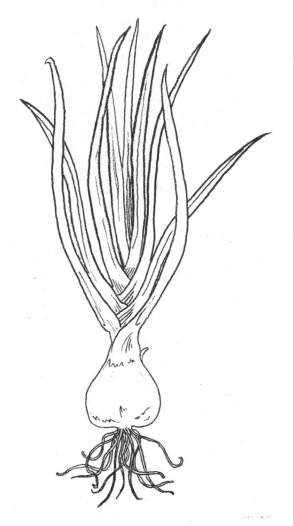

AN ONION CAN DO THAT?

Allium cepa

("W.F.")

Biennial

Medicinal Uses: *Antiseptic, antibiotic, antispasmodic, carminative, diuretic, expectorant*
Medicinal parts of plant: *Bulb*
Forms: *Raw plant poultice, cooked poultice, syrup*

WHAT IS ITS CHARACTER?

Onion spends most of its life looking rather plain with its emerald green shoots standing at attention. Somewhere along the way, it decides it needs a little something extra to perk up its personality. So it uses up all its energy to create a bulbous seed head. Unfortunately, in its desire to make a grand impression, the onion overlooked the fact that the seed head is a little bit too big for its body. While it does its best to hold its seed head high, eventually the onion breaks under the pressure and collapses, seed head and all. Sometimes I think it looks rather defeated with its seed head hung low. Then there are other times I look at it and think that it's just taking a little nap. After all, the plant has been busy.

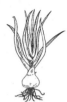

WHERE DO I FIND IT?

From sea level to approximately 9,000 feet in sunny fields, meadows and cultivated areas. Different varieties require different regions.

HOW DO I GROW IT?

From either seeds or sets.

If you prefer seeds, plant as soon as the soil is warm and frost-free. Sow 1/4" to 1/2" deep, spacing plants six to twelve inches apart in soil that is well drained. Cover seed completely with soil since onions need darkness to germinate. Water lightly to keep soil moist but *never* drown seed or you will get a low germination rate. Some growers get impatient waiting for the 14 to 21 day germination and over water thinking that will speed things up. However, onion seeds will not tolerate being drowned. To eliminate that "trigger finger" on the garden hose, one grower I know mixes a few radish seeds in with the onion seeds. Radish seeds usually germinate within five to seven days. Once you see the wide leafed radish seedlings appear, you will know that the soil conditions are right and that the thin, green onion seedlings should appear within seven to fourteen days. When the onion seedlings appear, wait one full week and then carefully pull out the radish seedlings.

If you purchase onion sets, cover with one-inch of soil as you place them firmly into the ground. Within one to two weeks, new shoots should be pushing up.

The Walla Walla Sweet is an easy variety to grow and is widely adapted to many regions. The only drawback is that it has a short storage life. If you are looking for a good long-term storage variety, try the New York Early, favored for years by many New York onion farmers. Onion is another plant that has many hybrid varieties. To ensure a steady supply of viable seeds from one season to the next, choose open-pollinated varieties over hybrids (also called "Heirloom" seeds) that always grow true from seed year after year.

HOW DO I HARVEST IT?

If you are gathering wild onions, do not pick plants that are growing near heavily traveled areas such as roadways or around places that are obvious toxic dumping grounds (mines, railroads, leech fields). The reason is that plants in the *allium* species (which includes garlic) are known as soil purifiers and soak up everything from lead to mercury. Always go as far away from the road as possible and look around the area to determine if it is a healthy environment.

For the backyard herbal gardener, two weeks before the anticipated harvest, *stop watering*. When the onions have begun to develop skins and the tops have fallen over, they are ready to harvest. To create better storage onions, pull up the entire plant and lay them down in the field to "cure" for one week under the hot sun. This way they harden up and produce a tougher skin. After one week, cut off the seed head. When you are certain they are dry, store them in shallow boxes or mesh "onion bags" at near freezing temperatures with an optimum 65°-70° humidity.

HOW DO I USE IT?

Back in the late 1800's, my great grandmother Perry was known for two things. First, she apparently lived in the cleanest dugout in Kansas. That's not easy since we're talking about a dirt house.

The second thing she was known for across those wheat-filled plains was her cough-stopping, congestion-clearing onion syrup. This concoction was legendary, apparently having the ability to stop a cold dead-on and scare away the mightiest of coughs.

Yes, my great grandmother Perry was into herbs. Then of course, back in the 1800's, before the drugs of today, everyone turned to nature whenever they felt sick. And because onions grow so plentifully, they were a first choice for many pioneers.

In addition to being the base of a great cough syrup, **onion also helps to lower blood pressure when taken internally in its raw or cooked form**. It can be turned into a **very soothing chest poultice whenever you need to draw out respiratory congestion**. It also acts as a **healing poultice for bruises, external inflammation in joints** (i.e. **"water-on-the-knee," "tennis elbow,"** sprained ankles and **sore wrists**), and works as an awe-inspiring **natural antiseptic as it reduces the redness and pain of a bad bug bite or bee sting.**

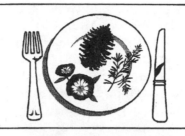

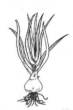

Wild Food Facts

There's something wonderful about wild onions. I think they taste a little sharper than their backyard counterparts. If you can properly identify this wonderful wild edible, it can work as a pungent seasoning to those outdoors dishes. When you are cooking other wild edibles such as burdock root and nettle leaves, adding one or two chopped wild onions to the food can provide a nice touch of flavor. You can also mix them into chickweed salads as well as toss them into stew, chile and soup. Since wild onions vary in pungency based on where they grow and the particular variety, do a taste test before adding too many of them to your food. Some varieties are so strong that it takes only a few slices to overpower the food.

SAVED BY THE SULPHUR

What makes it work? Sulphur compounds are one major ingredient responsible for onion's antiseptic abilities. These same compounds work wonders at pulling the toxins out of your body that are causing you grief.

That "pulling" action can actually **break up fluid congestion in tissues and lymph glands, taking with it the toxins that are clogging your system**.

This reminds me of a movie that came out in the early 1970's called *Where The Lilies Bloom*. In the story, an Appalachian family takes in this fellow who is suffering from the most awful respiratory illness. He's near death but they "ain't gonna let him croak." One of the family members hollers out, "Boil me up some onions!" Then they dump the sick feller into this big ol' bathtub and pack steaming layers of stewed onions all over his chest, neck and back. He figures they're trying to kill him, but when he starts to breathe easier, he realizes they have saved his life.

While that "backwoods cure" might sound strange to some people, it's not so far off the mark. Basically what those hillbillies were doing was making a hot poultice which activated the sulphur compounds in the onion that broke up the fluid on the guy's chest. It's something that has been done for hundreds if not thousands of years.

That onion bath scene from the movie came to mind when *I* was the one suffering from one of those awful respiratory illnesses. However, I didn't have enough onions to fill a bathtub. So, I fashioned the next best thing: a hot chest poultice. I chopped two large white onions (yellow will also work) into thumb-size pieces. After adding just enough olive oil to a pan so the onions would not stick, I placed the chopped pieces into the pan. Keeping the flame on low, I covered the pan and let the onion gently sauté until soft. This takes anywhere from five to ten minutes. After turning off the heat, I added one-half cup of cider vinegar and stirred it into the soggy pieces. The vinegar gives the poultice an extra spurt of "pulling" action. Using a square piece of cotton flannel that was cut to cover my chest, I layered the onions onto the top half of it and pulled the bottom half of flannel up and over the steaming onions (i.e., I made a "sandwich" of the flannel with the onions in the middle). I secured the open sides of the flannel with safety pins and carefully placed the hot pack over my chest. Sometimes the onions have a tendency to clump to one side so make sure they are evenly distributed. I then laid an old towel over the onion for better insulation. Over the towel, I placed a very hot water bottle to generate as much heat as possible and encourage the necessary pulling action from the onions.

Literally, within minutes, I could feel a definite release of pain in my chest and I was able to get some rest. As it turns out, I ended up keeping the pack on for 12 hours. You can leave an onion pack on for several hours, but the longer it remains the better. When I took the pack off the next morning, there were deep red blotches on my chest located at the exact spots of congestion. Those splotches gradually disappeared within a day. However, one day later, after placing that one and only onion pack on my chest, I woke up to find tiny pimples emerging from the area where the onion poultice had been placed. The pimples—or pustules—developed pin-point size blisters on their heads. I attributed this to the extreme toxicity within my respiratory system which was partially being released through the pores of my skin. Within less than two days, the pustules were completely gone.

AN ONION AND SALT ANTI-INFLAMMATORY POULTICE

A raw onion poultice—with the addition of sea salt—works wonders on **inflamed joints**. The sea salt really jazzes up the drawing action and pulls out the inflammation. To make this onion poultice, finely chop up one cup of raw onions and add one-half cup of sea salt. Pour the salty onions into a flannel cloth, secure with safety pins and place the poultice against the inflamed area. (I have found that if you put raw onions directly against your skin for a long period of time, surface redness can occur as well as tiny water blisters. This is especially true for those with fair or sensitive skin). Cover the onion poultice with a hot water bottle, keeping it on for one to three hours. This poultice can work for **minor**

arthritis and **bursitis** pain as well as **sports-related sprains** and **muscle strain**.

For **surface bruises or cuts due to minor scrapes and falls**, a fresh, raw onion can help speed the healing process. In this case, it is okay to place the onion directly on the skin. However, if it starts to feel as if the area is on fire, immediately remove the onion and thoroughly wash off any of the residue from the juice. The poultice is easy to make: simply cut a section of the onion off and place the wet side over the cut or bruise. The raw juice starts working immediately on the swelling and also acts as an **antiseptic**. This little herbal helper is good to remember if you are on a picnic and someone takes a spill. There will usually be an onion or two near the grill—and maybe one that's already cut for you.

AN INCREDIBLE ANTIBIOTIC

Onion's ability to act as an emergency antiseptic is only outdone by its **supreme antibiotic activity**. Recent research has shown that the common onion is **active against Staphylococcus aureus, Brucella abortus, Escherichia coli, Pseudomonas pyocyaneus, Salmonella typhi, Salmonella typhimurium, Bacillus subtilis, Bacillus communis, T. glabrata** and **Candida albicans**. What is truly amazing is that studies have shown onion to be effective against **Staphylococcus aureus** and **Brucella abortus** when the onion was highly diluted.

THAT WONDERFUL ONION SYRUP

And what about that famous onion cough syrup my great grandmother Perry whipped up in her clean little Kansas dugout? Well, sadly to say, she never wrote down the recipe. But I do have one very good recipe that great grandmother Perry would probably approve of.

Finely chop one cup of onions and place them in a stainless steel or glass pot. Chop up several tablespoons of *fresh* ginger root and add it to the onions. Add the juice of a fresh lemon and, if the lemon is organic, cut up the peel and toss it in the pot. Pour two cups of distilled water over the herbs and simmer the concoction on a very low flame with the lid on. Stir the mixture every few minutes, taking care not to burn the bottom of the pot. Continue simmering until the onions become very soft—usually around 20 to 30 minutes. Strain the onions, ginger and lemon and measure how much liquid remains. Double that amount and that will give you the correct quantity of honey that needs to be added to the liquid. Place the strained liquid back onto the stove and gradually stir in the honey, bringing the mixture just to a boil. Pour the syrup into dark, amber glass bottles and store it in the refrigerator. It should keep for up to six weeks. Use a cork stopper instead of a screw top on the bottle since some syrups have been known to ferment and explode. For a nasty cough, take up to a tablespoon every half hour (a teaspoon for young children).

Onions have no known toxicity. The only caution I could uncover had to do with the herb's tendency to lower blood sugar levels. For this reason, those suffering from hypoglycemia need to moderate their onion consumption.

The common onion may not have the "headline" generating reputation of other herbs. But, I can assure you, it certainly goes above and beyond the call of duty whenever it is asked.

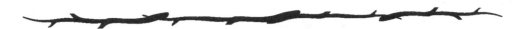

THE "DIRT" ON...ONION

Botanical ~	*Allium cepa*
Growth cycle ~	Biennial.
Medicinal uses~	Antiseptic, antibiotic, antispasmodic, carminative, diuretic, expectorant.
Part(s) used for medicine ~	Bulb.
Vitamins/Minerals ~	Vitamins C, B_1, B_2, protein, beta carotene, calcium, potassium, magnesium, manganese, copper, zinc, iron, tin, geranium, selenium.
Region ~	From sea level to approximately 9,000 feet in fields, meadows and cultivated areas. Different varieties require different areas.
Wild or Domestic ~	Both.
Poisonous look-alikes in the wild ~	Yes. The nodding wild onion (*Allium cernuum*) and the wild or prairie wild onion (*Allium stellatum*) and all other onion species are part of the large lily family. There are many lilies that can resemble *allium* species and some of those lilies are poisonous. Although the leaf structure and flower heads are different, common poisonous look-alikes to wild onions are fly poison (*Amianthium muscaetoxicum*), death camus (*Zygadenus spp.*) and star-of-Bethlehem (*Ornithogalum umbellatum*). There is one very easy way to clearly identify wild onions: their unmistakable odor. Lilies do not smell like onions.
Hardy or Delicate ~	Hardy once established.
Height of mature plant ~	One to two feet.
Easy or hard to grow ~	Generally easy.
Cultivation ~	From either seeds or sets. **Seeds**: as soon as soil is warm and frost-free, sow 1/4" to 1/2" deep. Cover seed com-

216

pletely with soil. Water lightly to keep soil moist but never drown seed. **Sets**: Cover with one-inch of dirt and place them firmly into the ground. Within one to two weeks, new shoots should be pushing up. Note: the Walla Walla Sweet is an easy variety to grow and is widely adapted to many regions. The only drawback is that it has a short storage life. If you are looking for a good long-term storage variety, try the New York Early, favored for years by many New York onion farmers. Onion is another plant that has many hybrid varieties. To ensure a steady supply of viable seeds from one season to the next, choose open-pollinated varieties over hybrids (also called "Heirloom" seeds) that always grow true from seed year after year.

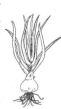

Plant spacing ~	Six to twelve inches apart.
Pre-soak seeds ~	No.
Pre-chill seeds ~	No.
Indoor seed starting ~	Yes. Use seed cells instead of dirt flats. Some growers feel that onions do better when they are started indoors. If you live in areas that experience freezing temperatures, start seeds in mid to late January and transplant out in mid-March to mid-April.
Light/dark seed requirements ~	Dark. Make sure seed is completely covered with dirt.
Days to germinate ~	14 to 21 days.
Days to full maturity ~	This depends completely on the type of onion that is planted. It can range from 90 to 150 days.
Soil type ~	Medium to sandy soil with excellent drainage.
Water requirements ~	Keep soil moist but do not over water.
Sun or shade ~	Full sun.
Propagation ~	Seed, if plant is allowed to go to seed after first year of growth.
Easy/hard to transplant ~	Easy.
Pests or diseases ~	Set-grown onions are more prone to disease than those grown from seed. If you plant both sets and seeds, separate the two to avoid any disease from spreading to the seed-grown varieties. If onions are over watered they develop a soft neck and browning of the outer skin which gives them a mushy consistency.
Landscape uses ~	If planted close together, could work as an interesting border.
Gathering ~	If you are gathering onions in the wild, do not pick plants that are growing near heavy traveled areas such as roadways or around places that are obvious toxic dumping grounds (mines, railroads, leech fields). The reason is that plants in the *allium* species (which include garlic) are known as soil purifiers and soak up everything from lead

to mercury. Always go as far away from the road as you can and look around the area to determine if it is a healthy environment. For the backyard herbal gardener, two weeks before the anticipated harvest, stop watering. When the onions have begun to develop skins and the tops have fallen over, they are ready to harvest. To create a better storage onion, pull up the entire plant and lay them down in the field to "cure" for one week under the hot sun. This way they harden up and produce a tougher skin. After one week, cut off the seed head. When you are certain they are dry, store them in shallow boxes or mesh "onion bags" at near freezing temperatures with an optimum 65°—70° humidity.

Best fresh or dried ~   Fresh.

Drying methods ~   Onions are used fresh for medicinal purposes.

Amount needed ~   That depends upon how often you will need them. Normal medicinal use might require 10 to 20 plants.

Seed collection ~   Allow clipped off seed head to completely dry out, then store in breathable bag in dark area. Some growers allow a few plants to go to seed in the field and let nature take its course when the seed head falls to the ground.

Companion planting ~   Chamomile is an excellent companion to onion. Planting onions next to most other plants helps repel certain garden pests.

Container planting ~   No.

Common mistakes ~   When planting from seed, some growers get impatient for germination and over water thinking that will speed things up. However, onion seeds will not tolerate being drowned. To eliminate that "trigger finger" on the garden hose, one grower I know mixes a few radish seeds in with the onion seeds. Radish seeds usually germinate within five to seven days. Once you see the wide leafed radish seedlings appear, you will know that the soil conditions are right and that the thin, green onion seedlings should appear within seven to fourteen days. When the onion seedlings appear, wait one full week and then carefully pull out the radish seedlings.

Interesting facts/tips ~   Keep onions well weeded. Once the bulb begins to develop and can be seen, "hill" the plants (i.e., pack dirt around the base of the plant). This keeps the bulb from drying out.

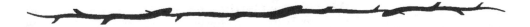

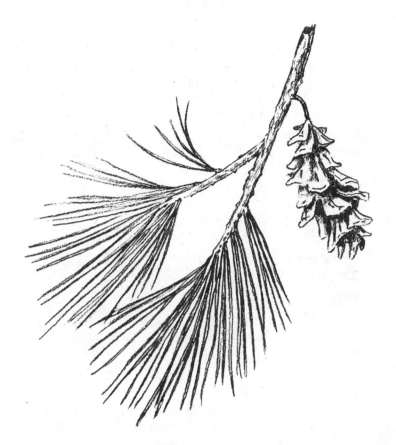

Chapter 26

PINE
EUELL GIBBONS WAS RIGHT

Pinus strobus (white pine—considered the best species for medicine)

Pinus sylvestris (scotch pine—a good alternative when you can't find white pine)

("W.F.")

Hardy perennial

Medicinal Uses: *Expectorant, demulcent*
Medicinal parts of plant: *Needles, bark, sap (resin)*
Forms: *Tea, salve, syrup, steam inhalation, pure essential oil*

WHAT IS ITS CHARACTER?

The words "dependable" and "reliable" were created to describe pine trees. The white pine tree, in particular, with its soft bundles of heavenly scented needles, is like an old friend. If the white pine tree were human, I'm pretty sure it would be the kind of friend who would use his one day off each week to help you move. The kind of friend that you could call at midnight to come pick you up at the airport. The kind of friend that brings you homemade chicken soup when you're ill. You get the point.

WHERE DO I FIND IT?

The white pine tree is found from above sea level to around 3,000 feet in the eastern part of the United States. White pine is distinguished by its bundles of five soft needles held together at their base by a paper-like sheath called a "fascicle," dark, deeply furrowed bark and long, slender cones that can range from five to eight inches long.

HOW DO I GROW IT?

From nursery stock. Reproduction of the white pine tree (as well as all other pines) begins in the spring when the male "flowers" appear, which are actually compacted clusters of dense pollen. This pollen is blown by the wind and lays a thin coating of yellow "dust" on everything in its path, including the waiting stigmas of the pistillate blossoms. When fertilization takes place, the commonly known pine cones appear. They require a full two to three years to mature before casting their winged seeds into the wind.

HOW DO I HARVEST IT?

In the spring, harvest the *inner* bark of the *branches only* since stripping the trunk can kill the tree. Strip off outer bark using a knife or, if it is soft enough, use your fingers. Peel the inner bark off, taking care to not include any of the dark, outer bark. The inner branch bark can also be stripped in the fall but you spend a lot more time to get less bark. The needles can be gathered directly off the tree or, if you want to keep them as fresh as possible, cut off a small branch and store it in a dark, cool area. The needles can remain viable for as long as three weeks this way. Needles are best harvested February, March and April for optimum medicinal value. As for the sap (resin), it can be gathered from the trunks of trees throughout the year. The best time for gathering sap is during the early morning or evening since that is when it hardens up and is less messy. If you live in regions that experience freezing temperatures, use those cold days to pick the sap chunks off the tree trunk since they are solid and easily removed from the bark.

HOW DO I USE IT?

When I think of pine, I think of two things: soap and Euell Gibbons.

The soap is pine tar. More specifically, *Grandpa's Wonder Pine Tar Toilet Soap*. Grandpa's soap has a distinctive odor that can shrivel nose hairs. It's the color of dark, rich earth and lasts a very long time. This latter quality is either a positive or a negative depending upon how much you like *Grandpa's Wonder Pine Tar Toilet Soap*. I happen to love the stuff. Most people do not. My aunt Monie's favorite way to describe something that smelled like an open sewer was to say, "It was almost as bad as Grandpa's Pine Tar Soap."

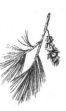

The second thing that pine brings to mind is Euell Gibbons. That gardening gourmet. That tree eating trail blazer. That fellow who turned the words "Ever eat a pine tree? Many parts are edible" into a successful cereal ad campaign. In one of Euell's many books on eating his way through the forest, he wrote "When I was a boy, I enjoyed chewing on the inner bark of ponderosa pine. But now I dislike it, finding it to taste too much of turpentine to be good." Yes, you may think that Euell was a few pine cones short of a full bag, but I liked the guy. He wasn't afraid to go out on a limb and grab some bark, crush it to see if he could make bread. If his idea didn't work (i.e., if he had to take a day off due to "complications"), he was open about it and even laughed at himself.

But when Euell said that "Many parts are edible," he wasn't yanking your chainsaw. Pine may just be a popular Christmas tree to you, but to Indians, pioneers, mountain men and hikers, the tree has been a source of nutrition, medicine and at times, a lifesaver.

There are somewhere around 300 species of trees that fall under the pine label. There are pines named after places where they are found (Pond Pine, Sand Pine), pines with weird names (Blister Pine, Poverty Pine) and pines that sound as if they came from a phone book (Jack Pine, Rosemary Pine, Walter Pine). They all fall under the general *Pinus* genus and they all share the same medicinal qualities.

The main medicinal species and the one that is recommended in most formulas is white pine (*Pinus strobus*). If you are not near where white pine grows, a good medicinal alternative is Scotch Pine (*Pinus sylvestris*). In a pinch, it doesn't really matter which of the dozens of species you choose since they all share almost identical healing qualities in different degrees. However, if you want to use the essential oil–which we'll talk about later in the chapter—make sure the label on the bottle indicates it is distilled from the *Pinus sylvestris* variety. For the purposes of this chapter, unless otherwise noted, I will be discussing the medicinal benefits of white pine.

WHY ARE THE EVERGREENS SO EVER GREEN?

Here's a great little story about how all the evergreen trees were given that name. It seems that in the beginning of time, God was looking down upon the earth and realized He had a lot to accomplish in less than seven days. He created all the plants first and then asked if they could lend Him their energy to get Him through until he finished creating the world. The plants and trees agreed, but as each day came to a close, more and more of the plants and trees gave up due to exhaustion. By the time God was finished, the only plants that made it through to the final hour were the conifers. To reward them for their loyalty and enduring energy, he proclaimed that they would be "ever green" for eternity. That should give you something to think about the next time you pass a conifer.

To paraphrase Euell Gibbons, "Many parts of the pine tree are medicinal." Those would include the needles, inner bark and sap (also called "resin" or "tar") of all pine trees. While the needle tea is a "woodsy" tasting beverage you can drink just for the sheer thrill of it, you might be interested to know that pine needle tea is high in vitamins A and C. The fresh green needles have five times the amount of vitamin C found in one lemon. Throughout the centuries, people have literally survived on pine needle tea as well as cured themselves of scurvy (a vitamin C deficiency) by drinking both the needles and inner bark of the pine tree. It is ironic that many of the pioneers died of scurvy along the trail—often within reach of the healing pine tree.

As for the medicinal qualities, they fall into three categories: **the respiratory system, the skin and the urinary tract.**

RESPIRATORY RESCUE

Far and away, white pine is considered an excellent remedy for **any ailment having to do with the throat, sinuses and lungs**. A heaping tablespoon of the fresh green needles (or a heaping teaspoon of dried) can be broken into small pieces and tossed into an eight ounce cup of boiling water, steeped for 15 minutes, strained and then used as an **antiseptic gargle for sore throats**.

A heaping handful of those same needles can be placed into a pasta-sized pan of boiling water, allowed to steep covered for 10 minutes, and then used **as an effective steam inhalation for clogged sinuses**.

The inner bark, boiled for 10 minutes in distilled water (a heaping teaspoon of the dried bark to 10 or 12 ounces of distilled water) makes **a good expectorant tea to drink after the infectious as well as feverish edge of the cough and cold have passed**. You can also simply **chew on the inner bark or boil it and get a nutritious, vitamin C-packed burst of energy**.

Perhaps the most effective way to use white pine bark is in a cough syrup. Not only does it work quickly to **break up and expel trapped phlegm**, it **helps kill infection and reduces inflammation in the upper respiratory tract due to its natural antiseptic and anti-inflammatory properties**. Euell Gibbons gives a nice little "White Pine, Whiskey and Honey Cough Syrup" recipe in his book *Stalking the Healthful Herbs*. Put one-half cup of coarsely ground white pine bark in a mason jar and cover it with two-thirds cup of boiling water. When cool, add one-half cup of whiskey, seal the jar and let it set overnight. Shake the jar vigorously a few times to make sure the contents mix. The next day, strain the bark and add one cup of honey to the liquid. Shake the jar thoroughly to make sure the honey dissolves into the tea and whiskey. The dose, according to Euell, is one tablespoon for adults and one teaspoonful for children as needed. My own personal preference would be to slightly warm the tablespoon first before swallowing the cough syrup. I think this helps to give the syrup a more soothing effect. Of course, with that much the whiskey in it, it'll probably go down pretty smoothly whether it's warm or cold.

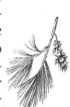

URINARY TRACT INFECTIONS

Since white pine has such tremendous antiseptic abilities, it works as a disinfectant as it courses through the urinary system. For serious or persistent **urinary tract infections,** get a medical opinion. But for occasional problems, you can try a tea made from equal parts fresh pine needles, dried buchu and dried uva ursi. Two to three cups of this blend taken each day for no longer than five days should get things moving down there. If the problem persists or worsens during that time, discontinue using the tea and seek medical attention.

THE GUM THAT'S NOT REALLY GUM

The fresh or dried resin (sap) that "bleeds" from the tree trunk is often referred to in old herbal books as "gum." This is misleading since some people expect the sap to actually have the consistency of commerical chewing gum. If you tried to chew pine "gum," you would have a hard time releasing your upper teeth from your lower teeth. Instead of chewing pine sap, it is better to take a very small piece (less than half the size of a marble) and attach it to the inside of your front, lower teeth. It will take hours to dissolve. Why would you want to do such a thing? Well, if you are camping in the woods and feel a **sore throat** coming on, sucking on pine sap can gradually coat your throat with an antiseptic layer of protection as well as fill your body with natural vitamin C.

A SAPPY SALVE

Pine sap is excellent for soothing skin conditions such as **psoriasis**, **eczema** and **fresh wounds**. If you are in the wild and scrape your skin, for instance, you can use the fresh, dripping sap to cover the wound. Pine sap acts as a **natural antiseptic** and forms a "band-aid" over the skin to protect it from infection.

Since pine sap is not always accessible, I wondered if I could make it into a salve and still get the same healing effect. To my delight, it was a huge success.

The salve is made differently than other herbal ointments. There are only three ingredients: Equal parts sap and castor oil and just a touch of beeswax shavings to give the salve a soft consistency. You can use the sap from *any* conifer, including fir or spruce. In experimenting with this "sappy salve," I've found that spruce sap works best and adds a lovely natural scent.

Place a measured amount of the sap into a one or two ounce, wide mouth glass jar and set the jar in a 400° oven. Melt the sap slowly, using a toothpick to pick out any bugs, bark or dirt that might have gotten trapped. Once the sap is completely melted and bubbling, add equal parts of castor oil. Allow the castor oil to blend with the sap, occasionally stirring the mixture with the toothpick. When it is bubbling hot, stir in beeswax shavings until completely melted. Check for proper consistency by removing the toothpick and allowing one drop of the hot mixture to fall on a plate. If it feels smooth and is easy to spread, you don't need to add further beeswax. If it seems rather runny, add just a few more shavings of beeswax. Take the jar out of the oven and set it aside to cool. When the salve is cool, cap the jar and store in a cool, dark place. It should keep for several years.

By the way, recognizing the "band-aid" action of the salve, I decided to see if it would work as an **effective lip balm for chapped lips**. It not only worked wonders, it stays on for hours!

BACKWOODS SPLINTER REMOVAL

Pine sap can come in handy when you have a **sliver of wood or some other small foreign object under your skin**. Basically, it's the same process as sticking a piece of gum on the end of a stick and attempting to retrieve a lost object. The only difference is instead of soft, cool gum you'll be dripping hot, molten sap over your bare skin. I can see that many of you are already grimacing at the thought. You'll need to hold the piece of sap over the area you are treating, light a match and allow the hot resin to drip directly onto your skin. Can you see where this might hurt? I tried it to get a sliver out of my toe. The sliver was really bugging me but once two drops of that hot, liquid sap hit my skin, I had other, more important concerns. Like, how to stop screaming. But I've got to tell you, once that sap dried to a rock hard mass (which took a mere two or three seconds) and I gently lifted up the resin, out came the trapped splinter. It doesn't always work this well. **The trick is to first uncover a piece of the trapped object and get the hot sap to adhere to it, thus allowing a firmer grip**. However, if you're a sap novice, you can rip off a top layer of skin and/or get a minor blister from the melting sap.

Another more industrial use for sap is as **"nature's super glue."** Someone once told me that pine resin would hold "anything together." Anything, eh? Okay, I thought, how about that metal file attachment that kept coming apart from the wooden cabinet? I must have burned three large chunks of pine sap between that metal holder and the wood and it never stayed stuck. However, when you have a crack in a piece of wood furniture, pine sap can be dripped into the crevice and it works remarkably well to increase the integrity of the area. In a case such as this, the sap is like a natural epoxy that dries hard and shiny to the touch.

THERE'S NOTHING LIKE A PINE NEEDLE BATH

You can benefit from pine's skin-comforting abilities by soaking in a needle bath. To make the bath, gather several large handfuls of fresh pine needles and boil them in a large pot of water for 10 minutes. Pour the entire mixture directly into a warm bath. You don't need to strain the needles since they are too big to slip down the bathtub drain and cause plumbing problems. A 30 to 45 minute soak in this heavenly scented bath does wonders for many skin ailments. It also serves to reduce some rheumatic pain and other forms of joint discomfort. One point to remember is that a pine bath is considered to be stimulating to the body. Thus, it may not work at night if you want to drift off to sleep right away.

IT'S LIKE BRINGING A PINE TREE INTO THE HOUSE

Now, onto pine tree pure essential oil.

Remember to buy only the pure essential oil that has been distilled from the *Pinus sylvestris* tree. All essential oils have both an emotional as well as physical effect on the body. On the emotional side, taking a whiff of pine essential oil or diffusing it into the room via a lamp ring is said to promote a **sense of peace and balance**. It can be a **comforting fragrance while at the same time, invigorating to the senses**. It is **useful for people who struggle with apathy, lethargy, loss of concentration and nervous depression**.

As other oils that fall into the "forest" group (spruce, fir, cedar), it is **very grounding to the senses**. This means that if you're the kind of person who tends to have your feet firmly planted in mid-air, the smell of

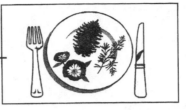

Wild Food Facts

Pine trees offer some of nature's most popular wild foods.

For example, if you're stuck in the woods and for some reason feel the need to make bread, you can apparently accomplish this task by grinding the inner bark of most pine trees into a fine powder. When someone told me about this, the first thought that came to mind was that if I were lost in the woods and nearing starvation, there are about 27 other things I would do to get out of the woods before I said, "Hey, let's make some bread." But if that's your priority, go for it.

A more reasonable and far more tasty use of the pine tree are the seeds, or "nuts." These are typically available August through October. While all pine cones hold these nuts, the pinyon pine of the southwest (*Pinus edulis, P. monophylla, P. quadrifolia*) is considered the best of the bunch. Pinyon nuts are available in cycles that run every four to seven years. They can be found scattered on the ground beneath pinyon pines or vigorously shaken from the cones. Eaten raw or roasted, pinyon pine nuts are highly nutritious and make a high energy, protein-rich food

pine can help draw you back down to earth. A wonderfully grounding, clean smelling, antiseptic room spray is made by combining 25 drops *each* of the essential oils of pine, spruce and fir into a bottle filled with three ounces of distilled water. I'm not saying that simply smelling pine will make a "flake" turn into a dependable human being. It just might be an aid for those in need of "cloud rescue."

Pine essential oil works very well for respiratory conditions via a **soothing chest rub**. I make this concoction by adding three drops *each* of the following essential oils: pine, thyme, eucalyptus, tea tree and lavender to one tablespoon of apricot kernel or grapeseed oil. Rub the mixture briskly on the chest and then place a hot water bottle or moist heat pad over your chest to allow the oils to penetrate into your skin. In my opinion, this combination works much better than store-bought chest balms and smells 100 times better.

Ten drops of pine essential oil can be added to a bowl of hot water and used as a steam inhalation for **sinus congestion**.

If you dislike using chemical floor and toilet bowl cleaners, combining a tablespoon *each* of pine and eucalyptus essential oils into a three quarts of water will give you **a healthier alternative to toxic household cleansers**.

Two cautions: **never use pine essential oil undiluted since it can irritate sensitive skin**. Also, **if you are taking homeopathic remedies, refrain from using any essential oils since many can eradicate the remedy's effectiveness**.

Obviously Euell Gibbons was ahead of his time when he chowed down on this forest favorite. One sip or sniff of this perennial treasure and you might be surprised how much *you* pine for it.

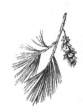

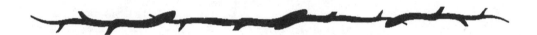

THE "DIRT" ON... WHITE PINE

Botanical ~	*Pinus strobus*
Growth cycle ~	Perennial.
Medicinal uses~	Expectorant, demulcent.
Part(s) used for medicine ~	Needles, bark.
Vitamins/Minerals ~	Vitamins A and C, phosphorus, iron, thiamine. The fresh green needles have five times the amount of vitamin C found in one lemon.
Region ~	From above sea level to around 3,000 feet in the eastern part of the United States. White pine is distinguished by its bundles of five soft needles held together at their base by a paper-like sheath called a "fascicle," dark, deeply furrowed bark and long, slender cones that can range from five to eight inches long.
Wild or Domestic ~	Both.
Poisonous look-alikes in the wild ~	No.
Hardy or Delicate ~	Very hardy.
Height of mature plant ~	150 feet.
Easy or hard to grow ~	Very easy from sapling.

Cultivation ~	Purchase nursery stock.
Plant spacing ~	16 to 20 feet.
Pre-soak seeds ~	Not applicable.
Pre-chill seeds ~	Not applicable.
Indoor seed starting ~	Not applicable.
Light/dark seed requirements ~	Not applicable.
Days to germinate ~	Not applicable.
Days to full maturity ~	White pine is considered a "fast grower," adding one foot or more of growth each year. If grown from an established sapling, tree can be ready to harvest for medicine in eight to twelve years.
Soil type ~	Moderate to moist, fertile soil is best.
Water requirements ~	Needs moderate watering to establish itself as a sapling. Once mature, let nature take its course.
Sun or shade ~	Full sun to partial shade.
Propagation ~	In the spring, the male "flowers" appear, which are actually compacted clusters of dense pollen. This pollen is blown by the wind and lays a thin coating of yellow "dust" on everything in its path, including the waiting stigmas of the pistillate blossoms. When fertilization takes place, the commonly known pine cones appear. They require a full two to three years to mature before casting their winged seeds into the wind.
Easy/hard to transplant ~	From sapling, easy if you follow nursery directions.
Pests or diseases ~	Virtually pest and disease-free.
Landscape uses ~	Makes great shade tree as well as effective windbreak.
Gathering ~	In the spring, harvest *inner bark* of branches only since stripping the trunk can kill the tree. Strip off outer bark using a knife or, if it is soft enough, use your fingers. Peel the inner bark off, taking care to not include any of the dark, outer bark. The inner branch bark can also be stripped in the fall but you spend a lot more time to get less bark. The needles can be gathered directly off the tree or, if you want to keep them as fresh as possible, cut off a small branch and store it in a dark, cool area. The needles can remain viable for as long as three weeks this way. Needles are best harvested February, March and April for optimum medicinal value. As for the sap (resin), it can be gathered from the trunks of trees throughout the year. Best time for gathering sap is early morning or evening since that is when it hardens up and is less messy. If you live in regions that experience freezing temperatures, use those cold days to pick the sap chunks off the tree trunk since they are solid and easily removed from the bark.

Best fresh or dried ~ **Bark**: fresh or dried; **Needles**: fresh or dried; **Sap**: fresh or dried.

Drying methods ~ **Inner branch bark**: Lay the strips in an air dryer away from direct sunlight. The thinner the strip, the less time it will take to dry. **Needles**: Scatter across large cloth out of direct sunlight. Ideally, you still want the dried needles to have an aromatic scent to them. **Sap**: Since you should gather already dried sap, storage is the only concern. Do not store sap in paper bags since it can stick like glue to the sides if it is exposed to heat. Better to store sap in glass bottles or empty cans.

Amount needed ~ One tree.

Seed collection ~ Not applicable.

Companion planting ~ I've seen patches of blue violets, chickweed and mullein all around white pine trees.

Container planting ~ No!

Common mistakes ~ Thinking that when people say "Gather white pine bark" that they are referring to the trunk and not the branches.

Interesting facts/tips ~ Use the needles to acidify soil. Layer them two to four inches deep in the dirt and around plants. Don't place them near plants that cannot tolerate acid. If you don't live where the white pine grows but you have friends who do, ask them to clip off several small thin branches into eight inch lengths and mail them to you. Take it from someone who has done this very thing, the branches will remain viable for harvest even after a week or so. Your friends may wonder if you've gone off the deep end. But tell them not to worry—you read about it in a book called *Plant Power*.

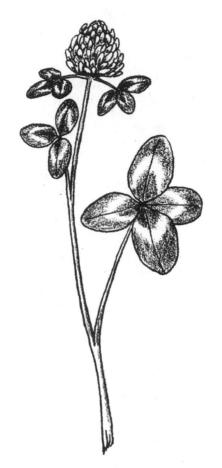

Chapter 27

I'M LOOKING OVER THE HERB RED CLOVER

Trifolium pratense

("W.F.")

Biennial

Medicinal Uses: *Depurative, alterative, anti-tussive, diuretic, mild sedative*

Medicinal parts of plant: *Flowers*

Forms: *Tea*

WHAT IS ITS CHARACTER?

Although it might sound presumptuous, I think red clover likes to be picked. Perhaps it's the way the globe-like flowers stand up from the makeshift calyx at their mid-summer peak, rocking to and fro in the slightest breeze, trying to get your attention as you walk by. I don't think it has any idea that most people regard it as "just a weed." Deep down in its heart, red clover clearly understands its miraculous healing power and it wants more than anything to share that gift with those who are ready to listen.

WHERE DO I FIND IT?

Found in the wild at 6,000 feet and below. Look for red clover growing in farm and livestock fields where there is lots of moisture and manure.

HOW DO I GROW IT?

Broadcast seed in spring or fall, barely covering with dirt. Soil can be light, sandy and even rocky but you will get a better medicinal plant if you seed it into fertile, rich, lightly composted dirt. Press the seed firmly into the soil and barely cover with dirt. Red clover needs light to germinate which means you don't want to bury it. Lightly spray with water without drowning the seeds. This is a fast germinating plant, with seedlings breaking through the soil in as little as two days. Thin excessive growth, spacing plants six to eight inches apart.

HOW DO I HARVEST IT?

Harvest the purple flowers at full bloom which is anywhere from June to August. Choose flowers that are full of moisture, have a pretty pink-purple color and show no signs of brown, dried edges. **Important note:** According to botanist and herbalist Dr. James Duke, do not harvest flowers that bloom in late fall (often referred to as "the second bloom"). These have been known to cause toxic reactions in cattle and some humans. Red clover can be used for medicine either fresh or dried. To dry the flowers, place them on a piece of cloth or in an air dryer *away from direct heat*. When you cannot feel any more moisture in the flower, they are ready to store in airtight glass containers.

HOW DO I USE IT?

Once upon a time in the 1930's, an ex-coal miner named Harry Hoxsey told folks he could cure cancer. It seems that Harry's great grandfather had a cancer-stricken horse who recovered after eating a specific combination of grassy herbs and weeds. The story really stuck with Harry and when he was old enough to know better, he put the combination together in a formula and called it "The Hoxsey Cancer Formula."

He opened a clinic and folks came from miles around to partake of Harry's herbal heavyweight formula. It didn't help everyone, but hundreds swore it cured their cancers.

Then the FDA closed down Harry's clinic because they said a bunch of herbs could not cure something as complicated as cancer. In the end, all the people who didn't like Harry got the last word when he died of prostate cancer. Harry tried his own formula, but alas, it didn't work for him.

Harry's cancer formula is still being used today in Mexico. Just as it was true 60 years ago, the Hoxsey formula does *not* have a 100% "cure" rate. But those who *have* been "cured of cancer," beg to differ. They might also tell you that of the ten herbs in the formula, one is considered the "main ingredient."

That herb is red clover. Some folks even dubbed Harry's formula "the red clover combination." Harry's great grandfather wasn't the first person to consider the clover as a **cancer remedy**. Over 33 cultures have used the herb for treating the disease with some referring to red clover as "the prize herb."

The pretty purple-flowered weed (not to be confused with the famed "lucky four leaf clover") has a long history of being the "one herb to keep on the shelf"—and not just for cancer. Frontier folk who lived 100 miles from the nearest doctor were always within reach of red clover blossoms to take care of everything from **bee stings** to **chronic degenerative diseases**. When spring arrived, farmers drank cup after cup of the tea to **cleanse their body and build physical strength** for the planting season.

When red clover's pink-purple, round-headed flowers are at their absolute peak (usually around mid-summer), they have always reminded me of very large gumdrops. That candy comparison is not so far off in that red clover tea is a very pleasant tasting beverage. I think that many people tend to underestimate red clover since it looks mild, tastes mild and doesn't produce body-jolting sensations. What people don't realize is that this incredible herb weaves its healing power through your body in very subtle ways. It **nourishes**, **detoxifies** and **rebuilds whatever needs to be strengthened** and it does it all using the most delicate brush strokes.

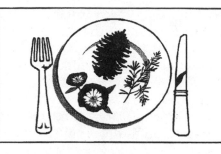

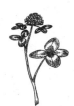

Wild Food Facts

Eating raw, uncooked red clover flowers and leaves is questionable since too much of it can cause terrible bloating. If you are out in the woods and are starving, you can munch on a small handful of fresh flowers and leaves. But don't overdo it. Red clover is a rich protein source. The dried flowers and leaves can easily be crushed and sprinkled into cereals, soups and stews to give you a nutritious burst of energy. Fresh blossoms and leaves, when steamed, do not produce the same bloating effect and can be safely consumed. Steam them for five to ten minutes to retain as much of the vitamin content as possible. Save the water and add it to soups or drink it as a healing beverage. Fresh seeds have been soaked in water overnight and then pounded into a nutritious "mush." Unfortunately, the name "mush" doesn't exactly make a person want to run out and taste this wild food. Seeds can be added to soups and stews as flavoring. Dried seeds are ground into a fine powder and added to regular flour in one-third proportions as a high-protein boost.

A "SPECIFIC" FOR SOLITARY, SWOLLEN GLANDS

Red clover tea **purifies the blood**, as it **gently drains toxins from the liver**, **lymph and lungs**. In addition, it works as a natural remedy for **sinus infections**, allowing the pressure to drain from the head. Unlike other liver cleansers, red clover's action is not as jarring to the system. In other words, toxins are gradually released without the cathartic, sometimes purging effect that strong liver detoxifiers such as dandelion root can produce.

Red clover has **four antitumor compounds** as well as an **anti-cancer** compound called "genistein." In addition, this common weed is loaded with the antioxidant chemical *tocopherol*—a form of vitamin E—which has helped prevent breast tumors in animals.

While red clover is good for so many different ailments, it is considered **a "specific" herb when one is suffering from a single, hard swollen gland**. This could be located in the neck, the groin, the armpits or around the upper chest area. Research shows that red clover can be effective whether that single swollen gland is benign or malignant. Can red clover take that a step further and reverse a malignancy? History has proven that for some people, red clover tea can reduce the size of malignant tumors as well as make it more difficult for them to spread. This is as far as the available literature will go in the discussion of cancerous tumors. If you want to hear more of the "miracle cancer reversals," you will have to rely upon word-of-mouth, personal experiences from those who have used the herb. As with *any* serious health condition, I believe that the healing process takes place using a special *combination of therapies* which are customized for each individual. Red clover tea may indeed be *one* of those modalities.

By the way, even though red clover is a specific for single glandular swellings, I would still consider the herb a valuable remedy for multiple swellings, if only for the fact that it helps clean and purify the lymphatic system.

AN AID TO SKIN DISEASE

Red clover not only purifies the blood, it enriches it. Because of this, the tea is renowned for its beneficial effect on **psoriasis** as well as **adult and childhood eczema**. Thanks to red clover's **natural diuretic ability**, it helps to flush toxins quickly out of the body. When one cup of the tea is taken three times a day, red clover tea has gradually brought relief and positive results within two to three weeks. If the skin disease is considered chronic, add equal parts of yellow dock root to red clover to enhance the systemic cleansing action. When you are taking the tea, it's a grand idea to stay off fried foods, dairy products, meat, potatoes, soft drinks and alcohol. If the skin condition creeps back when you start consuming any of the above, your body is obviously telling you something.

HEY, IT'S GOOD FOR HAY FEVER

Red clover tea, taken three times daily, has been known to help those suffering from **hay fever** and **pollen allergies**. The idea is that when the bloodstream is kept flowing and impurities are continually being removed, those nasty foreign invaders will be swept out with the rest of the debris. The sooner you start drinking the tea before the official start of the hay fever season, the better. In other words, one might start the daily tea dose in early February and carry it through early May. You don't need to be gulping down three cups each and every day, but daily consumption of one cup is recommended.

WHOOP THAT WHOOPING COUGH

This gentle giant of an herb has been used successfully to treat **whooping cough** and **bronchitis**—especially when it affects children. Thanks to its mild sedative and gently restorative capabilities, red clover soothes any respiratory rawness as it calms the constant need to cough. For cases such as this, the tea can be taken freely throughout the day, as often as one needs it.

LOVE THAT "FLESH PRODUCING" TEA

Red clover used to be credited as a "flesh producer." That's a turn-of-the-century way to say the tea works as **a tonic to restore the health of those suffering from debilitating, "wasting" diseases**. A cup of red clover tea can be taken up to four times a day as an energy boost for those with **mononucleosis**, **hepatitis**, **month-long colds and flu** and even **tuberculosis**.

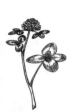

Regarding **tuberculosis**, red clover was scientifically shown to fight against the bacteria that causes the illness. As red clover rebuilds the body, the herb also fights off invading viral and fungal infections that would further weaken the body. Another advantage of drinking red clover tea during an illness is that it has a tendency to **relax the body and release tension**, thereby providing a clearer channel to accept the healing process.

INFECTION FIGHTING

You don't have to be ill to enjoy the benefits of red clover tea. This amazing beverage can be taken daily to **combat infection** and **gain greater immune strength**. One cup in the morning and one after dinner is a good idea when the cold and flu season are upon you.

MENOPAUSAL MANAGEMENT

The herb has estrogen-like compunds in its little blossoms which have led herbalists to suggest it as **a tonic tea for menopause**. It is highly nourishing and has a calming effect during moments of anxiety and energy loss. In order to benefit the most from the tea, you will have to drink at least two or three cups a day. There is a tendency for red clover to be a natural blood thinner, so if you're still menstruating, you may experience an increased flow.

A GREAT GARGLE

Red clover tea, made double strength, is a good gargle for **sore throats** and mouthwash for **mouth sores**. Place four heaping teaspoons of dried red clover flowers (or eight teaspoons of the fresh flowers) in eight ounces of hot water. Cover and let the mixture steep until it is cool. Strain and use as often as needed.

INSECT BITES/BEE STINGS

If you get bitten in a field of red clover (or you're near *fresh* red clover), grab one of the blossoms, moisten it with your saliva and press the blossom into the bite or sting for five to ten minutes. The herb acts as a natural antibiotic, helping to draw out the poison.

DOSE AMOUNTS

Instead of the typical one teaspoon of dried herb or two teaspoons of fresh herb to eight ounces of hot water, red clover requires *double those amounts*. Since you are dealing with flowers, remember to make sure you don't use boiling water since it will reduce and sometimes even eliminate the herb's healing power.

BE AWARE OF...

Most herbalists will tell you that red clover is nearly caution-free and that you can drink the tea for as long as two months nonstop. *However*, if you are using the herb as part of a cancer treatment, be aware that **red clover is not suggested for cancers diagnosed as "estrogen-dependent" (often with breast and gynecological tumors) because of the estrogen-like compounds in the herb**. I will say, though, that the jury is still out on how these estrogen-like compounds interact within the body. One thing is for sure, they do not react the same way on every individual. Due to these natural estrogenic compounds, some herbalists question how the herb might interact with the use of birth control pills. Again, the reaction on the body will be different for every woman. Finally, it is known that pregnant cows that overgraze on fields of red clover (and other clovers) have had spontaneous abortions. The *Botanical Safety Handbook* rates red clover as an herb that **"should not be taken during pregnancy due to its uterine stimulation."**

The red clover "cure" may not be everyone's cup of tea. But for some, it might be the greatest discovery of their life. And every time that happens, I'm sure ol' Harry Hoxsey looks down and says "I told you so."

THE "DIRT" ON...RED CLOVER

Botanical ~	*Trifolium pratense*
Growth cycle ~	Biennial.
Medicinal uses~	Depurative, alterative, mild stimulant.
Part(s) used for medicine ~	Flowers.
Vitamins/Minerals ~	Vitamin C, B-complex, calcium, potassium, niacin, magnesium, iron.
Region ~	Found in the wild at 6,000 feet and below. Typically in farming and livestock fields where there is lots of moisture and manure.
Wild or Domestic ~	Both.
Poisonous look-alikes in the wild ~	No.
Hardy or Delicate ~	Hardy.
Height of mature plant ~	One to three feet.
Easy or hard to grow ~	Very easy.
Cultivation ~	Broadcast seed in fall or spring, barely covering with dirt. Press seed firmly into soil. Lightly spray with water and expect to see sprouts in a few days.
Plant spacing ~	Six to eight inches.
Pre-soak seeds ~	Yes, it sometimes helps.
Pre-chill seeds ~	No.
Indoor seed starting ~	No.
Light/dark seed requirements ~	Light.
Days to germinate ~	Two to four days.
Days to full maturity ~	Approximately 90 days.
Soil type ~	Light, sandy, rocky soil will work but you will produce a better medicinal plant if soil is fertile, rich and lightly composted.
Water requirements ~	Likes regular moisture without being drowned.
Sun or shade ~	Full sun to partial shade.
Propagation ~	Seed.
Easy/hard to transplant ~	Fairly easy but it is better to direct seed red clover.
Pests or diseases ~	Virtually pest and disease-free.
Landscape uses ~	Excellent ground cover for fields and meadows.
Gathering ~	Harvest the flowers at full bloom which is anywhere from June to August. Choose flowers that are full of moisture, have a pretty pink-purple color and show no signs of

237

brown, dried edges. Important note: According to Dr. James Duke, do not harvest flowers that bloom in late fall (often referred to as "the second bloom"). These have been known to cause toxic reactions in cattle and some humans.

Best fresh or dried ~ Fresh or dried.

Drying methods ~ Dry flowers away from direct heat in an air dryer or on a piece of cloth. Once you cannot feel any more moisture in the flower, they are ready to store in airtight glass containers.

Amount needed ~ Moderate use: 20 plants; Regular use: 25+.

Seed collection ~ Allow the flowers to dry completely on the plant. Depending upon the region you live in, this could be as early as August or as late as November. When harvesting flowers for seed, it is a good idea to tap the flowers before picking them to see if the light tan seeds fall out. If this is the case, the remaining flowers on that plant should be nearing or at the same stage of seed development and can also be harvested. Place them into a brown paper bag, crush the dried petals between your hands and winnow out the seed.

Companion planting ~ Plantain, alfalfa, mullein.

Container planting ~ It can be done but you will never get enough flowers for medicinal use.

Common mistakes ~ Not allowing the harvested flowers to dry out completely before storing in airtight glass containers. Due to the naturally-occurring water within the fresh flowers, the stored flowers can turn brown as well as attract mold.

Interesting facts/tips ~ Red clover makes an excellent cover crop to improve poor soil and draw nitrogen into the ground. To use it in this manner, plant seed in the fall and turn the crop under in early spring. If your soil is particularly poor, use the appropriate inoculant (which can be purchased at any nursery or seed supply company) which encourages red clover to take better advantage of the available nitrogen in the soil.

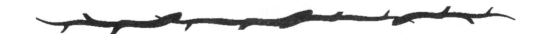

238

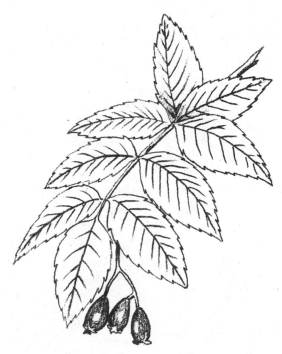

Chapter 28

TRY ROSE HIPS &
"C" WHAT HAPPENS

Rosa canina ("dog rose")
R. villosa ("apple rose")
R. gallica ("apothecary rose")
R. rugosa ("Japanese rose" or "wrinkled rose")
R. centifolia ("cabbage rose" or "provence rose")
R. carolina ("pasture" or "wild rose")
R. eglanteria ("sweetbrier rose")
R. damascena (used to make Bulgarian rose essential oil)
("W.F.")

Hardy to delicate perennial

Medicinal Uses: *Sedative, anti-depressant, antispasmodic, digestive stimulant, expectorant, anti-bacterial, anti-viral, antiseptic, anti-inflammatory, menstrual regulator, aphrodisiac*

Medicinal parts of plant: *Hips (fruits), petals*

Forms: *Tea, jam (made from hips), pure essential oil*

WHAT IS ITS CHARACTER?

Wild roses seem to know that they are special. When they bloom in early summer, they radiate an elegance that must make the weedier herbs feel a bit self-conscious. Wild roses don't care what the other plants think. For three to four weeks during that period, they reign supreme in the wild, thrilled to be the center of attention. However, I've always felt roses were a bit of a tease. They attract you with their incredible crimson and soft pink flower debut and when you move closer to pick a flower or two, you are greeted with a stem that is riddled with thorns. "Admire me all you want, but don't touch," should be the rose's motto. Come late fall and early winter when the flowers have long disappeared, the rose once again stands out from the rest of the plants. Against the stark background of October and November's brown and gray landscape, the wild rose is still very much alive, offering a brilliant scattering of vibrant red hips (fruits) and urging you to approach the shrub. You still have thorns to contend with, but by this time of year, the rose's "don't touch me" attitude has softened. It welcomes—even yearns—to be picked and enjoyed. The rose knows it has captured your heart and that you'll return. I can't help but think that as you turn to leave, it is grinning from hip to hip.

WHERE DO I FIND IT?

Wild roses are usually found thriving along roadsides, near streams and in meadows where there is moderate moisture and some organic matter around the base.

There are many wild rose species—so many that seasoned botanists admit to having a difficult time distinguishing them. One of the reasons for this species confusion is that bees have a hey-day cross-pollinating the flowers, causing new varieties to pop up across the land. The only common thread that runs through most wild rose species is that they all have five petals. Cultivated or hybrid roses, on the other hand, have numerous petals.

HOW DO I GROW IT?

I encourage everyone interested in growing their own "wild roses" to pay close attention to the Latin names when purchasing nursery stock. **Use only medicinal rose varieties, not garden hybrids**.

It is important to understand that some species are known for having larger hips (fruits) and some are known for having more fragrant flowers. For example, *Rosa canina*, also known as "dog rose," is the most commonly used medicinal rose and the one often referred to in herb books. It can grow up to 18 feet tall and makes a stunning addition to the backyard.

It has small to medium sized leaves, small pink flowers and medium sized rose hips that hold a great number of seeds.

Rosa gallica, also referred to as the "apothecary rose," has highly fragrant petals that retain their aroma when dried. Because of this, it is the "approved rose" for making rosewater.

The traditional "wild rose" known as the "pasture rose" (*Rosa carolina*) is the two to five foot variety you often find growing in the wild. In my opinion, this variety is not worth growing in your yard—*especially* if you are looking for a rose species that has large hips. The hips on the traditional wild rose are smaller than the hips on those million dollar "super models." (They are about the size of a pea).

When you're looking for big rose hips, choose the *Rosa villosa* ("apple rose") or *Rosa rugosa* ("wrinkled rose" or "Japanese rose") species. I am particularly fond of *Rosa villosa*. This five to seven foot shrub with light pink flowers features some of the largest, sweetest, most scrumptious rose hips I have tasted. **The secret to good rose hips is finding ones that have more of the fleshy inner pulp than seeds**. *Rosa villosa* and *Rosa rugosa* fit that criterion. Trust me, after you have spent the better part of your day scooping out bowls of seed only to end up with microscopic amounts of rose hip pulp, you will make a concerted effort to either locate better hips the next time around or decide to grow a variety that is more "hippy."

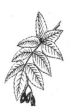

If you want the best of both worlds (i.e., large rose hips and large flowers), *Rosa rugosa* is the plant for you. Its large crimson flowers are wonderfully fragrant as well. The only drawback is that you have to contend with a very nasty bunch of stems that are densely covered with large, medium and small thorns.

Wild roses can be cultivated from seed, cuttings or buddings—all of which require the patience of Job and the skill of a florist. I have tried and failed miserably to grow a plant from seed and always ended up wondering how nature managed to accomplish this challenging task. Take my word for it, save yourself hours of misery and purchase nursery-grown plants.

Most medicinal roses prefer a heavy, loamy soil that has a fair amount of composted matter added to it. While they like a clay consistency, roses do not enjoy standing in water. Make sure your garden site is well-drained so this does not happen. Provide roses with a half sun/half shade location, spacing plants about three to four feet apart to allow for future growth and to avoid crowding since this makes the plant susceptible to mildew. When you purchase dormant stock (as opposed to potted rose plants) from nurseries or catalogs, you will need to put them into the ground immediately. Roses do best when planted in the springtime. If you purchase roses in pots, they can be purchased during the winter months and kept indoors until early to late spring (or until the weather permits outdoor planting).

One or two weeks before purchasing the dormant stock, prepare their planting bed by digging down one foot and removing the dirt. Mix that dirt with compost and any other soil conditioners that will provide enrichment. Replace the soil and soak the spot with enough water until it becomes quite soggy. Allow this to settle for seven to ten days before planting the dormant rose. The same soil preparation can be made for potted roses.

When placing either the dormant rose or potted plant into the prepared hole, always give the roots plenty of room so that they are not packed too tightly. Set the plant firmly into the dirt and, once in place, pack the soil tightly around the base. Water no more than once a week unless the soil becomes excessively dry.

Roses need a certain amount of maintenance to provide years of healthy growth and superior flowers. Between late spring and early summer when the flowers bloom, it is a good idea to feed the plant an "herbal manure" tea (such as the one described on page 12) once a week. When the flowers fade, use the herbal manure tea every two to three weeks until fall when a good layer of manure or organic mulch should be applied. You may also want to consider using an organic, balanced, fish-based plant food that includes ingredients such as fish bonemeal, bloodmeal and sulfate of potash. Applied every two to three months, this type of natural additive breaks down in the soil and feeds the roses gradually. To repel aphids—which have been known to infest wild roses—plant garlic and chives underneath the shrub. One natural pest spray that roses love is made by soaking 20 juniper berries (*Juniperus communis*) in two cups of water. Let them sit overnight in a covered container. The next day, add one quart of water to the mixture and spray the whole amount all over the plant. Toss the juniper berries around the base of the trunk. Reapply the juniper tea twice a week and after rain storms, especially if you have a bad bug problem.

HOW DO I HARVEST IT?

Rose petals are harvested in late May to early June, depending upon the region. Petals should be gathered in early morning before the sun shines on them and before the flowers burst open. Separate the petals from their white base (sometimes referred to as a "claw") which can contribute a rather bitter flavor. Use the petals fresh or dry them on a cloth, out of direct sunshine, but in a room where there is plenty of heat and low moisture. Petals need to be dried quickly and then stored immediately in an airtight glass container and placed in a dark cupboard to preserve their healing and aromatic power.

Rose hips (which is what forms after the flower has died) are harvested between early October and late November when the fruit is bright red. If it has turned ruby red, it is too ripe and will be sour. If the hips are orange in color, leave them because they are not ripe.

Many skilled rose hip pickers suggest waiting for at least three good frosts before harvesting the fruit. Some even say that the fruit should have snow or ice on the branch before it is worth using. In my quest to wait until the "perfect rose hip picking moment," I have been beaten to the hip by families of deer who apparently value this herb as much as I do. More important than finding the right moment is making sure the rose hip is ripe. If you taste the hip and it's a good one, forget about the frost or ice on the branch and start harvesting!

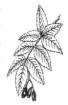

ROSE ESSENTIAL OIL ~ A PRICEY PETAL

It takes about 60,000 rose petals to produce just one ounce of the pure essential oil. For this reason, rose pure essential oil is one of the most expensive healing oils. To give you an idea, 45 *drops* of Bulgarian rose (*Rosa damascena*) can cost about $35.00. That comes to approximately *78 cents per drop*. Rose essential oil prices vary depending upon availability of supply, the type of rose that is used and the cost of production.

Unfortunately, rose oils are often adulterated or cut with a base oil, such as apricot kernel oil, and sold as "rose oil." This confuses an unsuspecting public who think they are buying the real thing. Price is one way to know if you are getting the pure stuff. If you see a one ounce bottle of "rose oil" selling for $5.00, you are getting mostly a base oil that has one or two drops of the essential oil added to it for fragrance.

Always check the wording on the bottle to see if it says "pure essential oil" or "100% pure essential oil." While this is not a fail-safe way to determine purity, it is a start. If the bottle simply says "rose oil" or "rose fragrance," it is *not* a pure essential oil.

Fortunately, it only takes one or two drops of pure essential oil of rose to initiate a healing effect. For example, many people place a single drop of the oil on their forehead to enhance meditation and to relieve headache pain. Inhaling the aroma from the bottle is good for depression, anxiety, and is soothing during periods of shock or grief.

Used on the skin, rose essential oil acts as a cell regenerator, similar to the herb comfrey. Five drops stirred into a two ounce jar of face cream can help to smooth fine lines and wrinkles, gradually heal scar tissue, protect sensitive skin and provide nourishment right down to the cellular level. Best of all, all day long you will be exposed to the aromatic healing benefits of this heavenly scent.

Rose hips pack their biggest medicinal punch when they are eaten fresh off the branch (minus the top and bottom stem attachments) or made into a non-heated jam so they can retain their outstanding vitamin content. (For a tasty and mighty healthy rose hips jam recipe, turn to the end of the chapter and find the "Wild Foods Facts" box). To dry them for later use, you'll need to carefully slice the top and bottom stem attachments off and cut the hips in half. Completely remove the abundant seeds before drying. Try to retain as much of the fleshy pulp inside the hip since that is where most of the vitamins are located. Lay the fruit out singly, fleshy side upward on an ungreased cookie sheet. Do not heap one hip on top of another since that tends to attract mold. Allow them to dry naturally in a covered, warm place. The hips are ready when they are slightly shriveled and hard to the touch. This can take anywhere from two to three weeks. Never put rose hips in the oven and turn on the heat to speed the drying process since this greatly reduces the healing benefits. Store dried rose hips in an airtight, glass container and keep the jar away from heat.

HOW DO I USE IT?

Let's get one thing straight: I do not go out into the woods, blithely pick berries off bushes and trees and eat them. Lots of berries look alike to the untrained eye. Pick the wrong one and the results can run the gamut from vicious vomiting to an early meeting with your Maker. Neither appeals to me.

This brings me to one snow-covered November many, many moons ago. A friend and I were hiking through the Colorado Rockies. At that time, I was still a west coast city dweller and not familiar with the high altitude plant life. We came upon a spindly bush with juicy bright red berries. My friend was thrilled and announced that we were in the presence of the wild rose.

"Are you sure?" came my response.

She didn't respond. She was too busy plucking several "hips" off the bush and plopping them into her mouth like peanuts at a carnival. I waited to see if her eyes rolled back into her head or if she broke out in a profuse sweat. She didn't. In fact, she kept picking the rose hips off the branches like a woman with a mission. Obviously, she knew the plant well and had done this before.

I leaned forward and picked a single "hip" from the bush and popped it in my mouth. As I bit down, I experienced the sweetest, most delectable taste sensation. I picked another and another, and before I knew it, a full blown party was breaking out in my mouth. This was heaven. Life was good. Nature was king.

And then I picked a "hip" that tended toward more of a ruby red tone than the bright red cast of the others. As I bit into this one, the most awful taste engulfed my mouth. The party was over. It only took one bad hip to ruin the whole bunch. But up to then, I wanted to homestead that property.

POUR YOURSELF A CUP OF ROSE PETAL TEA

For centuries, people have imbibed rose petal tea and discovered amazing results.

These delicately fragrant flowers act as a **gentle blood purifier** as well as a **heart** and **nerve tonic**. They are also effective as a gentle aid to **diarrhea**. Externally, rose petal tea makes **a good eyewash for inflamed eyes** or when you have **redness due to eyestrain**.

There are those who say that rose petal tea might have **aphrodisiac qualities**, although that fact hasn't been proven by science…yet. It is known that one cup of rose petal tea can be **beneficial for a woman to drink after going through labor since it tends to ease residual pain and calm both mind and body**.

Pour eight ounces of hot water over one heaping teaspoon of dried petals (or two heaping teaspoons of fresh petals). Cover and allow to steep for 10 to 20 minutes. If the petals are fresh, you don't need to strain them and might even enjoy chewing them after you are finished with the tea. The recommended dose is anywhere from one to three cups a day. It makes a pleasant tea either hot or cold.

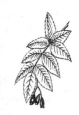

"GETTING HIPS" WITH THE BRITS

Apparently I wasn't the only one in history who imbibed rose hips with such passionate abandon. Over a thousand years before Christ, rose hips were considered "Food of the Gods." In England during World War II, there was a shortage of citrus fruit, among other things. The British needed their vitamin C to prevent scurvy and contagious diseases. When it was discovered that rose hips had plenty of "C" to go around, the government advised everyone from the local youth groups to the happy homemakers to go out into the fields and pick those hips. Within months, thousands of tons of rose hips were picked, eaten and made into syrups, preserves and teas.

I'm sure many of those British people would tell you today that the natural "C" found in the rose hips was the magic bullet that kept them healthy. Today, scientists tend to debunk that statement. They argue that one would have to eat or drink "a dangerously high volume" of rose hips to get the amount of vitamin C that is recommended.

But herbalists, nutritionists and holistic health practitioners strongly disagree. We know that **fresh rose hips straight off the bush have 60 times more vitamin C than citrus fruit**. A single rose hip approximately one inch in width is equivalent to 500 milligrams of vitamin C. One cup of fresh rose hips equals the vitamin C content found in *twelve dozen oranges!* The syrups, preserves, extracts and teas don't pack the same punch as the fresh fruit due to the cooking and drying process often needed to make them. However, they still retain around 30 to 40% of the initial levels of natural vitamin C found in the fresh fruit. That is still a fair amount of "C" compared to what you might be getting in the typical synthetic-based vitamin C tablet. (For an excellent rose hips jam that does not need to be cooked, check out the "Wild Foods Facts" box at the end of this chapter).

It is known that in order for vitamin C to really be effective it must be combined with bio-flavonoids. **In plants and berries that are known for their inherent vitamin C count, bio-flavonoids naturally occur together with no synthetic, lab-created "middle man."** Those bio-flavonoids are considered essential nutrients when it comes to **building and sustaining a strong vascular system**. This, in turn, helps those who suffer from **problems associated with veins and capillaries**. **What's more, when bio-flavonoids and vitamin C are in combination, they enhance the body's ability to absorb vitamin C and use it more efficiently**.

"C" WHAT IT'S GOOD FOR

So what's all this "C" good for? Plenty.

The obvious benefits of rose hips' strong "C" association are its ability to **treat infections**, **stimulate the immune system** and **prevent contagious disease**. Along with vitamin C, rose hips also have a healthy dose of vitamins A, B, E and K as well as iron, selenium, manganese, calcium and B-complex.

Rose hips tea acts as a **gentle blood purifier, cleansing the body of toxins which are eliminated through the kidneys**. This kidney connection is important since rose hips have been used **to prevent and even treat kidney stones and bladder infections by breaking up "gravel" (a.k.a., uric acid deposits)**. They do this without irritating the kidneys as many diuretics have been known to do.

When one is suffering from **colds and/or fevers**, rose hip tea can be a gentle and tasty drink that both **replenishes the system with much needed vitamins as well as supports the immune response and soothes the body**. For those who enjoy making homemade cough syrups, rose hips can be a nice addition to the brew. Besides the natural value of vitamin C, the hips coat the throat and add a sweet flavor to the syrup.

An infusion of rose hips tea taken three times a day is a **wonderful tonic when you have that "running on empty," exhausted feeling**. Furthermore, **one cup taken before bedtime is said to ensure a restful night's sleep**. You can thank rose hips' high vitamin C content for this feat since it works directly to **soothe the nervous system**.

If you suffer from **migraine headaches**, there has been great success with stopping the attacks when one takes three 100 milligram vitamin C tablets *which include natural rose hips*. **The secret to this "cure" is that you take the three 100 milligram tablets at the very beginning of the migraine attack**.

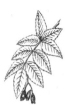

One to three cups of the tea each day are strongly recommended for those who have scheduled **minor or major surgery**. Start drinking the tea one to three weeks before the date of surgery. Not only does the herb **help prepare the body for trauma**, it also **works to repair cell damage where the skin has been cut**. Furthermore, drinking one to three cups after surgery has been known to help fend off possible post-operative infection. If you feel you need a bigger boost of infection-protection, one herbalist friend of mine suggests combining equal parts of dried rose hips with hibiscus (*Hibiscus sabdariffa*).

WATCH OUT FOR THOSE FADED HIPS

If you buy dried rose hips from the local herb/health store, their appearance should be bright red and not overly cracked from intense dryness. If they are pale, faded, yellow, orange or uneven in their appearance, they were harvested at the wrong time or dried improperly and are probably not very effective.

When making a tea from the rose hips, **DO NOT BOIL THEM**! This destroys their medicinal value. Place two teaspoons of dried hips (four teaspoons of fresh) into a cup and pour eight ounces of very hot water over them. Cover and let the hips steep for 20 minutes. Drink up to three cups a day for as long as four weeks. Even children under the age of two can enjoy the tea, although you'll want to cut the amount of rose hips in half.

The only caution is that **high doses of rose hips (or vitamin C alone for that matter) can cause diarrhea and put a strain on the kidneys. However, it takes a lot of rose hips for this to occur**. If you experience diarrhea or kidney strain from the rose hips tea, simply reduce your intake or stop taking it altogether.

You might be tempted to say that a rose hip is a rose hip is a rose hip. But once you partake of this "Food of the Gods," life may never be the same again.

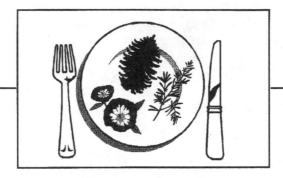

Wild Food Facts

Fresh rose petals—especially those that are highly fragrant—can be added in small amounts to salads. Chopped finely, the petals make an interesting addition to pancake batter, pudding, muffins and omelettes.

As mentioned earlier in this chapter, rose hips are always more nutritious when they are eaten fresh and uncooked. Here is a recipe for a tasty jam that works great on muffins or eaten alone as a sweet, vitamin-rich confection.

ROSE HIPS JAM RECIPE

Cut off both the stem and blossom ends of each rose hip. Make a slit down the middle of each hip and carefully remove all the seeds.

Put one cup of firmly-packed, prepared (unseeded) hips, 3/4 cup water and the juice of one lemon in the blender and blend until perfectly smooth.

Gradually add three cups of raw or brown sugar, running the blender all the time. Blend together for about five minutes more, so all the sugar is completely dissolved.

Dissolve one tablespoon of apple pectin powder in three-quarters of a cup of water. Bring the water to a boil and then boil hard for one minute. Add this to the puréed rose hips and blend for one minute more.

Pour mixture immediately into small, sterilized, screw-cap jars and store in the refrigerator. If it is to be kept for more than one month, store it in the freezer. Being uncooked, all the rich vitamin C content is retained and a tablespoon of this really tasty jam will give you your minimum daily requirement of vitamin C!

THE "DIRT" ON... WILD ROSE

Botanical ~
Rosa canina ("dog rose"), *R. villosa* ("apple rose"), *R. gallica* ("apothecary rose"), *R. rugosa* ("Japanese rose" or "wrinkled rose"), *R. centifolia* ("cabbage rose" or "provence rose"), *R. carolina* ("pasture" or "wild rose"), *R. eglanteria* ("sweetbrier rose") and many others.

Growth cycle ~
Hardy to delicate perennial, depending upon species and region where it is grown.

Medicinal uses~
Sedative, anti-depressant, antispasmodic, digestive stimulant, expectorant, anti-bacterial, anti-viral, antiseptic, anti-inflammatory, menstrual regulator, aphrodisiac.

Part(s) used for medicine ~ Hips (fruits), petals.

Vitamins/Minerals ~
Extraordinary amounts of vitamin C (one cup of prepared fresh rose hips have the vitamin C content found in 12 dozen oranges). Also, bioflavonids, iron, selenium, manganese, calcium, beta carotene, B-complex, D, E, K and zinc.

Region ~
Different varieties of wild roses are found in various areas around the United States. Wild roses are usually found thriving along roadsides, near streams and in meadows where there is moderate moisture and a good dose of organic matter around the base. Some species do best when they are exposed to seasonal freezing.

Wild or Domestic ~
Both.

Poisonous look-alikes in the wild ~
No.

Hardy or Delicate ~
Hardy.

Height of mature plant ~
Depends upon the variety. Wild roses vary from two feet to eighteen feet.

Easy or hard to grow ~
Moderately easy if maintained correctly. I think potted nursery plants are your best bet if you want to start off on the right foot.

Cultivation ~
Seed, cuttings, buddings or nursery stock (either dormant roots or potted plants). By far, you should choose nursery stock to make life less frustrating. (For more detailed instruction, refer to information at the beginning of this chapter under the heading "How Do I Grow It?")

Plant spacing ~
Three to four feet.

Pre-soak seeds ~
No.

Pre-chill seeds ~
Yes, but germination is very erratic. (That's why it is best to buy nursery stock).

Indoor seed starting ~	Not applicable.
Light/dark seed requirements ~	Light.
Days to germinate ~	Erratic. A lot depends upon the variety of rose.
Days to full maturity ~	Depends upon the variety and at which stage you planted it.
Soil type ~	Roses enjoy a fairly heavy loamy soil or a well-drained, compost-enriched soil bed.
Water requirements ~	Water once a week unless soil becomes excessively dry. Never drown or allow plant to stand in pools of water.
Sun or shade ~	Full sun to partial shade.
Propagation ~	Seed, but only under very specific natural conditions that involve temperature and weather patterns.
Easy/hard to transplant ~	Fairly easy either from dormant roots or potted plants. Follow directions in chapter under the heading "How Do I Grow It?"
Pests or diseases ~	Organically grown roses are more resistant to pests and disease. However, sometimes you encounter a few persistent pests such as aphids, leafhoppers, Japanese beetles, red spider mites and an array of slugs. Planting garlic and chives underneath each plant is said to help repel aphids. Wild roses can also attract mildew, canker, rust and blackspot. One of the easiest ways to prevent these is to keep the plant pruned so as to avoid dense foliage overgrowth.
Landscape uses ~	Excellent windbreak and "privacy" hedge between neighbors.
Gathering ~	**Rose petals** are harvested in late May to early June, depending upon the region. Petals should be gathered in early morning before the sun shines on them and before the flowers burst open. **Rose hips** are harvested between early October and late November when the fruit is bright red. If it has turned ruby red, it is too ripe and will be sour. If the hips are orange in color, leave them because they are not ripe.
Best fresh or dried ~	**Hips**: best fresh, but can be used dried; **Petals**: fresh or dried
Drying methods ~	**Petals:** Separate the petals from their white base (sometimes referred to as a "claw") which can contribute a rather bitter flavor. Use the petals fresh or dry them on a cloth, out of direct sunshine, but in a room where there is plenty of heat and low moisture. Petals need to be dried quickly and then stored immediately in an airtight glass container and placed in a dark cupboard to preserve their healing and aromatic power.

Rose hips: carefully slice the top and bottom off and cut the hips in half. Completely remove the abundant seeds before drying. Try to retain as much of the fleshy pulp inside the hip since that is where most of the vitamins are located. Lay the fruit out singly, fleshy side upward on an ungreased cookie sheet. Do not heap one hip on top of another since that tends to attract mold. Allow them to dry naturally in a covered, warm place. The hips are ready when they are slightly shriveled and hard to the touch. This can take anywhere from two to three weeks.

Amount needed ~

Three to five plants are sufficient for moderate use; five to fifteen plants might be necessary for more regular use.

Seed collection ~

Simply save the seeds that are gathered when you dry the rose hips. As mentioned earlier, planting roses from seed is a challenge.

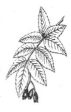

Companion planting ~

Usually, roses should be kept to themselves. The only exception to this rule would be to plant garlic and/or chives underneath the plant to help repel aphids.

Container planting ~

No. You can, however, temporarily keep the plant in a container for a few months before planting them outside in the spring.

Common mistakes ~

Simply not taking the time to maintain the plants so that they can flourish. Allowing too many plants to encroach around the roses which can choke off its development.

Interesting facts/tips ~

Pruning helps prevent diseases from attacking roses as well as promoting a better sized bloom the following year. Keep the surrounding area weeded to provide an optimum growing environment for the roses. Look for organic, balanced, fish-based plant food that includes ingredients such as fish bonemeal, bloodmeal and sulfate of potash. Applied every two to three months, this type of natural additive breaks down in the soil and feeds the roses gradually.

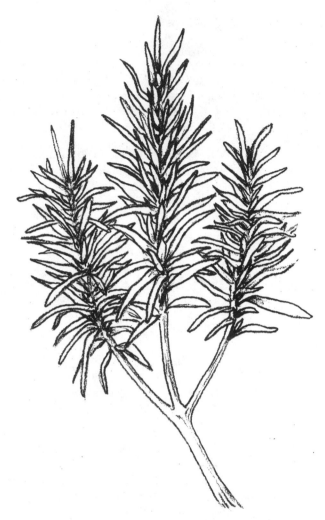

Chapter 29

A ROSEMARY TO REMEMBER

Rosmarinus officinalis
("W.F.")
Perennial

Medicinal Uses: *Antispasmodic, cholagogue, emmenagogue, stimulant, diuretic, stomachic, antiseptic, antirheumatic, anti-bacterial, antioxidant*

Medicinal parts of plant: *Leaves*

Forms: *Tea, tincture, pure essential oil*

WHAT IS ITS CHARACTER?

Rosemary is truly an independent soul. You can't tell this herb what to do. It will grow when and where it wants and likewise, *not* grow where it doesn't feel comfortable. Similar to independent human beings who prefer to live alone and dislike social interaction, rosemary tends to revolve in its own little circle, quite happy to perk along at its own speed. It also has developed a single-mindedness (very much like some independent humans) which overrides everything else. Rosemary's singular purpose in life is to produce a highly aromatic needle-like leaf. My best advice is not to bother rosemary too much. Say "hello" to it occasionally but never dote on it. Always remember, rosemary grows because it wants to—not because *you* want it to.

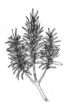

WHERE DO I FIND IT?

Different varieties are found from sea level to 9,000 feet. Some of the wild varieties are found growing in the foothills and hillsides of the southwestern United States as an erosion-control plant. Rosemary can tolerate most climates. However, it cannot live through weather that drops below 15°F.

HOW DO I GROW IT?

Rosemary is grown from seed, cuttings and established plants that are three years old or older. Of the three, I would choose established plants simply because they are more hearty and less trouble. Cuttings are erratic, slow growing and can take as long as six months to take hold. Seeds have a *very low* germination rate—about 20 percent. They require a steady temperature of 70°F to germinate, which can take 21 days or longer. Barely cover seed with soil. When seedlings reach three inches, transplant into larger pots, maintaining the 70°F temperature. When they reach six inches, transplant them into a pot or outside in a permanent location if you do not experience temperatures below 15°F. Plants grown from seed will not bloom for three years and should not be harvested until that point.

Established plants require about one good watering every seven to ten days. However, if you notice the soil drying out quickly, you may need to water more frequently. I've gone as long as three weeks between watering rosemary plants that were planted in the shade. If you wait too long and the leaves start to droop or curl, one good soaking normally perks up the entire plant within 12 hours. Be aware of pests such as scale which can destroy rosemary. If planted in a container, remove all the branches with scale and locate it away from the suspected host source. Container plants of rosemary are susceptible to aphids, whiteflies, spider mites and various fungus diseases. Young seedlings are prone to damping off disease if over watered.

HOW DO I HARVEST IT?

Harvest fresh leaves as needed from plants three or more years old. Gather no more than one-third of a plant since it takes awhile for rosemary to regenerate. Rosemary is best used fresh but you can also use the dried leaves. To dry, gather together three to five of the woody stalks, tying them together at one end with a piece of string or a rubber band. Hang them in a dry, warm area with a cloth underneath to catch any of the dried leaves as they fall. For moderate use, one medium-sized shrub is sufficient. For regular medicinal and culinary use, you might require three or more medium-sized shrubs.

HOW DO I USE IT?

A friend once told me she was having trouble remembering things. "Try some rosemary," I told her. "That should spark the ol' noggin." I saw her a few days later and asked her if she'd tried the herb. "No," she said, "I keep forgetting to pick it up."

If she can ever remember to get the plant, I know she won't be disappointed. Rosemary is considered to be one of the best brain stimulants and memory enhancers. This popular herb has always had a reputation for preserving your memory...and meat. Long before Mr. Frigidaire invented his refrigerator, folks discovered that if they packed their meat in layers of crushed rosemary leaves, the meat stayed fresh longer. Rosemary's preservation reputation had them leaping to the conclusion that rosemary could also "preserve" the memory. Greek students were soon wearing garlands of rosemary around their neck while they studied, convinced that the aroma of the fresh leaves would improve their learning skills. (I know a few students today who swear that diffusing rosemary pure essential oil into the air while they study helps them remember facts and figures). By the 16th century, rosemary took on another meaning in England. If the herb was growing outside the home, it signaled that the woman of the house—not the man—was in charge. This, of course, led to the men trampling, cutting and uprooting the plant to send out their own message.

ALZHEIMER'S ALLY

The message being sent these days is that rosemary is an herb which deserves serious attention. One of the most promising studies on rosemary involves its possible positive effect on Alzheimer's disease. Botanist, author and herbalist Dr. James Duke strongly believes that rosemary herb and essential oil might be effective in reducing the mental deterioration of the brain. Duke explains that the enzyme "acetylcholine," which is considered critical to nerve-impulse transmission, is often deficient in the brain of those with Alzheimer's. Its continued breakdown tends to parallel the mental decline of these patients. Rosemary has been shown to contain around 24 known antioxidants (i.e., compounds that slow the aging process at the cellular level). This is why rosemary works so well as a natural meat preservative. According to Duke, oxidative damage "plays a role in Alzheimer's." Several of the antioxidant compounds in rosemary have "proven equal in strength to synthetic antioxidants such as BHA and BHT." Thus, Duke put an herb and an illness together and encourages those with Alzheimer's to drink one or two cups of rosemary tea each day. If you prefer the tincture, I would suggest using one made from the fresh plant and combine 25 to 30 drops of the tincture in several ounces of hot water. This could be taken once or twice a day.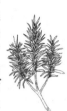

Dr. Duke doesn't stop there. He says that many of the antioxidant compounds that retard the breakdown of acetylcholine can be absorbed through the skin and may even cross the blood-brain barrier. Because of this, he theorizes that regular use of a rosemary shampoo could ostensibly have a similar effect on the brain. The effect might not be astounding but it could help some people. Your best bet is to buy a plain castile shampoo and add 25 drops of rosemary tincture for every ounce of shampoo. I would also add an additional five drops of rosemary pure essential oil to every ounce of shampoo. Not only does this give the shampoo a lovely aroma, it adds lots of shine to hair—especially dark hair. Feel free and add the essential oil (five drops per ounce) to your conditioner as well. I wouldn't add the tincture to the conditioner because that might alter the effectiveness of it. Since many popular conditioners have an array of chemical ingredients, try a brand from a health products store. *Aubrey Organics* is a good brand to consider.

WAKE UP! IT'S ROSEMARY!

Consider rosemary an herbal "wake up call." The tea as well as the pure essential oil are very stimulating to the body and to the senses. Because of this, you don't want to use rosemary in any form if your main objective is rest. Rosemary **stimulates circulation**, **metabolism**, **digestion** and **menstruation**. If you want to churn it up, call rosemary.

Got a **headache**? Reach for rosemary. Combine one teaspoon of the dried leaves or two teaspoons of the fresh plant for every eight ounces of hot water and steep for 10 to 20 minutes in a covered container. Strain and drink one-half to one cup of the tea at the onset of the headache pain. The tea is **good for tense, nervous headaches that are often brought on by stress**.

I've found that simply mixing one or two drops of the pure essential oil with about a teaspoon of almond, olive or castor oil and applying it to the temples and nape of the neck can give quick relief. This is especially **good for tension headaches and migraines where you are so upset you can hardly see straight**. If you have a tendency to grit your teeth during this stressful bout, you can apply the same mixture to your jaw line to release the tightness. To "juice up" the effect, add one drop of peppermint essential oil. This will add a cooling sensation that never fails to give at least moderate relief.

MUSCULAR & JOINT ROSEMARY RUB

Rosemary essential oil mixed in a base of apricot kernel oil or peanut oil can **help relieve sore or strained muscles**. If you're a long distance runner, an intrepid mountain biker or someone who just loves to test the limits of your muscular power, try rubbing rosemary oil mixed with one of the above "base" oils into your body *before* starting out. It may not stop the pain but it can cut down on the strain. The formula is two tablespoons of the "base" oil with 30 to 35 drops of rosemary essential oil mixed in. For **arthritis** and **rheumatism**, add an additional five drops *each* of juniper essential oil and lavender essential oil for a soothing rub that can temporarily reduce minor pain.

Rosemary tea, made from the fresh or dried leaves, is recommended for **arthritic** and **rheumatic joint pain** due to its **natural diuretic abilities**. The tea is thought to remove excess uric acid from the joints, thereby allowing more fluid movement. One or two cups a day is sufficient.

A DIVINE DINNER TEA

This fragrant leaf tea makes an excellent beverage to **promote better digestion**. Rosemary improves liver function which, in turn, increases the flow of bile. Bile helps break down fat and prevents putrefaction in the intestines. I would either drink one cup of the tea with a meal or as an aromatic after-dinner libation.

FEELING DEPRESSED? GIVE ROSEMARY A CALL

A rosemary bath can **clear your head and stimulate your senses** and **increase circulation**. It's a great bath to take if you're feeling **depressed**, **mental fatigue**, **lethargy** or **apathy**. Best of all, the scent will linger throughout the house for several hours. Steep a handful of dried leaves (two handfuls of fresh) in several quarts of very hot water. Cover the container and let the mixture sit for 20 to 30 minutes. Strain the tea into the bath water and soak for as long as you wish. If you really want to perk up this experience, put 15 drops of rosemary essential oil into a tablespoon of apricot kernel oil and swish it into the bath water. I can't guarantee it, but when you get out of that tub, you should feel much more alert than when you got in. Since this is a stimulating bath, I would refrain from trying it at night when your goal is a good night's sleep.

A rosemary foot bath (using half the measurements mentioned above) is a **terrific pick-me-up for tired feet**. To boost the circulation properties, add a few drops of either rosemary essential oil or lavender essential oil to the water. This is a wonderful foot bath for the elderly or infirmed— especially if they tend to have "cold feet" due to lack of activity and circulation.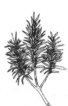

Another effective way to **beat the "blues"** is to diffuse the aroma of rosemary essential oil into the air. I like to use a brass or *glazed* ceramic lamp ring that fits either directly on top of the light bulb or rests directly above the bulb on the lamp shade's metal support bars. Place no more than 10 drops of rosemary essential oil into the ring and adjust it on an *unlit* light bulb that is between 40 and 60 watts. Once it is firmly in place, turn on the light. Within several minutes, the soft aroma should be wafting through the air. Adding an additional 10 drops of lavender essential oil makes a truly **anti-depressant, nerve-soothing** aromatic treatment for the senses. If you just need to feel a little more lively, a classic combo is 10 drops *each* of rosemary essential oil and peppermint essential oil. I've seen this light a fuse under folks who were running on empty. My only advice is not to expose hyperactive kids to this very energizing formula. I tried that once just to see what would happen and they nearly levitated off the ground.

YOUR ANTISEPTIC, WOUND-HEALING FRIEND

Arabs used to sprinkle dried rosemary leaf powder on the umbilical cord of newborns to act as an astringent and natural antiseptic agent. Modern research has found that rosemary indeed has natural antiseptic as well as anti-bacterial qualities. For this reason, you might want to keep a small jar of dried leaf powder in the medicine cabinet to sprinkle on **minor scrapes and cuts**. Topical use of rosemary has also been shown to **promote the healing of wounds**. This makes the herb very valuable since it allows new skin growth while inhibiting any possible infection within the wound.

Thanks to rosemary's natural antiseptic qualities, a double strength tea makes an **excellent gargle for a sore or inflamed throat**.

STIMULATING RECOVERY TEA

A cup or two of rosemary tea (fresh or dried) makes an excellent beverage for those who are **recovering from an illness and are having a difficult time regaining their strength**. I've found it especially good **when a person feels sluggish or "logy" and finds it hard to remember simple words in conversations**. Adding approximately 25 drops of ginkgo biloba tincture to the tea can pump an additional shot of oxygen into the head.

FLEA AND BUG PROTECTION

Rosemary essential oil works as **an effective bug repellant** when five to ten drops are mixed into a tablespoon of apricot kernel oil. Some people promote the topical use of rosemary essential oil on dogs and cats to prevent and repel fleas. I think this is a questionable practice since I don't believe essential oils should *ever* be taken internally. Since dogs and cats lick themselves, there's a good chance they would ingest some of the essential oil. I have seen instances where animals had a negative reaction to the topical use of essential oils—either rubbed into their coat or added to their collar. Because of this, I cannot recommend the use of rosemary essential oil as a flea repellant. However, it would be safe to wash your pet in rosemary tea, use rosemary soap or rub 10 drops of the tincture into their fur.

"HAIRS" TO ROSEMARY

You can also sprinkle two to three drops of the essential oil into your hair brush to **stimulate hair growth and add shine without making your hair oily**. And three drops mixed into the palms of your hand and rubbed into dry hair helps **combat dandruff**. I discovered another scalp-related use for rosemary essential oil. During a summer camping trip, I awoke one morning to find that I had been bitten across my scalp by fleas and mites. I couldn't stop scratching my head. What did I do? I poured one tablespoon of castile shampoo into my hand and added about 15 drops of rosemary essential oil and vigorously washed my hair, allowing it to stay on my head for about 10 minutes. I placed the same amount of essential oil into the conditioner, letting it sink into my scalp for about five or ten minutes. After only one treatment, the itching was reduced by about 80 percent. Another shampoo and conditioning treatment finally did the trick and those bites dried up within a day.

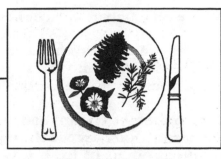

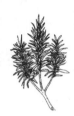

Wild Food Facts

Toss fresh or dried rosemary leaves into soups, stews and omelettes to add a stimulating flavor.

Thanks to rosemary's amazing antioxidant qualities, it has been used effectively as a temporary preservative against food spoilage—especially with meat. The oils in rosemary prevent the fats in meat from going rancid. For this reason, I've used them on picnic and hiking food. For example, I've pressed fresh leaves into sandwich meat, mixed them into cottage cheese, sour cream, potato salad and anything else that could spoil due to exposure to heat. You can pick off the leaves when you eat the food or leave them on. While history shows us that this method of food preservation was meant for months instead of hours, I have no experience using rosemary as a preventative against spoilage on a long-term basis.

A TEA SOAK FOR TIRED EYES

A cotton pad dipped into a cup of cool rosemary tea can be the perfect natural answer to **tired eyes**. Just lay the soaked cotton pad over your closed eyes and rest for 10 to 15 minutes.

YOUR FRIENDLY ANTI-FAINTING HERB

Because it has a stimulating aroma, rosemary tea and essential oil are good to have on hand **if someone faints**. A whiff or two of rosemary essential oil is a lot gentler than smelling salts. Once the "fainter" has come back to life, one cup of strong rosemary tea should help them remain vertical.

SOME CAUTIONS TO REMEMBER

Rosemary essential oil and the tea can bring on menstruation. Sometimes, simply rubbing the oil around your hip region will encourage your period to begin. For this reason, **pregnant women should not use rosemary in tea or oil form**. A sprig or two to season your food is okay as long as the meat isn't packed with the herb. **The essential oil can burn the skin of some people and therefore should always be di-**

luted using a gentle base oil (such as apricot kernel oil) before being applied to the skin.

If you have high blood pressure, it's not a good idea to use rosemary essential oil—either diffused into the air or in a massage formula. It has a tendency to aggravate the condition since it is such a stimulating aroma.

Also, **excessive internal doses for anybody can cause stomach cramps and even poisoning. Don't exceed the typical one teaspoon of dried leaves (or two teaspoons of fresh leaves) for every eight ounces of hot water**.

For all this herb can do, it's definitely worth remembering.

THE "DIRT" ON...ROSEMARY

Botanical ~	*Rosmarinus officinalis*
Growth cycle ~	Perennial.
Medicinal uses~	Antispasmodic, cholagogue, emmenagogue, stimulant, diuretic, stomachic, antiseptic, antirheumatic, anti-bacterial, antioxidant.
Part(s) used for medicine ~	Leaves.
Vitamins/Minerals ~	Loaded with natural antioxidants (compounds that slow the aging process).
Region ~	Different varieties are found from sea level to 9,000 feet. Some of the wild varieties are grown in the foothills and hillsides of the southwestern United States as an erosion-control plant. Rosemary can tolerate most climates. However, it cannot live through weather that drops below 15°F.
Wild or Domestic ~	Both.
Poisonous look-alikes in the wild ~	No.
Hardy or Delicate ~	Hardy.
Height of mature plant ~	Three feet.
Easy or hard to grow ~	Hard from seed, tricky from a cutting, easy from established seedlings or three-year-old plants and older.
Cultivation ~	Rosemary is grown from seed, cuttings and established plants. Of the three, I would choose established plants simply because they are more hearty and less trouble.

Cuttings are erratic, slow growing and can take as long as six months to take hold. Seeds have a very low germination rate—about 20 percent. They require a steady temperature of 70°F to germinate, which can take 21 days or longer. Cover seed barely with soil. When seedlings reach three inches, transplant into larger pots, maintaining the 70°F temperature. When they reach six inches, transplant them into a pot or outside in a permanent location if you do not experience temperatures below 15°F. Plants grown from seed will not bloom for three years and should not be harvested until that point.

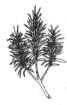

Plant spacing ~	One to two feet.
Pre-soak seeds ~	No.
Pre-chill seeds ~	No.
Indoor seed starting ~	Yes.
Light/dark seed requirements ~	Light.
Days to germinate ~	21 days or longer.
Days to full maturity ~	From seed, three years.
Soil type ~	Light, sandy, well-drained.
Water requirements ~	Needs light spray of moisture as a seedling. Once mature, requires little water, perhaps once a week if soil dries out. If the leaves begin to droop, I've found that a good soaking will bring the plant back to life within 12 hours.
Sun or shade ~	Full sun.
Propagation ~	Seed, underground roots.
Easy/hard to transplant ~	Easy from seedlings or small established plants; from firmly established garden plants five years old or older, difficult.
Pests or diseases ~	Scale can destroy rosemary since it latches onto it and sucks the oils from the leaves. If planted in a container, remove all the branches with scale and locate it away from suspected host source. Container plants of rosemary are susceptible to aphids, whiteflies, spider mites and various fungus diseases. Young seedlings are prone to damping off disease if over watered.
Landscape uses ~	Wonderful aromatic hedge that can eventually become quite dense. South-facing placement in yard is best. One of the best varieties for a tall hedge is called "Miss Jessopp's Upright Rosemary" which can grow as tall as six feet.
Gathering ~	Harvest fresh leaves as needed from plants three or more years old. Gather no more than one-third of a plant since it takes a while for rosemary to regenerate.
Best fresh or dried ~	Best fresh, however dried works fine too.
Drying methods ~	Gather together three to five of the woody stalks, tying them together at one end with a piece of string or a rub-

ber band. Hang them in a dry, warm area with a cloth underneath to catch any of the dried leaves as they fall.

Amount needed ~

One medium-sized shrub for moderate use. Regular use might require three or more medium-sized shrubs.

Seed collection ~

Rosemary seed is very small and can be difficult to gather from the flower heads. Wait until the flower heads begin to dry and shake them into a white cloth. If possible, plant the fresh seed immediately as long as the growing requirements are right.

Companion planting ~

Planting nettles nearby can increase the aromatic oil content of rosemary.

Container planting ~

Yes. This is your best bet if you live in regions that experience 15°F or lower since you can bring the containers indoors. Keep in mind that rosemary needs room to grow. Choose a deep, wide container that allows for future growth.

Common mistakes ~

The tendency to over water rosemary can be a strong one, especially with young seedlings. Only water when the soil is completely dry and/or the plant shows signs of drooping.

Interesting facts/tips ~

When rosemary does decide to die, it dies and nothing can bring it back to life. To ensure a healthy plant, it should ideally be replanted or replaced every five to six years. The fresh leaves are said to repel moths. Dried rosemary and juniper branches were burned in sick wards in French hospitals during World War II to clean the air and act as a natural antiseptic against infection.

Chapter 30

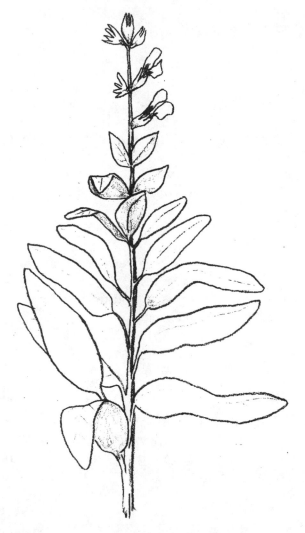

SAGE ADVICE

Salvia officinalis (garden sage)

Salvia sclarea (clary sage)

Hardy perennial

Medicinal Uses: *Astringent, antihydrotic, antispasmodic, antiseptic, circulatory stimulant, bactericidal*

Medicinal parts of plant: *Leaves*

Forms: *Tea, tincture, pure essential oil*

WHAT IS ITS CHARACTER?

I've always felt rather sorry for garden sage. When the other plants are at their height of bloom and color, there sage sits, looking rather dowdy and plain with its "army green" leaves. It tends to get lost amidst the greens, blues, yellows and reds that cover the summer landscape. Somehow, I think sage has come to terms with the fact that it's never going to be the bell of the ball. It faithfully returns year after year, happy to lend a medicinal hand or content to simply stand in your garden and take a backseat to other more attractive herbs. Because of this, whenever I see garden sage, I always go over and say "hello." Funny thing is, it always thinks I'm talking to the plant behind it.

WHERE DO I FIND IT?

If you happen to be traveling along the Mediterranean coast, you will find the so-called "garden sage" growing wild. Everywhere else, this plant is cultivated. Garden sage is usually found growing in dry to semi-arid regions from sea level to 7,000 feet.

HOW DO I GROW IT?

Sage can be difficult to grow from seed. If you don't think you have a "green thumb," consider purchasing established seedlings or plants instead.

Broadcast seed in early spring in *moist, cool ground,* barely covering seed. *It really helps if the seed can be exposed to a period of 35°-45°F temperatures for one or two weeks.* Without this special handling, germination can be very erratic. The typical germination time is seven to twenty-one days.

To ensure better germination, you might want to start the seeds indoors in either cells or dirt flats. Expose them to one or two weeks of moist, cold temperatures that range from 35°-45°F. Seedlings require consistent moisture to get started. Never drown them with water or they will dampen off. When seedlings are two inches high, carefully transplant into larger containers or outside if weather permits. Space plants one to two feet apart.

HOW DO I HARVEST IT?

Harvest the leaves just before plant flowers, which is usually in midsummer. Gather only from plants that are two to four years old to ensure optimum medicinal effect. Cut stems four to five inches above the ground. Gather together five to eight leafy stems and secure base with a piece of string or a rubber band. Dry in a cool, dry environment, away from direct sunlight. Once leaves are brittle to the touch, strip them from the stems and store in airtight glass containers. Never overdry leaves since they will lose their aromatic value.

HOW DO I USE IT?

There's nothing like walking through a field of sagebrush after a hard rain has drummed that heady fragrance into the air. The bittersweet aroma sweeps across the summer wind, allowing the most wonderful scent to filter into the valleys and through the corridors of brush. Ah, sagebrush. To smell it is to know heaven.

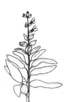

To *eat* sagebrush, however, is to know nausea. So let's make it clear: when I talk about sage, I'm talking about *garden* sage—the stuff you grow in the garden, NOT the common sagebrush that layers the hillsides.

Garden sage is first and foremost an **astringent** and **disinfectant**. One of the active ingredients in sage is *thujone* which gives the herb its antiseptic qualities. However, thujone taken in large doses and over a long period of time can be potentially toxic to your system. Because of this, **sage is not a long-term tea**. Drink it for only seven to ten days at a time with about two weeks off in between. During that seven to ten day period, you can drink up to three cups a day.

"THE MOUTH HERB"

One of the time-honored uses for sage is as a **gargle for a sore throat**. It's **the "mouth" herb** to many herbalists because it does such a bang up job on **gums and the mucous membrane of the mouth**.

To use sage as a gargle, make a tea using either fresh garden sage leaves (two heaping teaspoons) or the dried variety (one heaping teaspoon). Let the leaves steep for five to ten minutes in eight ounces of hot water and then cool until warm. Strain the leaves and use up all the liquid in the cup, allowing each "gargle" to last as long as possible. After several "gargles," you might notice a slight constriction in your throat and even a numbing effect. This is the strong astringency in sage doing it's work. To speed the healing of your sore throat, you'll want to keep gargling about every two to three hours. The advantage is that not only does sage **numb the soreness in your throat, it also works as a disinfectant, killing any nasty bacteria that are causing you grief**.

Sage is great for **relieving bleeding gums, reducing canker sores** and even **diminishing pressure sores caused by dentures or braces**. It also works as a **mouthwash to eliminate bad breath**. To use sage for these symptoms, make a tea as mentioned above and, while still warm, swish the liquid in your mouth for as long as possible. The only unpleasant effect you may experience is a kind of dry mouth sensation. Once again, this is sage's astringent ability literally pulling all the tissues together and soaking up excess liquid. If it bothers you, dilute the tea with more water and/or swish it in your mouth for less time.

DON'T FORGET SAGE

Like the herb rosemary, sage tea is **helpful in improving concentration and memory**. This is not some new-fangled idea. Back in the 17th century, famed herbalist John Gerard wrote that "sage helpeth a weake braine or memory and restoreth them...in a short time."

Recent studies have shown that sage activates the brain in various ways. First, similar to rosemary, sage has many powerful antioxidants (anti-aging compounds) which could prevent "spoilage" of brain tissue. Identical to rosemary, sage—specifically the *oil* in the plant—inhibits the breakdown of acetylcholine in the brain. Lack of this enzyme has been found in patients suffering from **Alzheimer's** disease. In addition, sage supplies oxygen to the cortex of the brain which acts to revitalize the brain and help bring one's thoughts into better focus. Further, its **natural ability to feed the nerves makes it a good tea when you are burned out or suffering from mental fatigue**.

Everyone from students and lecturers to actors have employed sage tea at specific times to "tune up" their brain and sharpen their memories. In the case of students who are cramming for tests and trying to remember more than seems humanly possible, one cup of sage tea taken before studying can help bring the facts into focus. By the way, please don't fall into that "more is better" mentality and think that if one cup will help sharpen your memory, *six cups* will make you a genius. Remember that the ingredient *thujone* is often toxic in large amounts.

NATURAL ANTIPERSPIRANT

With its strong astringent properties, sage is excellent for people who suffer from **excessive perspiration**. By soaking in a sage bath for up to 30 minutes, three times a week, you should notice a change in your body. However, this bath can be awfully drying to the skin since it pulls out surface moisture. If you are already prone to dry skin, I wouldn't do the bath since it really does suck out every drop of moisture. To make the bath, place one cup of dried sage leaves in two quarts of very hot water. Cover and let it steep for 20 minutes. Strain and add to a hot bath. If you have dark hair, **soak your locks in the water as well to bring out the dark highlights**. In fact, rinsing your hair with sage tea on a regular basis is said to **encourage hair growth**. However, the tea tends to dry out the hair over time. Because of this, follow up the rinse with one of those "leave in" conditioners.

Women who are experiencing **night sweats during menopause** have found almost immediate relief by drinking a *lukewarm to cool* cup of sage tea before bedtime. The effect usually kicks in about two hours later and, for some women, it can last for *days*. Since sage tea is not recommended for long term use, try alternating the internal tea with a sage bath as long as the bath water is not too hot.

WEANING WONDER HERB

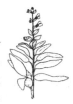

For years, **nursing mothers have turned to sage tea when they wanted to dry up their breast milk**. The herb's slight estrogenic properties are thought to play a part in this as well as that strong astringent ability. If you would like to try this, use *only cold sage tea* and drink no more than three cups a day. You should note the effect within one week.

NIP THAT COLD BEFORE IT NIPS YOU

Sage's latin genus "Salvia" means "to save." Throughout history, sage has been thought of as "the savior herb," capable of doing anything. Some writers in the Middle Ages went so far as to say that sage "rendered Man immortal." I never really understood the romance with sage until I met a family from Canada who kept telling me about this great herb they relied upon whenever they felt as though they were **catching a cold**. When I asked them to show me the plant, one of their children led me over to garden sage. "Sage?" was my response. It wasn't the first herb I would grab when I was feeling sick. But these folks considered it a "miracle plant." The mother explained that the minute anyone felt sick, she would give them one or two cups of hot sage tea within the space of two hours. She followed this by a hot bath and then rest in a warm bed with plenty of blankets. If the cold was still present, another two cups were given. I asked if this process worked once someone was already sick and she enthusiastically told me sage worked either way. I'd say ol' sage is worth a try the next time you feel a cold coming your way.

AN ANTISEPTIC WOUND & BITE HEALER

Here's another good reason to plant sage in your garden. The next time you are **bitten by an insect, stung by a bee** or get a **minor scrape**, grab a fresh sage leaf, crush it between your fingers to release the oils and press it into the area. Hold it in place with either your hand or a piece of masking tape. The antiseptic qualities help to reduce the pain and cleanse the area of any possible infection. You can also bathe the area in sage tea

267

or sprinkle a fine powder of the dried leaves over the skin to achieve the same results.

TRIGGER THAT CYCLE

If your period is irregular or late, drinking a very hot cup of sage tea can often **bring on a menstrual cycle** within a day or two. Once again, those estrogenic properties in sage work to balance a woman's body and allow it to come back into balance.

CONSIDER THE ESSENTIAL OIL

Sage is available in a highly concentrated essential oil which should be used sparingly. There are two different sage essential oils: *Salvia officinalis* (also known as "dalmatian sage") which is used in lots of soaps, colognes and natural deodorants and *Salvia sclarea* (more commonly called "clary sage.")

Let's take dalmatian sage first. Just as sage dries up excess water in the body, it also pulls out oily secretions. This makes the essential oil valuable if you have **overly oily skin**. Add no more than five drops of the essential oil for every ounce of facial or body moisturizer. If you feel a slight burning sensation on your skin, reduce the amount of essential oil.

Place eight to ten drops of sage essential oil in a lamp ring and diffuse the aroma into the room as a **natural disinfectant** and **deodorizer**. The scent is uplifting for many. However, it can be depressing for others. As always, people respond to essential oils in very individual ways based upon their past positive or negative experience with a particular fragrance. One reaction that seems to be the most consistent is that **sage essential oil uplifts those who are buried under too much book work, schoolwork or are mentally exhausted**. Give it a try. It's amazing what a little aroma can do for you.

Clary sage essential oil is known for its incredible ability to **knock the blues out of the bluesiest beast**. Sometimes if you're feeling down, just taking a whiff of clary sage essential oil is enough to perk you right up. If you're feeling fine and you take a whiff of clary sage oil, you might feel a bit of a rush. Too much of this, though, will make you feel a tad woozy and can give you a headache.

Postnatal depression is a reality for many women. While clary sage oil may not mellow the melancholy completely, it can certainly **lift the spirits**. Keep a bottle of clary sage nearby and take a sniff whenever you are feeling low. You can also soak in a hot bath to which you've added five to ten drops of the oil *right before you get into the tub*. Let the warm aroma fill the bathroom and take deep, long breaths of the scent.

A clary sage essential oil bath is also **good for kids when they're grumpy or throwing tantrums**. Getting the kid in the bath is half the battle, but many mothers have relied on this approach when all else failed.

Clary sage essential oil also has the ability to lessen or eliminate **jet lag**. I heard this and decided to try it when I traveled to Egypt since I suffer from terrible jet lag. I carried the bottle in my purse and sprinkled a few drops of the oil on a cotton ball which I kept tucked into my shirt pocket. In order for clary sage to work, I was told to consistently sniff the aroma at least twice an hour. I did just that and you know what? I didn't have any jet lag. Was it the clary sage or was it mind over matter? I don't know. But I do know that every time I smell clary sage, my "aromatic memory" catapults me back to that airplane, sniffing the cotton ball.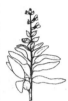

The only caution for clary sage essential oil is that it tends **to strengthen the effects of alcohol**. In other words, if you've had a few martinis and smell clary sage aroma or soak in a clary sage bath, the effects of the alcohol can be deepened. Thus, stay away from clary sage if you've had a little too much of the bubbly.

IMPORTANT CAUTIONS

One important point: **DO NOT DRINK SAGE TEA IF YOU ARE PREGNANT**. The *thujone* content and the uterine stimulating qualities in the herb are too strong.

Both sage tea and dalmatian sage oil have been known to bring on epileptic seizures. If you suffer from epilepsy, stay away from this herb in all forms.

Those with high blood pressure should also not use the herb or essential oil since they can aggravate the condition due to their stimulating properties.

As always, never ingest either of the essential oils.

Now that you know what this herb and essential oil can do, you can truly offer your friends and family some solid sage advice.

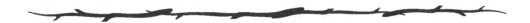

THE "DIRT" ON...GARDEN SAGE

Botanical ~	*Salvia officinalis*
Growth cycle ~	Hardy perennial.
Medicinal uses~	Astringent, antihydrotic, antispasmodic, antiseptic, circulatory stimulant, bactericidal.
Part(s) used for medicine ~	Leaves.
Vitamins/Minerals ~	Calcium, potassium, vitamin A, B_1, B_2, B-complex, zinc, magnesium, sodium, iron, niacin.
Region ~	Garden sage can be found growing in dry to semi-arid regions from sea level to 7,000 feet.
Wild or Domestic ~	Wild along the Mediterranean coast; domestic everywhere else, although some plants may escape to wild settings.
Poisonous look-alikes in the wild ~	No. However, some people assume that sagebrush (*Artemisia tridentata*) and wormwood (*Artemisia vulgaris*) are the same as garden sage due to their similar odor and common name of "sage." These are two completely different plants and should never be used as a "replacement" for garden sage.
Hardy or Delicate ~	Hardy.
Height of mature plant ~	One to two feet.
Easy or hard to grow ~	Can be difficult from seed. If you don't think you have a "green thumb," consider purchasing established seedlings or plants instead.
Cultivation ~	Broadcast seed in early spring in moist, cool ground, barely covering seed. It really helps if the seed can be exposed to a period of 35°-45°F temperatures for one or two weeks. Without this special handling, germination can be very erratic.
Plant spacing ~	One to two feet.
Pre-soak seeds ~	No.
Pre-chill seeds ~	Yes. Specifically, planting seeds in a moist, cold soil can ensure better germination.
Indoor seed starting ~	Yes. Start seed in either cells or dirt flats, exposing them to one or two weeks of moist, cold temperatures that range from 35°-45°F. Seedlings require consistent moisture to get started. Never drown or they will dampen off. When seedlings are two inches high, carefully transplant into larger containers or outside if weather permits.
Light/dark seed requirements ~	Light.

Days to germinate ~	Seven to twenty-one days.
Days to full maturity ~	Approximately 90 to 120 days.
Soil type ~	Light, sandy, rocky, well-drained, slightly alkaline.
Water requirements ~	Seedlings need regular moisture in well-drained soil. Once the plants are established, sage needs very little water.
Sun or shade ~	Full sun.
Propagation ~	Seed, roots.
Easy/hard to transplant ~	Easy, once seedlings are two inches and have developed good root systems.
Pests or diseases ~	Plants that are left to stand in pools of water are prone to root rot and wilting.
Landscape uses ~	Hardy filler or border. Good in desert gardens where other dry soil loving plants such as cacti abound.
Gathering ~	Harvest leaves just before plant flowers, which is usually in mid-summer. Gather from plants that are two to four years old to ensure optimum medicinal effect.
Best fresh or dried ~	Both.
Drying methods ~	Cut stems four to five inches above the ground. Gather together five to eight leafy stems and secure base with string or rubber band. Dry in cool, dry environment, away from direct sunlight. Once leaves are brittle to the touch, strip them from the stems and store in airtight glass containers. Never over dry leaves since they will lose their aromatic value.
Amount needed ~	Moderate use: 15 plants; Regular use: 20 to 35.
Seed collection ~	Sage seed does not store well. Because of this, the fresh, tiny seed is most viable. That means that when sage flowers and goes to seed in late summer, shake the flower heads into a white paper bag (white makes the dark seed easier to see) and plant immediately, following the cultivation directions.
Companion planting ~	Sage is thought to repel cabbage moths and carrot flies. Interspersing sage between these two vegetables may be beneficial.
Container planting ~	No.
Common mistakes ~	Confusing garden sage (which is in the *Salvia* genus) with sagebrush (which is in the *Artemisia* genus).
Interesting facts/tips ~	Sage is most medicinally active when it is between two to four years old. After that, the medicinal value begins to sharply decline. When you replant new seeds or seedlings, choose a different location in your garden since sage does not do well when replanted in the same soil.

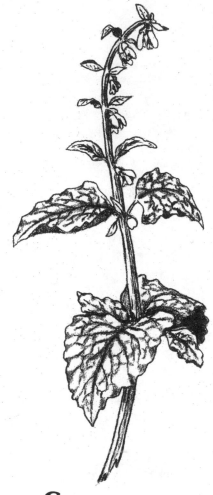

Chapter 31

SKULLCAP

~

SOOTHING SOLACE WITHOUT SEDATION

Scutellaria lateriflora

Hardy perennial

Medicinal Uses: *Antispasmodic, diuretic, nervine, anodyne, whole body tonic*

Medicinal parts of plant: *Entire above ground plant*

Forms: *Tea, tincture (made only from the fresh plant)*

WHAT IS ITS CHARACTER?

If skullcap could talk, I think it would speak softly. When you find it in the wild—which is rarely—it tends to quietly make its presence known. It's not that it doesn't want to be found, it just isn't into advertising its appearance in neon lights. I will say that it always seems delighted to see people and be appreciated for its value. The funny thing about skullcap is that as the flowers open, each one looks like a wide open mouth, held high and on the verge of singing. It makes me think it's a rather carefree little plant, happy as a lark to be alive and eager to be your friend.

WHERE DO I FIND IT?

Originally, skullcap was native in the eastern states. It has since moved westward and can be found in moist meadows and along streams from 1,000 feet to 10,000 feet.

HOW DO I GROW IT?

Skullcap can be grown from seed, root cuttings and root division. Of the three, I think root division is the easiest. The trick is finding someone who (a) grows skullcap and (b) is willing to let you dig up their crop. Your second best method is to grow the herb from seed. Broadcast skullcap seed into wet, fertile, well-drained soil in early spring when you know all chances of a hard frost are over. Press the seed into the moist earth and keep it well watered without drowning. I have had luck with pre-chilling the seeds in a flat for one week prior to exposing the flat to heat. However, I have also tossed the seed into late spring soil once the temperature warmed up and had a nice crop.

For indoor seed starting, I think seed cells work best over dirt flats since it is easier to transplant the individual cells into the garden. Make sure the soil stays moist without drowning the seed. I had *great* results when I covered the seed flat with a plastic dome and allowed the interior to become hot and humid. My only suggestion is that you will want to transplant the seedlings into the garden before they become root-bound in the cells. If that happens, skullcap starts to fade quickly and may not survive the transplant.

HOW DO I HARVEST IT?

Always wait until skullcap is fully in bloom before harvesting. This is usually around August to September, depending upon your region. After several years of the plant successfully proliferating in your garden, you should be able to develop a rather dense patch of skullcap. If you live in regions that allow for year-round growing, it is conceivable to get as many as three cuttings each year from that one planting.

Skullcap is always best used *fresh*—either as a tea or made into a tincture from the freshly picked plant—due to the fact that the herb loses medicinal power quickly in the dried form. However, history has shown that the dried plant is effective if properly stored in airtight glass jars and kept away from any heat source.

Cut skullcap several inches above the ground. Place the plant on a drying rack or on a clean cloth *in the shade and completely away from any direct heat.* If skullcap is exposed to excessive heat in the drying process, most of the medicinal action is lost. Check the plant frequently to chart progress. Once it is dry to the touch, crush up the entire plant—leaves, stems and flowers—and store it in an airtight, glass jar. If kept in this manner, dried skullcap should be medicinally viable for six to nine months.

HOW DO I USE IT?

During one of my classes several years ago, a woman asked me to name my favorite calming herb. Without hesitation, I said, "That's easy. Skullcap."

"Are you trying to be funny?" she said with a skeptical look.

"No," I said, "I would use skullcap if I needed to relax."

"And where would you put it?" she asked pointedly.

"Where would I put it?" I said, getting a little bemused. "Well, since I'm making a tea or a tincture out of it, I'd—"

"You'd make a tea or tincture out of it?" she interrupted. "I've heard enough!" She turned on her heels and headed for the door. "I came here to learn about *herbs*. And now you're telling me that whenever I need to calm down, I'm supposed to make a tea out of a Judaic religious head covering! You're *crazy!*"

If she had stayed around a little longer, I would have assured her that the skullcap *I* referred to was indeed an actual plant from the common mint family. While the name "skullcap" might sound weird, I assure you the herb is not.

Skullcap—named after the small "cap" that shrouds its mauve/purple flowers—is first and foremost **a tonic for the nerves**. It received its biggest press buzz over 200 years ago when a New England doctor discovered it could prevent "the mad dog's bite": a.k.a. **rabies**. A Dr. Vandesveer claimed to stop 400 people and 1000 cows from "going mad" after they were attacked by a pack of wild dogs by giving them copious doses of skullcap. Word got out and the good doctor quickly became the town hero. He nicknamed the herb "mad dog-weed," a name that has stuck to this day. But, alas, the medical community scoffed at Dr. Vandesveer's nonscientific approach. For years afterwards, skullcap wasn't given much attention by the medical community who deemed this plant "useless."

However, Chinese and American herbalists pressed on and finally uncovered skullcap's real potential. And that was as a **gentle, non-addictive sedative**.

A "SPECIFIC HERB"

Skullcap is considered to be **a "specific herb" for anyone suffering from a nervous condition brought on by emotional distress, worry and, thanks to its antispasmodic ability, accompanying digestive problems**. One old herbal book states that skullcap "quiets frantic, neurotic women." They may have been referring to the fact that **skullcap helps women during PMS**. However, might I add that skullcap can also quiet those frantic, neurotic men, as well. You can replace the word "neurotic" with "easily excited" as in the case of someone who sees life more as a continual melodrama rather than a long play with occasional action sequences. Skullcap won't sedate or tranquilize you into a stupor. Instead, it will, over time, **nourish the nervous system and gently restore balance**. However, the operative words here are *over time* because it takes skullcap many consistent doses before users will see any lasting benefits.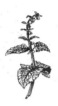

As skullcap feeds the nerves, it gradually builds a support system that will help sustain the body, allowing greater productivity without that "nervous edge." Skullcap is considered the herb of choice for **workaholics who force themselves to put in long days, only to end up with complete mental exhaustion**.

THE INSOMNIAC'S BEST FRIEND

The most common use for skullcap is as a gentle, non-addictive sleep aid. More specifically, **if your insomnia is caused by pain, skullcap could be your best friend due to its slight anodyne (pain-killing) effects. Skullcap has been used to take the edge off of pain that has resulted from a nerve related injury or disease**.

As a sleep remedy, skullcap can be made into a tea or taken in tincture form. Remember, the *fresh* herb is more medicinally active than the dried plant which rapidly deteriorates. Because of this, it is best to make the tea from the freshly cut plant, with two heaping teaspoons of the herb for every eight ounces of hot water. I realize that the fresh plant may not always be available. For this reason, making or purchasing an alcohol tincture made only from fresh skullcap is an option. Some herbalists believe that the fresh plant alcohol tincture is actually more effective than a fresh plant tea. **If you choose the fresh plant tincture, the herb will be delivered into your bloodstream faster if you place the tincture in several ounces of warm water. This is true for all tinctures, not just skullcap.**

275

Skullcap works well when combined with other herbs. One of the classic calming blends is equal parts fresh lemon balm and fresh skullcap made into a tea. You could also make an alcohol tincture from both of these fresh plants if you don't have year-round access to the herb.

An excellent formula for both children and adults is made by combining one-half teaspoon of hops, one-half teaspoon of chamomile and a pinch of cloves in a large cup. Pour one cup of hot distilled water over the herbs and cover the cup with a saucer. Steep for 20 minutes, than strain the herbs and add 15 drops of skullcap *tincture* to the tea. If you wish to sweeten the brew, use honey instead of sugar. Sip this tea an hour before bedtime or whenever you need to relax. **This formula works well for nervous, high strung kids five years old and up who have a hard time going to sleep**. Cut the amount of herbs and tincture in half if the child is under 12 years of age.

This formula has worked wonders for knocking out the "un-knockable." However, I've made this exact blend for people and it has also failed miserably. Why the different reactions? There can be many reasons— everything from not drinking the whole dose to individuals who have too many drugs in their system. If someone has been dependent upon chemical over-the-counter or prescription drugs (such as antidepressants or Valium) or even narcotics and alcohol, herbs will take longer to work because they first have to combat the chemicals.

CONSIDER THE CONSTITUTION

Sometimes, the herbs will have the exact opposite effect on the body because of chemical dependency (i.e., they might keep you awake instead of putting you to sleep). If you want to try an herbal program, you first have to cleanse your body of the chemicals. If this is what you want to do, please, please, *please* only do a chemical detox through a qualified holistic practitioner who knows exactly what he or she is doing.

It is important to mention that some herbs can also react in the opposite way depending upon a person's "constitution." Chinese herbal medicine takes into consideration an individual's constitution and how well that constitution matches the inherent energy within each herb.

For example, herbs are classified on a cold to hot scale, with many falling into that neutral zone. Skullcap is considered to be a "cooling" herb. In other words, it is extremely beneficial for people who have "hot" or "warm" constitutions since it helps balance the energy. In natural medicine, you are always striving for that often elusive "balance." A "hot" or "warm" type person would be described as someone who is more aggressive than passive, speaks in a loud voice rather than softly, has strong opinions and is easily agitated or quick to anger. People who have a "cold" or "cool" constitution tend to be more passive, speak more quietly, are more reticent to voice their opinions and tend to "go with flow" without getting angry or uptight. *Keep in mind that these are very broad generalizations but they do follow in many cases.* If you were to give a "cooling" calming herb (such as skullcap) to someone who has a "cold" or "cool" constitution, it could dampen their energy and produce no effect. I compare it to tossing a wet, cold blanket on someone who has just fallen through the ice. All that would do is make the condition worse. Give them a warm blanket and you neutralize the situation. Thus, a person who is in the "cold" or "cool" constitution group needs a sedative herb that has more inherent "warm" or "hot" energy. The herb that matches that profile is valerian. Valerian—which is *not* used to make the drug Valium—is very effective for someone who has a "cold" or "cool" type constitution. Unfortunately, valerian is often promoted as a "safe, reliable sleep aid" for *everyone.* This is just not true. If you give valerian (either alone or in formula) to people who fit that "hot" or "warm" constitutional profile, it could easily react more like a stimulant and keep them up all night as well as make them *very* agitated.

ALL TWITCHED UP?

Skullcap is also well known for its effectiveness on a condition known as "St. Vitus Dance." Not to be confused with "The Tijuana Quickstep," **St. Vitus Dance (or chorea)** is a minor to major twitching or flailing of the arms and legs. Adults can have chorea but it's more common in children. It definitely requires medical attention to determine if the root problem is chemical, emotional, allergy-related or even diet-oriented. However, a strong infusion of *fresh* skullcap (i.e., four heaping teaspoons to eight ounces of hot water) can be extremely effective for calming the nerves. Adults can sip a cup of the tea while kids five to eleven years old should be given a tablespoon of the tea every 15 minutes or so.

SPINAL CORD SPECIFIC

Herbalist Dr. John R. Christopher writes that **skullcap is a specific herb for any disorder of the spinal cord or the motor nerves**. The motor nerves are housed in the medulla oblongata which is located at the base of the skull. Christopher notes that when the motor nerves are congested, "messages cannot reach the rest of the body." Skullcap, used over time, can help to gradually correct this problem. He suggests using the herb internally *as well as rubbing the tincture over the skin at the base of the skull several times* a day to facilitate the recovery.

CALMS THAT SHAKY WITHDRAWAL

Skullcap has been called into duty when it comes to **weaning people off of barbiturates, alcohol and nicotine**. It has been shown to lessen the latter stages of convulsions and manic activity. For years, folk healers gave skullcap to people who were going through the D.T.'s and it was often the only remedy that allowed them to get any rest. It has also come in handy **to calm those who are trying to get off of Valium**. I would definitely suggest using the fresh plant tincture at 15 to 30 drops, either under the tongue or placed into four ounces of hot water. If you are having a very difficult time during withdrawal, you can take this dose every one to two hours or as needed. If you are withdrawing from alcohol and are worried about using the alcohol tincture, place the tincture in several ounces of boiling water and let it sit until cool. This will burn off the alcohol but still retain skullcap's herbal benefit.

WHAT'S THE DOSE?

The recommended dose of the fresh herbal tincture is 15 to 30 drops—either under the tongue or diluted in several ounces of hot water—two to three times a day. When making a tea out of the fresh plant, use two or three heaping teaspoons for every eight ounces of hot water. Drink one to three cups a day. For the dried plant, use one rounded teaspoon for every eight ounces of hot water. Never boil skullcap since it can reduce its healing benefit.

THINGS TO CONSIDER

If you are suffer from chronic nervous exhaustion or stress which are causing insomnia, headaches, irritability and even involuntary twitches, it's going to take skullcap longer to work if you continue to take prescription drugs and/or eat refined sugar. As always, if your nervous condition begins to interfere with the quality of your life, contact a trusted holistic practitioner who can suggest not only specific herbs, but an overall program that addresses your entire body and lifestyle.

It takes more than a few doses of skullcap for it to sink into your nervous system. You should see some noticeable effect within two to three weeks of consistent use. **Long term use of skullcap (i.e., several months or longer) has been known to suppress sexual desire or stop it altogether**. If you want to avoid this possibility, but you still want a good sedative, I'd consider trying chamomile or only include skullcap as part of a larger calming herbal formula.

Don't take double or triple doses of skullcap to make it "kick in" faster. There's no way to rush this herb. Excessive use of skullcap can cause confusion, giddiness, twitching and even muscular spasms.

Skullcap should not be used in tandem with drug tranquilizers, sedatives and antihistamines since the herb can enhance their effect and cause a decrease in sensory function, alertness and reaction time when operating a vehicle.

The herb is classified as safe to use in small doses while pregnant.

Skullcap may have been burdened with an odd name, but its soothing effects may wipe any suspicion from your mind.

THE "DIRT" ON...SKULLCAP

Botanical ~	*Scutellaria lateriflora*
Growth cycle ~	Hardy perennial.
Medicinal uses~	Antispasmodic, diuretic, nervine, anodyne, whole body tonic.
Part(s) used for medicine ~	Entire above ground plant.
Vitamins/Minerals ~	Vitamins A, B$_1$, C and E with the minerals zinc, selenium, calcium, magnesium, potassium, manganese, silicon.
Region ~	Originally found throughout the eastern part of the United States, typically around water. It has since moved westward and can be found in moist meadows and along streams from 1,000 feet to 10,000 feet.
Wild or Domestic ~	Both.
Poisonous look-alikes in the wild ~	No. On the non-poisonous front, apparently some forest foragers mistake American speedwell (*Veronica americana*) with skullcap. I don't quite understand how this could happen since speedwell's leaf, stem and flower—while slightly similar—are diverse. Skullcap is a member of the mint family and one identifying marker is the typical square stem that all mint family plants share. Speedwell does not have a square stem.
Hardy or Delicate ~	Delicate in the formative stages. Once firmly established, can be hardy.
Height of mature plant ~	12 to 18 inches. In rich, moist soil with semi-shade, skullcap can grow up to four feet tall.
Easy or hard to grow ~	Easy.
Cultivation ~	Skullcap can be grown from seed, root cutting and root division. I think root division is the easiest. The trick is finding someone who (a) grows skullcap and (b) is willing to let you dig up their crop. Second best is to grow the herb from seed. Broadcast seed into wet, fertile, well-drained soil in early spring when you know all chances of a hard frost are over. Press the seed into the moist earth and keep it well watered without drowning. I have had luck with pre-chilling the seeds in a flat for one week prior to exposing the flat to heat. However, I have also tossed the seed into late spring soil once the temperature warmed up and had a nice crop.

279

Plant spacing ~	Six to twelve inches.
Pre-soak seeds ~	No.
Pre-chill seeds ~	Yes. However, as mentioned above, it is not required to ensure germination.
Indoor seed starting ~	Yes. I think seed cells work best over dirt flats since it is easier to transplant the individual cells into the garden. Make sure the soil stays moist without drowning the seed. I had great results when I covered the seed flat with a plastic dome and allowed the interior to become hot and humid. My only suggestion is that you will want to transplant the seedlings into the garden before they become root-bound in the cells. If that happens, skullcap starts to fade quickly and may not survive the transplant.
Light/dark seed requirements ~	Light.
Days to germinate ~	Seven to fourteen days.
Days to full maturity ~	Depends upon your region. I've seen it take as long as 120 days in higher altitudes.
Soil type ~	Rich, fertile and consistently moist. Remember, skullcap is part of the water-loving mint family and needs to be treated accordingly.
Water requirements ~	Requires a constant supply of water without being drowned.
Sun or shade ~	Does best when it is exposed to sun in the early or late part of the day with partial shade the rest of the time.
Propagation ~	Seed and underground roots.
Easy/hard to transplant ~	Easy from seedling as long as it is not root-bound in cell tray. Very easy from root division as long as you get it into moist soil as soon as possible.
Pests or diseases ~	Some people have no trouble with skullcap — others complain of aphids running wild over it. If aphids are your problem, poor soil may be the culprit. Try relocating the plant in better soil in a different part of the garden.
Landscape uses ~	Makes a beautiful border or filler, especially when the mauve/purple flowers bloom in late summer.
Gathering ~	Always wait until skullcap is fully in bloom before harvesting. This is usually around August to September, depending upon your region. After several years of the plant successfully proliferating in your garden, you should be able to develop a rather dense patch of skullcap. If you live in regions that allow for year-round growing, it is conceivable to get as many as three cuttings each year from one planting.
Best fresh or dried ~	Skullcap is always best used fresh—either as a tea or made into a tincture from the freshly picked plant—due

280

to the fact that the herb loses medicinal power quickly in the dried form. However, history has shown that the dried plant is effective if properly stored in airtight glass jars and kept away from any heat source.

Drying methods ~ Cut skullcap several inches above the ground. Place the plant on a drying rack or on a clean cloth in the shade and completely away from any direct heat. If skullcap is exposed to excessive heat in the drying process, most of the medicinal action is lost. Check the plant frequently to chart progress. Once it is dry to the touch, crush up the entire plant—leaves, stems and flowers—and store in an airtight, glass jar. Keep the jar away from any heat source. If kept in this manner, dried skullcap should be medicinally viable for six to nine months.

Amount needed ~ Moderate use: 20 plants; Regular use: 25+.

Seed collection ~ Skullcap's seed is carried in pods that burst open anywhere from late summer to early fall. If you pick the plant too soon, you will stop the development of the seeds; if you pick it too late, most of the seeds will have already been dispersed. Observation on your part will determine the perfect time. Look for plants that have several pods already open and others still closed. Clip them and place them into a paper bag, allowing plenty of ventilation. As the plant dries, the pods will spontaneously pop open and unleash their seeds into the bag. As always, fresh skullcap seed is more viable. If possible, collect the seeds from established plants in the yard and replant them immediately in the garden if weather permits.

Companion planting ~ Needs other water-loving plants. Because aspens, cottonwoods and willows grow near or over an underground water source, this would be a good place to plant your patch of skullcap. In fact, skullcap can often be found growing under these trees in the wild.

Container planting ~ No, you can't get enough for your medicinal needs.

Common mistakes ~ Ignoring the fact that skullcap requires constant water. It will soon dry up and die out if this happens. Also, do not transplant the seedlings outside if there is any chance of a late spring frost. Skullcap will not survive it.

Interesting facts/tips ~ The first year you plant skullcap, plant a little bit more than you think you'll need since some of it may not take. Once established, its underground roots will spread and push the plant into crevices and corners, similar to other members of the mint **family.**

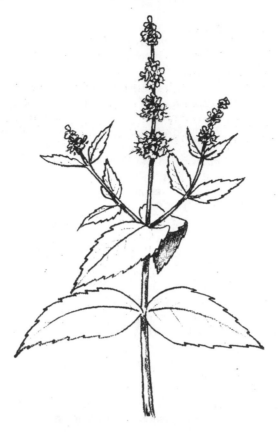

Chapter 32

SPEARMINT

~

LIKE CHEWING GUM WITH YOUR MOUTH OPEN

Mentha spicata
Mentha viridas (sometimes used for making spearmint essential oil)

Hardy perennial

Medicinal Uses: *Antispasmodic, digestive tonic, carminative, diuretic, stimulant, stomachic*

Medicinal parts of plant: *Leaves*

Forms: *Tea, fresh plant tincture, pure essential oil*

WHAT IS ITS CHARACTER?

Determined. That's the best way to describe spearmint's character. You think you've pulled the last root from the ground and it comes back better than ever. You can (literally) build a brick wall around it and it will find a way to grow under it, between it or *through* some small crack in the wall. You can't keep a good spearmint plant down and there's no reason you should. Whenever I feel like I'm hitting a brick wall, I think of this tenacious mint and look for the tiny "crack" that will lead me towards the solution.

WHERE DO I FIND IT?

Widely distributed in wet meadows, pastures and along river banks, at all elevations and in practically all regions except for dry, hot desert areas. When you stumble upon a patch of wild "mint," you are most likely looking at spearmint or a cross-pollinated species.

HOW DO I GROW IT?

Spearmint is grown from root division, stem cuttings and seeds. Root division is easiest. Stem cuttings are second best if you can establish a root system before the plant dies out. Some people have great luck with seeds and others fail miserably. I've fallen into both categories. I think the trick is to broadcast the seed into moist, rich, *warm* soil and gently press the seed into the dirt. Barely cover with dirt. A combination of heat and humidity tend to speed germination of seed. Keeping the soil moist but well-drained is also beneficial. Once established, thin seedlings approximately six inches apart.

HOW DO I HARVEST IT?

Spearmint can be used either fresh or dried. I tend to favor the fresh plant since you get more of a minty "kick" out of it. Cut the plant several inches above the ground in early to mid-summer *before* the plant flowers too much. Gather five to eight stalks, tie them together on one end with a piece of string or a rubber band and hang them in a dry, dark, moisture-free area. If you live in an especially dry region, leaves can be ready to store within several days. Do not over dry spearmint or the natural healing oils will gradually dissipate. For anyone who has grown this prolific plant, once it gets going, you never lack for enough spearmint.

HOW DO I USE IT?

In the late 1980's, when the distillers of pure essential oils started coming out with pamphlets listing the possible "mood changing," emo-

283

tional effects of their aromatic oils on the human brain, I could hardly wait to try them on my friends.

One of the first essential oils I bought was spearmint. I remember it well. Driving home with that tiny bottle clutched in my hand, I recalled what the pamphlet told me about this popular scent. "Helps to release emotional blocks—especially when they are hormonally related," the booklet stated. "Brings about a feeling of calm while stimulating the senses. Has been known to bring back happy childhood memories, allowing one to feel secure and safe." It all made sense except for the childhood memories part. The only connection I could figure out was that spearmint is used to flavor chewing gum. If someone had pleasant memories as a child chewing gum, well then hey, it might do the trick.

Three friends were coming over and so I dropped about 15 drops of the essential oil into a brass lamp ring and placed it over a 60 watt light bulb. My heart was beating with anticipation. As I greeted my friends at the door, I could hardly wait for them to start releasing emotional blocks —especially those that were hormonal. I wanted them to tell me how calm they were while stimulated at the same time. And, oh, I wanted to hear about all those happy childhood memories.

They cocked their heads, smelling the spearmint scent that was now wafting quite heavily through the air. "Are you cooking lamb?" one of them said. Without missing a beat, the other one said he had a sudden urge for a mint julep. The third announced that it smelled like a bunch of people were chewing gum in my house with their mouths open.

There was no emotional release—especially hormonal. No calm feelings and not one happy childhood memory. Their only aromatic association with spearmint came from the fact that the herb does season lamb, is the base for mint juleps and also flavors chewing gum.

So much for spearmint, I thought.

But a few years later, a friend gave me a large spearmint plant. I planted it in the garden and watched it take over my whole yard. Realizing I had to start using it before it decided to weave its way inside my house, I began looking into spearmint's proven medicinal uses. After that, I had a whole new appreciation for this spirited mint.

SPEARMINT VS. PEPPERMINT

I learned that United States growers plant over *28,000 acres* of spearmint each year. I'm sure much of that is for flavoring chewing gum and making all those mint juleps. For the herbal community, it means that there's plenty of it to go around. **Spearmint has similar medicinal uses to peppermint (*Mentha piperita*) except that it is rated as "milder."**

However, **spearmint can have a stronger diuretic (urine producing) and diaphoretic (sweat producing) effect than peppermint**.

How do you tell spearmint apart from peppermint in the garden? Well, there's the smell. Peppermint smells like peppermint and spearmint smells like chewing gum. Chew a peppermint leaf and then take a deep breath through your mouth. A cooling sensation should be felt on your tongue. This doesn't happen so much with spearmint. As for the leaves, peppermint's leaves are wider, shorter, smoother and take on a deeper shade of green—sometimes bordering on what looks like a deep purple. Peppermint's leaves also form on stalks. Spearmint's leaves have a sharper curve—like a "spear"—are more crinkled and boast a bright, cheerful green color. Instead of having a leaf stalk like peppermint, spearmint's leaves grow directly out of the main stem. What also distinguishes spearmint from peppermint is that **spearmint is safe and effective for children**, whereas peppermint can often be too strong and stimulating for youngsters.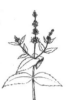

STEEP THOSE LEAVES!

The secret to successfully using spearmint as a medicinal is that you *never boil the leaves*. **Boiling completely strips every drop of healing potential from the plant**. When I make spearmint tea, I bring distilled water to a boil and then let the kettle sit covered for several minutes before I pour the water. The other thing about spearmint is that **it takes more of it—both fresh and dried—to get any effect**. If you are using the fresh plant—which I happen to think is the best form when you want to gain the most medicinal benefit—for every eight ounces of hot distilled water, you'll need about three, six to seven inch stalks or approximately 30 *fresh* leaves. Some people use as much as *1/2 cup of the fresh leaves* to eight ounces of water. You will need less of the dried leaves—about one to two heaping teaspoons for every eight ounces of hot distilled water.

Next to having spearmint growing outside your door, the *fresh* plant tincture is your best bet. Thirty to fifty drops of the tincture in several ounces of warm water equal one cup of the fresh plant tea.

Whether you choose the fresh plant or the tincture, here are some good reasons to keep spearmint close at hand.

GENTLE DIGESTIVE RELIEF

Spearmint is first and foremost a **digestive tonic**. It's effective for both children and adults at easing gas pains and calming any digestive upset that might be causing minor cramping. Some herbalists recommend **combining equal parts of chamomile flowers with the spearmint for extra soothing relief**.

The tea also works for **colic in babies**. However, the dose would be only two to three of the fresh leaves or 1/16 of a teaspoon of the dried leaves to 10 or 12 ounces of hot distilled water. The baby would not drink the entire 10 or 12 ounces—just baby-sized spoonfuls until the pain subsides.

STIMULATE THAT APPETITE!

Some say the very smell of the tea **arouses the taste buds**. I have also heard that the odor emitted from crushing the fresh leaves over food enhances the appetite. Try it to see what happens.

THE ANTI-NAUSEA & MORNING SICKNESS TEA

Ginger root is considered *the* remedy for both **nausea** and **morning sickness**. However, when you add spearmint to ginger, the taste is "softened" and less biting. The formula is one and one-half teaspoons spearmint to one-half teaspoon ginger root. Add a dash of cinnamon and pour eight ounces of boiling distilled water over the herbs, cover and let steep for up to 20 minutes. Strain and sip in small mouthfuls every few minutes until relief is felt. Some women feel that using *fresh* spearmint is the key. If you wish to do this, up the spearmint amount in the formula to three or four teaspoons.

PAINFUL, BURNING URINE

One of the oldest but little known uses for spearmint is as **a diuretic to relieve painful, burning urination**. You can use it alone or combine a teaspoon each of dried spearmint, juniper berries, cornsilk, marshmallow root and uva ursi into a teapot and pour five cups of hot distilled water over the plants. Cover and allow to steep for 25 minutes. Strain and drink one cup every hour for five hours. Repeat the same procedure for three days in a row. If there is no improvement, seek medical attention.

REPEL THOSE BUGS AND MICE

This is another old time use for spearmint. What's nice about it—besides the fact that it is non-toxic—is that it makes the house smell *so* good. You will need *freshly picked* spearmint for this purpose. Spread the stalks with leaves still attached in the areas where the rodents/insects usually reside. To "juice up" the **repellant potential**, in addition to the fresh spearmint, add equal amounts of *fresh* pennyroyal stalks and leaves and *fresh* tansy flowers. Typically, these plants are at their height between April and August—often the same period you may be experiencing those nasty pests.

TAKES THE PAIN OUT OF STINGS & BITES

The next time you get **stung by a bee or bitten by a bug**, pick several fresh spearmint leaves off the stalk, chew them into a juicy poultice and press them firmly into the sting or bite. Due to spearmint's **natural antiseptic, anti-inflammatory and anti-infectious abilities**, you could experience a quick and painless healing process.

CALM THAT FRETFUL CHILD

Spearmint is no "magic bullet" but between the scent and the taste, **some children have been known to be soothed by the tea**. For babies, steep two or three of the fresh leaves or 1/16 of a teaspoon of the dried leaves in 10 or 12 ounces of hot distilled water. For children between the ages of two and six, use 1/4 teaspoon to 1/2 teaspoon of the dried leaves.

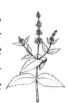

KEEP THAT ESSENTIAL OIL HANDY

The pure essential oil of spearmint may not be considered a "must have" by some aromatherapists and herbalists, but it's one of my favorites. Spearmint essential oil should be made from the flowering tops of the *Mentha viridas* species or from the standard *Mentha spicata* plant. When you purchase the oil, make sure one of these species is mentioned.

Spearmint essential oil is a wonderfully uplifting aroma. It doesn't have the "big bang" effect of peppermint or rosemary essential oils, but it does seem to lighten the environment and create a happy feeling. I use it either in a lamp ring or diluted in a spray bottle. For the lamp ring, figure eight to twelve drops; for the spray bottle, add 10 drops of the oil for every ounce of distilled water. It is always best to use a glass spray bottle (which can be purchased through herb suppliers or at a health/herb store) since concentrated essential oils have a nasty habit of actually *melting* the plastic bottles. A really nice aromatic combination that works for anxiety, mild depression or any time you want to inject a shot of "happiness" into the air is combining equal amounts of either tangerine or orange essential oil with spearmint essential oil. I've found this to be a good blend to use when you're having a party and you want to slip a little aromatherapy into the event without dealing with an overwhelming scent.

NURSING MOTHERS TAKE HEED

The only caution for spearmint is that, like peppermint, **the tea can suppress milk in nursing mothers**. Other than that, it is a safe, good tasting herb.

Spearmint's distinctive aroma may not make you release emotional blocks or even take you back to those happy childhood memories. At the least, it sure does smell good. In fact, after I place the essential oil in my lamp ring, I do feel more balanced. Yes, even calm—with a mix of stimulation and slight euphoria.

Then again, that might be from the mint julep.

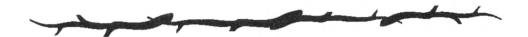

THE "DIRT" ON...SPEARMINT

Botanical ~	*Mentha spicata*
Growth cycle ~	Hardy perennial.
Medicinal uses~	Antispasmodic, carminative, diuretic, stimulant, stomachic.
Part(s) used for medicine ~	Leaves.
Vitamins/Minerals ~	Vitamin A, B-complex, calcium, magnesium, phosphorus, potassium, sodium, iron.
Region ~	Found in wet meadows, pastures and along river banks, at all elevations and in practically all regions except for dry, hot desert areas.
Wild or Domestic ~	Both. When you stumble upon a patch of wild "mint," you are most likely looking at spearmint or a cross-pollinated species.
Poisonous look-alikes in the wild ~	No. As for a non-poisonous (but somewhat irritating) look-alike, stinging nettle can easily resemble spearmint when it is young and immature. Both plants have square stems and lovely emerald green leaves. Then again, if you think young nettle is spearmint and reach down to pick it, you'll realize within one or two stinging seconds that you have the wrong plant.
Hardy or Delicate ~	Hardy.
Height of mature plant ~	Three feet.
Easy or hard to grow ~	Very easy from root division; can be difficult from seed.
Cultivation ~	Root division, stem cuttings, seeds. Root division is easiest. Stem cuttings are second best if you can establish a root system before the plant dies out. Some people have great luck with seeds and others fail miserably. I think the trick is to broadcast the seed into moist, rich, warm soil and gently press the seed into the dirt. Barely cover with

dirt. A combination of heat and humidity tend to speed germination of seed. Keeping the soil moist but well-drained is also beneficial.

Plant spacing ~ Six inches.

Pre-soak seeds ~ No.

Pre-chill seeds ~ No.

Indoor seed starting ~ Yes. However, I prefer direct seeding.

Light/dark seed requirements ~ Light.

Days to germinate ~ 14 to 21 days. Expect to see some seeds sprout well after that time period.

Days to full maturity ~ Approximately 90 days.

Soil type ~ Consistently moist, nutrient-rich, well-drained, slightly alkaline.

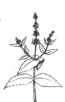

Water requirements ~ Requires constant moisture. Spearmint always does well near a natural water source or a dripping garden faucet.

Sun or shade ~ Partial shade will ensure a more fragrant plant.

Propagation ~ Seed and pervasive underground roots.

Easy/hard to transplant ~ Easy from established plants that have a strong root system. Don't become alarmed if your transplants fall over a few hours after transplanting. Give them a good watering and spray the drooping plants with water and they'll be upright within 24 hours.

Pests or diseases ~ Scale (that horrible plant-sucking menace) can attach itself to spearmint and destroy the plant in days. Since the bay laurel plant is a host for scale, keep spearmint away from it. If your plant becomes infected with scale, cut away all the affected parts and pour several watering cans of soapy water over what remains. Indoor or container-bound spearmint plants can be prone to aphids if the soil becomes poor. Once the aphids attack, you can try the soapy water routine but I've found it is more time efficient to cut away the affected parts and replant the roots in another pot that is filled with nutrient-rich soil.

Landscape uses ~ Makes a great aromatic filler around shade trees as well as a nice border plant against a garden wall.

Gathering ~ Cut the plant several inches above the ground in early to mid-summer before the plant flowers too much.

Best fresh or dried ~ Fresh or dried.

Drying methods ~ Gather five to eight stalks, tie them together on one end with a piece of string or a rubber band and hang them in a dry, dark, moisture-free area. If you live in an especially dry region, leaves can be ready to store within several days. Do not over dry spearmint or the natural healing oils will gradually dissipate.

Amount needed ~	Moderate use: 20 plants; Regular use: 35+. One thing about spearmint, when it gets going, you never lack for enough plants!
Seed collection ~	Wait until late summer when the flower heads are firmly established and the leaves begin to die back. I always tap the flower heads into my hand to see if any seed falls out before cutting the plant. Choose stalks that are tall, leafy and healthy for seed collection. Gather about 10 or 12 stalks, place them loosely in a white paper bag and set it in a warm, dry, shady spot. Occasionally reach in the bag and shake the seed heads to encourage the seeds to fall out.
Companion planting ~	Spearmint can take over a garden within two seasons of growth. Because of this, I think it is best to keep it by itself since other plants could easily get lost in the thicket. Stinging nettle has the reputation of increasing the volatile oil content of other plants. Because of this, you might want to consider a patch of nettle nearby. Remember, though, that young nettle can resemble young spearmint so keep them separated and under control once both are established.
Container planting ~	Yes. Some herb gardeners only plant spearmint in containers so they can control the rapid growth. Make sure the container is large enough to accommodate future root growth. Large whiskey barrels are perfect containers for spearmint. Either keep them above ground or sink the containers into the ground.
Common mistakes ~	Placing spearmint in poor, rocky soil that lacks moisture and nutrients. This produces leaves that have little medicinal value due to the reduction of volatile oils.
Interesting facts/tips ~	Cut spearmint frequently or it becomes woody after two or three years. As it dies back, always clip it to about two or three inches above the ground. Uproot sections when they become dense and overcrowded. If you can't bear to throw away the plants, stick them in a pot and give them to a friend so they can enjoy the wonders of spearmint.

Chapter 33

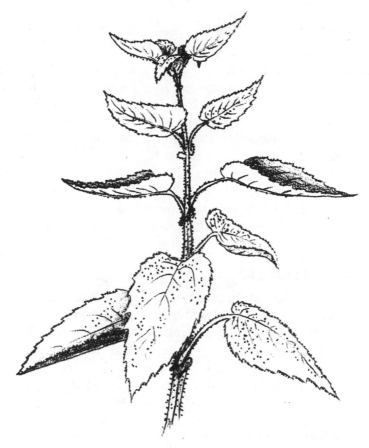

STINGING NETTLE

~

IT DON'T MEAN A THING IF IT AIN'T GOT THAT STING

Urtica dioica
("W.F.")
Hardy perennial

Medicinal Uses: *Diuretic, counterirritant, astringent, galactagogue, hemostatic, mineral tonic*

Medicinal parts of plant: *Leaves, root*

Forms: *Tea, root or whole plant extract, capsules, urtication*

WHAT IS ITS CHARACTER?

For most people, nettle is the "bad boy" of the wild. It's the "biker" plant, all geared up and ready to push the pedal to the metal and cause some serious trouble if you mess with it. Get in its path and nettle is going to get you...literally. But I don't buy into all that backwoods bravado. When I discover nettle in the wild, I don't run screaming from it — I race *toward* it, happy to find this exceptional herb. It can't fool me. Underneath that intimidating exterior lies a highly enlightened herb that holds tremendous healing power. After years of welcoming it rather than hating it, I discovered nettle's greatest irony. When you stop fearing nettle and truly appreciate its far reaching potential, it doesn't sting you as often. The "ominous" plant of the wild emerges as your protector and, ultimately, your greatest ally.

WHERE DO I FIND IT?

Some herb books say that nettle grows "anywhere." However, nettle requires a consistent source of water to ensure continued development. It can be found as low as sea level and as high as 10,000 feet in areas that are moist, dappled in shade and have rich to moderate soil. Nettle is not naturally found in desert areas where the soil is parched. There are approximately 50 species of nettle (*Urtica* species) in the world, all having similar properties as *Urtica dioica*.

HOW DO I GROW IT?

Nettle is grown from seeds, cuttings, nursery seedlings and root division, the latter best done in the fall after the leaves have died back. Cuttings can be challenging unless you have a "green thumb." If you live in areas that experience frost or freezing temperatures, direct seeding may be your best bet. Fall sowing is recommended with seedlings appearing in early spring. Seed must be exposed to a cold (freezing is best), moist environment in order to germinate. Plan to broadcast more seed than you think you will need since it is typical to have only 50-60 percent of the seed successfully germinate. While I have had some luck in starting the seeds in flats and following the cold, moist conditioning requirements, the seedlings unfortunately do not transplant that well since the young root structure is weak. Because of this, take great care if you purchase established seedlings that are three inches or larger. Space six inches apart. Nettles must be kept continually moist and have exposure to sunshine with partial shade. If you do not have these conditions available in your yard, don't waste your time or money on seed/plants since they will either never emerge or die before reaching maturity.

HOW DO I HARVEST IT?

Harvest the entire above ground plant with gloves in early to late spring when it is approximately eight inches to one foot in height. If you live in mountainous areas and have access to elevations as high as 8,000 feet, you could find young nettle in early stages of development as late as August. Where nettle grows in dense patches, you could possibly get three or four harvests each year since it will develop at various stages.

Wear gloves and, holding the tip of the plant in one hand, cut the stem two to three inches above the ground. If you are using the plant fresh, strip the leaves off the stem when you are ready to steam them as a wild green or make them into a fresh tea. If you are harvesting the plant to dry, tie several leafy stalks together at one end and hang upside down in a dry, dark, warm area. Don't rinse the leaves off with water before drying since this will make them turn brown or black as they dry. Dry leaves as quickly as possible without exposing them to artificial heat (such as a heat lamp or forced hot air). Leaves tend to turn under and become darkened if dried too quickly. Do *not* gather nettle after the drooping seed heads have formed since the plant becomes difficult for the body to assimilate at that point. If you are gathering nettle for external "urtication" purposes, the spring plants have the greatest "sting" potency. Mid-summer plants that are beginning to form seed heads can still be used for this, but the sting is less bothersome. Nettle is best used fresh. However, if the leaves are properly dried, they are very effective. Harvest the roots in the fall from plants that are two years and older since first year plants typically have less developed roots. Rinse off the dirt and allow them to dry in a warm, shady place.

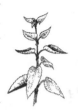

HOW DO I USE IT?

In the last few years, I've been doing something on my herbal field walks that could be considered rather strange. For some students, it has turned into the "highlight" of the day. For others, I think they leave the class wondering if I'm a few tacos short of a combination platter.

This "something" that I do is *purposely* sting my arm with a nettle plant. I don't just sting my arm a little, I sting it over and over and over again. It's rather fun to watch people's reactions. Many gradually step back and look around nervously, fearing perhaps that I'm going to turn the nettle stalk on them next.

I do this "stinging" demonstration to show two things: first, I want to take the "fear factor" out of this great plant and, secondly, I show people how they can easily and effectively remedy the nettle sting with one of the six plants that nature *always* grows around nettle (yellow dock, plantain, mullein, blue violet, hound's tongue and jewelweed). One or more of these plants grows within 15 feet of where nettle naturally occurs in the wild. The old adage is that the cure for the nettle sting is always within eyesight. Every time I think about that, I consider it a metaphor for life's problems—that the answer "or cure" is always close by and usually within eyesight.

NETTLE. NOT BULL THISTLE!

Before I go any further, let me make sure you understand that I'm referring to stinging nettle and *not* thistle. When I mentioned stinging myself with nettle in one class, I saw several eyes in the crowd get as big as saucers. I later found out they thought I was flailing myself with thistle which is covered with sharp, needle-like, one-half inch spikes. It makes me cringe just thinking about it.

Instead of thorny spikes, nettle's stem and leaves are covered with tiny "hairs" that are filled with sacks of formic acid, acetylcholine and histamine. It's the formic acid—one of the same compounds that makes red ant bites burn so badly—that contributes to the immediate "sting" of the nettle.

A MINERAL-RICH, PROTEIN-LADEN PLANT

Stinging nettle is loaded with iron and vitamin C which contribute to producing healthy red blood cells. Consider this herb to be a one-stop-shop when you need to flood your body with much needed minerals and vitamins.

Many herbalists suggest nettle tea to their patients who want to do a "Spring Cure"—a kind of recharging of the batteries that one can do in the springtime or anytime you are feeling a little droopy. It is an excellent herb to **prevent or remedy anemia**. If you are experiencing a sudden bout of **bad skin brought on my an overall sluggish system**, two or three cups of nettle tea each day can help wake up your tired organs and activate a cleanse.

Three cups of this tonic tea also help to gradually correct **physical fatigue or low energy**.

While nettle works just fine by itself, you might want to consider a combination of herbs that has been used for years to re-mineralize the system and tone up the organs. Combine one heaping tablespoon *each* of stinging nettle, red clover flowers, alfalfa, red raspberry leaves and burdock root in a large saucepan. Pour eight cups of boiling distilled water over the herbs and stir. Cover immediately and let the herbs steep for 20 to 30 minutes. Try to drink the entire amount over the course of one day.

Continue for as long as three weeks. You should expect a certain amount of purging (i.e., more frequent trips to the bathroom). This is a good thing. You might also feel much more energy and more clarity in your thought patterns. I like to drink this exact combination of herbs in the early spring when I'm feeling the cloistered effects of winter's cold temperatures and lack of physical activity.

Nettle's curative tonic ability can also be found in the young, supple, spring leaves. Wear gloves and pick 10 to 15 eight inch leafy stalks. Steam the leaves for no longer than one minute and eat them as you would spinach. For more information on how to use nettle as an incredible wild edible, turn to the "Wild Foods Facts" box on page 298.

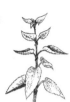

IT SMELLS LIKE WHAT?

Nettle does **a major cleansing job on the kidneys, dumping toxins through the urine as it purifies the blood**. Plain and simple, drinking nettle tea as a cleansing herb will make you urinate. Maybe not so coincidentally, some people say that the mature plant sometimes smells a tad like urine.

Acting as a whole body tonic, nettle **eliminates toxins and uric acid through the kidneys**. The removal of uric acid aids in the **relief of gout and arthritis** since uric acid can build up in the joints and contribute to pain and stiffness.

Folks who have **a predisposition to kidney stones** could benefit from drinking nettle tea on a daily basis—three weeks on with one week off—to flush the kidneys and eliminate waste.

The only caution here is that excessive consumption—which is defined as over four cups a day—of nettle tea can be irritating to the kidneys causing them to get overtaxed. For this reason, moderation is the key word. If you try this and you feel dizzy, flushed or weakened, by all means reduce your intake or stop drinking the tea.

TAKES THE SNEEZE OUT OF SPRING

Nettle is probably best known for being **a natural antihistamine**. Anyone who suffers from seasonal allergies, including **hay fever** and **pollen-related concerns**, might want to try a daily dose of nettle tea or up to five 500 mg. capsules each day. In a study conducted with allergy sufferers, over 50 percent reported that drinking three cups of nettle tea or taking three to five 500 milligram capsules each day significantly reduced their symptoms. Hay fever sufferers who start drinking one or two cups of nettle tea daily (or take two to four 500 milligram capsules a day) in November and continue through April when the pollen arrives have been happily rewarded with an allergy-free springtime. In addition, allergy sufferers also reported an **increased resistance to springtime colds**, possibly due to the high mineral and vitamin content in the plant.

The allergy benefits don't stop there. Thanks to the naturally occurring histamine in the plant, those who suffer from **minor allergies to lobster, shellfish and strawberries and develop hives** may find relief from the root extract. The leaf tea and freeze-dried leaf extract have been used but the root extract has proven more effective. Taking one or two 500 milligram capsules every two to four hours has been beneficial when the hives weren't critical. If you are susceptible to this kind of allergy, I would consider adding nettle to your diet when it is in season and drinking the tea or using the root/leaf extract for several weeks on and one week off to support the body and possibly increase its allergy resistance.

A SURGE IN CIRCULATION

Another important reason people use nettle tea is to **increase poor circulation**.

One way to do this is to use the tea in a bath or, more locally, as a foot bath. For either one, soak a generous portion (up to two cups) of nettle leaves in a bucket of cold water for 12 hours then heat the mixture, gently bringing it just to a boil. You can use either fresh or dried nettle. If you use the fresh plant, include the stalks along with the leaves and double the amount. Strain the liquid into a hot bath or footbath. If you're in the bath, keep your heart above the water so you don't overstimulate your body. For both the bath and footbath, stay in for a maximum of 30 minutes since it can be far too stimulating for many people.

In addition to increasing circulation, **the bath is also excellent for relieving rheumatism**. If this is the case, drink a hot cup of nettle tea while in the bathtub, stay in the bath 20 minutes, get out, pat yourself dry and climb into a warm bed. You'll start to sweat and as you do, your pores will excrete the acids that cause pain. While this is certainly no cure for rheumatism, it can ease the discomfort.

I've made this bath many times and had excellent results with it. Then one day I wondered what would happen if I put freshly picked nettles in the bath water along with the tea mixture. I figured it might be an extra stimulating experience. Yes, it was stimulating as well as *stinging*. I quickly discovered that the combination of fresh stinging nettles and warm water tends to escalate the stinging sensation against the skin. It wasn't until months later that I read an account of a woman in her late 60's who did the same thing to take the edge off of her arthritis pain. Apparently, it worked so well that she planted a huge patch of nettles along a stream that ran through her rural property and rolled naked in the nettles to keep her arthritis pain at bay. If you think that's a bit on the odd side, keep reading.

IT'S NOT SELF-ABUSE...REALLY, IT ISN'T...

My field class demonstrations of slapping my arm with fresh nettle stalks is dramatic but it isn't original. Roman soldiers discovered that by flailing their bare skin with fresh nettle stalks—especially in cold climates—the sting of the leaves warmed their skin and kept their circulation flowing. This practice has a name: *urtication.* "Uro" in Latin means "to burn." As strange as this sounds, it is still used in some approved therapies to **alleviate joint stiffness**, **muscular pain** and **sciatica**. There are folks in Europe who spend a great deal of money at retreats and spas to have someone lash their stiff joints with fresh nettle stalks.

Brushing up against a nettle stalk (i.e., as you would if you came upon the plant in the woods and it rubbed against your bare skin) is not the same as smacking yourself with the nettle stalk. Rubbing against the plant and getting "stung" is like getting a scratch—it just disturbs the surface layer of skin but goes no deeper. When you slap the fresh plant hard against your skin (i.e., urtication) you are literally delivering hundreds of "micro-injections" of nettle's formic acid, along with doses of acetylcholine and histamine. The implications of this are far reaching.

The first time I ever slapped a nettle stalk against my arm, the most amazing thing happened. The best way I can describe it is that it felt as if a million electrical sensations were ricocheting inside of me. I came to life, and not just because my arm was stinging, burning and starting to show signs of several dozen pin-pointed nettle welts. It was as though the compounds within the stingers were activating every cell in my body. I felt a surge of energy that lasted for hours as well as a definite increase in mental alertness.

Years later, I was reading an article by botanist and herbalist Dr. James A. Duke in which he spoke of the benefits of urtication in relationship to treating **Alzheimer's disease**. In the article, Duke mentioned that acetylcholine—which is one of the compounds that is released from the fresh stingers—is lacking in the brains of Alzheimer victims. Duke theorized that Alzheimer patients should drink nettle tea, eat the steamed greens and swat the nape of their bare neck with fresh nettle stalks in the hope of "shooting" the acetylcholine through the skin (via that "micro-injection") and into the head where the brain might absorb it. Mind you, this is only a theory and one that stretches the credibility of herbal medicine in the eyes of the medical profession.

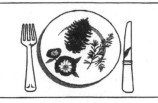

Wild Food Facts

When nettle is just popping out of the ground in early spring, harvest plants that are no higher than six inches and lightly steam them, stems and all, for no longer than three or four minutes. If you overcook this wild food, it tends to get extremely mushy and not very palatable. When cooked correctly, it makes a highly nutritious, spinach-like side dish. If you only want the leaves sans the stems, you will need many nettles since the leaves are greatly reduced in volume when they are steamed.

Tired of using plain ol' salt as a seasoning? Make your own healthy alternative that adds plenty of zip to the meal. Combine equal parts of sea salt, nettle leaf powder, basil powder and finely ground dulse into a salt shaker and sprinkle it over salads, vegetables, meat, fish and fowl.

One of my favorite reasons for picking nettles is to make nettle soup. There are dozens of recipes, many of which include milk. However, since nettles are a high protein food, I don't like combining them with milk. Here's a non-dairy, nettle soup recipe that will satisfy your taste buds and keep you healthy.

Nettle Soup Recipe

This soup is high in natural protein and works as a tonic for the whole body. Don't overdo on it since it can cause a loose bowel if you are not careful!

(Serves 4)

    1 large onion
    1 to 3 fresh garlic cloves (depending upon how much you like fresh garlic)
    2 large potatoes
    Olive oil
    2 large handfuls of FRESH, YOUNG nettle leaves
    One 14 ounce can of chicken or vegetable broth
    Salt & pepper
    Fresh thyme and rosemary to taste (optional)

Peel and chop the onion, garlic and potatoes. In a large, deep fry pan, add enough olive oil to coat and sauté the vegetables for three to four minutes. With gloved hands, trim the nettle leaves from their stems. Discard the stems. Gently wash any dirt off the leaves and add them to the saucepan, placing them on top of the vegetables. Try not to let the leaves get near the bottom of the pan since they might stick.

Heat the can of chicken or vegetable broth. Add the soup to the saucepan and bring to a rapid boil. Boil uncovered for 15 minutes or until the potatoes are tender enough to break with a fork.

Either add the entire contents of the saucepan to a blender or use a hand mixer to purée the mixture into a thick soup. If you wish, at this time add fresh rosemary and fresh thyme to taste and continue to blend. Serve immediately or place back into the saucepan and reheat for later use.

However, as a red-blooded, plucky herbalist who has a streak of adventure in her, I decided to try this. As you can probably guess, the nape of the neck is incredibly sensitive. After a few whacks with the nettle stalk, I waited to see if anything happened. It burned and stung but there was no immediate burst of mental revelations hitting my brain. I hit the back of my neck a few more times with the nettle before the stalk totally disintegrated and then I continued on my merry way. It wasn't until about an hour later that I noticed a slight improvement in my mental sharpness. Was it the nettles that did this or was it a lucky coincidence? Since this was probably the least scientific study ever done outside of a laboratory, I cannot make any concrete conclusions. But I will say that if you are adventuresome, whipping the nape of your neck with nettles can't hurt (in the long run, that is) and it may just inject a minor moment of clarity that wouldn't normally be present.

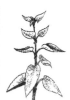

WHIP THAT SCIATICA!

One of the more extraordinary uses for urtication is to **alleviate sciatic pain**. It might sound as though it's some heinous act to sting someone who is already in pain, but I assure you it can really work wonders. The nettle sting is considered to be a "counterirritant," which is something that causes minor pain and allows the nervous system to ignore the deeper pain that is present. According to Dr. Duke, the compounds within the stingers that create the welts and burning sensations, "trigger the release of the body's natural anti-inflammatory chemicals." Says Duke, "The body's own medicine helps get rid of the sciatic inflammation."

To amplify the effect, after striking the skin with fresh nettle stalks, place a hot washcloth over the area for several minutes. Remove it and replace it with a cold washcloth for several minutes. Continue this hot and cold routine for 10 minutes and then allow the body to take over and start the healing process.

It may not work for everyone, but I have witnessed amazing recovery from sciatica using this exact method. For some, relief is temporary, lasting only a few days—for others, relief can last for weeks.

STOPS THE PAIN OF DEER FLY BITES, TOO

Another odd use I have found for urtication is to **take the itching and swelling out of deer fly bites**. After spending a long afternoon in the Colorado mountains one mid-summer day, I emerged from the thicket with large deer fly bites across my ankles. Within a day, they were terribly inflamed and forming tiny pustules which itched like mad. I was out picking nettles and getting very upset with the irritation these bites were causing when I mistakenly slapped a nettle stalk against my bare leg. I suddenly felt instant relief from the bites and decided to directly hit the bites a few more times with the nettle stalk. Several hours later, half the inflammation around the bites was gone, the pustules began drying up and the pain and itching were a distant memory. I've never read about using nettles in this way, but if you are ever unlucky enough to be bitten by deer flies, by all means, give nettle a try.

If you'd like to try urtication, start out slowly and only hit the area a few times with the nettle stalk. Wait an hour or so to see if you feel any relief. Often times, the "prickliness" and increased circulatory stimulation can be felt for up to 36 hours. I have noticed one unusual "side effect" of urtication and that is that it tends to increase urination. Since nettle tea affects the kidneys, it is interesting to note that topical "micro-injections" stimulate the same response. I suppose the healing compounds in the stinger really are penetrating through the skin and flowing into the system. But the sting itself was probably enough to convince you.

A WOMAN'S BEST BUDDY

Nettle is one of the best herbal allies a woman can have during all stages of her life. Chalk it up to nettle's high mineral content and top-notch cleansing abilities.

Those cleansing properties come in handy to tone and detoxify the liver of built-up estrogen which can contribute to symptoms of **PMS**. Drink two to three cups of the tea at the beginning of ovulation and continue until the menstrual cycle begins. If you have a large amount of stored estrogen "stuck" in your liver, you may experience a few days of emotional outbursts as the nettle tea works to cleanse the liver. If you have been having PMS symptoms for many years, I strongly suggest moderating your nettle tea dose so that you don't aggravate an already overly sensitive system. In the mind/body paradigm, the liver represents the place where you hold emotions—specifically anger. Thus, when you take herbs to clean out the liver, you release stored "anger" along with stored estrogen. For this reason, I'm not a big fan of cleansing programs that detoxify the liver too quickly and expect the individual to dump and deal with all that "emotional garbage" in an abbreviated time frame.

Thanks to nettle's natural knack of **stopping excessive internal bleeding**, a leaf tea can be taken by women to **reduce flooding during their menstrual cycle.**

Pregnant women can benefit from nettle when used in combination with red raspberry leaf. This is one of the oldest **pregnancy mineral tonics**, providing the body with much needed iron, calcium and other necessary nutrients. For every three tablespoons of dried red raspberry leaves, add one tablespoon of dried nettle leaves. Mix the herbs together and place one tablespoon of the blend into a container. Pour two cups of boiling water over the herbs and cover, allowing it to steep for 20 to 30 minutes. Strain and sip the tea throughout the day.

Once the baby is born, nettle tea comes to your aid again as a mineralizing **postpartum tonic**. Not only does this feed much needed minerals and vitamins to the mother, nettle tea helps to **increase breast milk**. To get the most benefit from the herb, nursing mothers need to drink the tea one hour or less before breast feeding.

There's another herbal rumor about nettle tea. Supposedly, it helps women **develop a more "ample breast"** over time. If this is something that sounds intriguing to you, try drinking one to three cups of the tea a day for several weeks with one week off.

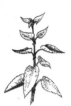

NETTLE TO THE RESPIRATORY RESCUE

Another classic use for nettle is an aid to **treating respiratory ailments such as bronchitis, tuberculosis, whooping cough, asthma and hay fever**. The root is considered the strongest part of the plant. You can use the liquid root extract or make a decoction by simmering one heaping teaspoon of the dried root in 10 ounces of distilled water for 20 minutes. Strain and sip the root tea, drinking several cups a day. The dried or fresh leaves are also viable as a tea. Make an infusion using two teaspoons of the dried leaf or four teaspoons of the chopped fresh leaves for every eight ounces of hot water.

PROSTATE HELP

A concentrated root extract of stinging nettle is being used successfully in Germany to treat **benign prostatic hypertrophy (BPH)** — an enlarged prostate gland. BPH affects half of men over the age of 50 and causes frequent trips to the bathroom during the night to urinate. Studies with 67 men over the age of 60 showed that two or three teaspoons of the root extract taken each day reduced their need to urinate at night.

HAIR RAISING RINSE

Nettle has been used as **a wonderful hair rinse to promote lots of shine while preventing hair loss and dandruff.** Some even say that regular rinses with the tea **may eventually bring back your natural hair color**. (Now I've got your attention.) Make up a big batch of nettle tea—figure one cup of the dried herb to two quarts of water. Boil the water, pour it over the dried plant and let it steep for eight to twelve hours. When ready, strain the herb and use part of the tea to wash your hair and the remaining part to rinse your hair. Don't rinse out the nettle tea.

For **dandruff**, steep one tablespoon of the dried leaves in a warm brew made from one-half cup apple cider vinegar and one-half cup water for 45 minutes. When cool, massage the mixture into the scalp. You can make up a big batch of this "tea" and keep it in the refrigerator for up to a week. It may take six months before you see any change, but there are people who swear by this hair raising recipe.

THINGS YOU SHOULD KNOW

Some herb books will tell you that once the herb is dried there is no chance of getting stung. This is not always true. I have touched one year old, bone-dry nettle stalks and received a sharp sting for the effort.

Only harvest the leaves from young plants that have no developed flowers (seed clusters). **Older plants that are brimming with tiny blooms are fine for urtication but not for eating or medicinal use. At that time, the leaves are known to develop gritty particles—known as "cystoliths"—that can cause severe kidney and urinary tract irritation**. I've known a few herbalists and nature lovers who make a habit of eating *fresh* nettle leaves, stingers and all. I'm always up for an adventure but I draw the line at eating fresh nettles.

You may have felt that nettle was not your cup of tea. But now you know that when you need a tingling tonic for your tired body—either internally or externally—it will be more than happy to oblige.

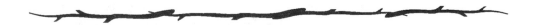

THE "DIRT" ON...STINGING NETTLE

Botanical ~	*Urtica dioica*
Growth cycle ~	Hardy perennial.
Medicinal uses~	Diuretic, counterirritant, astringent, galactagogue, hemostatic, mineral tonic.
Part(s) used for medicine ~	Leaves, root.
Vitamins/Minerals ~	High in iron, calcium, chlorophyll, potassium, magnesium, manganese, silica, silicon, boron, serotonin, protein, vitamins A, C, D.
Region ~	Found as low as sea level and as high as 10,000 feet in areas that are moist, dappled in shade and have rich to

moderate soil. Nettle is not naturally found in desert areas where the soil is parched.

Wild or Domestic ~ Both. There are approximately 50 species of nettle (*Urtica* species) in the world, all having similar properties as *Urtica dioica*.

Poisonous look-alikes in the wild ~ No. As for non-poisonous plants, immature nettle plants can be confused with wild spearmint. Both have square stems, but only the nettle has the sting. Some people also confuse stinging nettle with "dead nettle" (*Lamium album*), a member of the mint family. Dead nettle does not sting and, when mature, has white flowers that grow in the axils of the leaves.

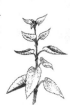

Hardy or Delicate ~ Very hardy.

Height of mature plant ~ Two to seven feet.

Easy or hard to grow ~ Can be difficult if the growing conditions are not optimum. Once established, nettle reproduces quite well as long as soil and water requirements remain present.

Cultivation ~ Grown from seeds, cuttings, nursery seedlings and root division, the latter best done in the fall after the leaves have died back. Cuttings can be challenging unless you have a knack for this. If you live in areas that experience frost or freezing temperatures, direct seeding may be your best bet. Fall sowing is recommended with seedlings appearing in early spring. Seed must be exposed to a cold (freezing is best), moist environment in order to germinate. Plan to broadcast more seed than you think you will need since it is typical to have only 50-60 percent of the seed successfully germinate. While I have had some luck in starting the seeds in flats and following the cold, moist conditioning requirements, the seedlings unfortunately do not transplant that well since the young root structure is weak. Because of this, take great care if you purchase established seedlings that are three inches or larger. Nettles must be kept continually moist and have exposure to sunshine with partial shade. If you do not have these conditions available in your yard, don't waste your time or money on seed/plants since they will either never emerge or die before reaching maturity.

Plant spacing ~ Six inches.

Pre-soak seeds ~ No.

Pre-chill seeds ~ Yes. Cold, moist conditioning required.

Indoor seed starting ~ No.

Light/dark seed requirements ~ Light.

303

Days to germinate ~ Once seed is exposed to cold, moist conditioning, germination can occur in 10 to 14 days.

Days to full maturity ~ Nettle can be harvested while still young (at six to eight inches). This can take about 50 to 70 days depending upon soil and water conditions. Full maturity (i.e., when seeds are well formed) can take a total of 120 days.

Soil type ~ Consistent moisture, rich, well-drained, composted.

Water requirements ~ Requires regular moisture without being drowned.

Sun or shade ~ Partial shade with full sun part of the day.

Propagation ~ Seed, underground roots.

Easy/hard to transplant ~ Hard. Direct seeding is best.

Pests or diseases ~ Virtually pest and disease-free.

Landscape uses ~ Dramatic background border. You could always put it in areas where you don't want visitors trespassing since they will be wary of it.

Gathering ~ Harvest the entire above ground plant with gloves in early to late spring when it is approximately eight inches to one foot in height. If you live in mountainous areas and have access to elevations as high as 8,000 feet, you could find young nettle in early stages of development as late as August. Where nettle grows in dense patches, you could possibly get three or four harvests each year since it will develop at various stages. Wear gloves and, holding the tip of the plant in one hand, cut the stem two to three inches above the ground. If you are using the plant fresh, strip the leaves off the stem when you are ready to steam them as a wild green or make them into a fresh tea. If you are harvesting the plant to dry, tie several leafy stalks together at one end and hang upside down in a dry, dark, warm area. Do not gather nettle after the drooping seed heads have formed since the plant becomes difficult for the body to assimilate at that point. If you are gathering nettle for external "urtication" purposes, the spring plants have the greatest "sting" potency. Mid-summer plants that are beginning to form seed heads can still be used for this, but the sting is less bothersome.

Best fresh or dried ~ Fresh is best but if properly dried, nettle is very effective.

Drying methods ~ Dry leaves as quickly as possible without exposing them to artificial heat (such as a heat lamp or forced hot air). Leaves tend to turn under and become darkened if dried too quickly. Do not rinse the leaves off with water before drying since this will make them turn brown or black as they dry. As for the roots, rinse off the dirt and dry them in a warm, shady place.

Amount needed ~ Moderate use: 25 plants; Regular use: 50+

Seed collection ~

Nettle seed is very small. Collection method is similar to spearmint. Wait until the tiny, green flower clusters are dried on the stalk (usually around August or September). Gather five or eight stalks and place them loosely into a paper bag. Keep the bag in a dry, warm place away from sunlight or extreme heat. Shake the plants occasionally to release the seed. Note that nettle has both male and female flowers. The female flowers grow down on the plant and in clusters; the male flowers grow upward and appear on dangling "strings" or racemes.

Companion planting ~

Nettles tend to increase the natural oil content of neighboring plants. For this reason, herbs such as anise, peppermint, spearmint, lemon balm, rosemary, thyme and yarrow could benefit. In the wild, nettles are often found growing amongst chickweed, lamb's quarters, hound's tongue, yellow dock, mullein, plantain, jewelweed and, occasionally, blue violet.

Container planting ~

No, you would never get enough to make it worthwhile.

Common mistakes ~

Planting nettle in a location that is too dry and/or rocky to support the herb. Nettles must be planted in rich soil and have a constant supply of moisture with an underground source being preferred. Also, many people are under the impression that nettles lose their sting an hour or so after they have been cut. This is absolutely not so. Nettles remain quite active in the "sting department" for days, even if they have been placed in a paper bag.

Interesting facts/tips ~

When added to compost piles, nettles set the decomposition motion in action. Nettle fiber—which can be pulled from the center of the dried stalks—is an incredibly durable thread that is woven into material that feels as fine as silk. The only drawback is that production of nettle fiber is labor intensive. Wilderness experts rely on nettle stem fiber to produce "cordage" that can be made into fishing line, a strong rope or twisted into a "backwoods bracelet" that is resistant to water.

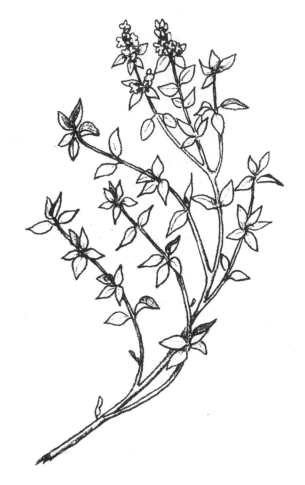

Chapter 34

IT'S ABOUT THYME

Thymus vulgaris (garden thyme or English thyme)

Thymus serpyllum (wild thyme or mother of thyme)

Hardy perennial

Medicinal Uses: *Expectorant, anti-bacterial, anti-viral, antiparasitic, antispasmodic, antifungal, antiseptic, antioxidant, carminative, diaphoretic, mild sedative*

Medicinal parts of plant: *Leaves*

Forms: *Tea, fresh plant tincture, pure essential oil, extracted oil*

WHAT IS ITS CHARACTER?

I had always looked on thyme as a rather genteel plant since I associated it with manicured, fragrant herb gardens. But after closer examination, I saw another side of this herb. Upon finding it in a well-manicured garden where all the plants look as though they are on their best behavior, I noticed that one of the many thyme plants was straying from its designated plot. Like a plant with a mission, it wandered purposefully across the pathway. I'm sure if the gardener hadn't seen it, the plant would have successfully escaped and kicked up its heels outside the garden gate. Thyme might look all buttoned up and ready for church when it is forced to conform to a stringent garden protocol. But underneath, it's a wild child, eager to roam and be free.

WHERE DO I FIND IT?

Thyme is a native plant to the western Mediterranean. It can be grown from sea level to 8,000 feet. However, the higher the altitude, the more likely thyme will need to be an inside plant due to low temperature sensitivity. Thyme is hardy to temperatures as low as 30°F and as high as 110°F.

HOW DO I GROW IT?

Thyme is easy to grow from either seed, root cuttings or established plants. While many herb books recommend stem cuttings, novice gardeners may have trouble with them since they can take several months to take hold. The seed *must* have warm soil and warm temperatures that hover around 70°F or higher in order to germinate. Place seed in 1/4" drills and barely cover with soil. Do not scatter seed too thickly. Thin seedlings to give plants plenty of room to grow. Space plants six inches to one foot apart.

HOW DO I HARVEST IT?

Harvest the plant just before it blooms, cutting it several inches above the base. The volatile oils, including *thymol*, are most active in the fresh plant. However, if thyme is dried and stored correctly, it can work just fine. Thyme has a tendency to clump together when harvested. If this happens, pull the plant apart as much as possible and lay it on a drying screen or clean piece of cloth *out of direct sunlight*. Thyme should be dried in a warm, dry area and checked daily. Don't over dry thyme since you will lose some of the oils that make it such a valuable remedy. Once ready, immediately strip the leaves from the stems and store them in an airtight glass jar.

HOW DO I USE IT?

With apologies to Willie Nelson, "If you've got a little money, honey, you can have the thyme." "Little" is the operative word because, like most herbs, thyme is inexpensive to maintain and oh-so good in the medicinal department.

Today, most people look at thyme and think "culinary herb." But a long time ago, this warmly aromatic garden favorite was considered to be a holy herb, believed to have supernatural healing powers. Thyme even caught the attention of Hippocrates who regarded it as an herb that was worth much more than a passing glance. Yet, as the centuries rolled on, thyme shuffled out of the medicinal loop and moved over to the cooking section. Thyme will still make your meat marvelous, your poultry positively perfect and your stuffing stupendous. But I believe it's thyme you should know the power behind this classic herb.

THE "ANTI-HERB"

Call thyme the "anti" herb–as in **antiseptic, antifungal, anti-viral, anti-bacterial, antioxidant, antiparasitic** and **antispasmodic**. Thank the major ingredient "thymol" for much of this action. "Thymol" is thought responsible for fighting a host of gram negative and gram positive bacteria, including **staphylococcus aureus** and **e. coli**. The fact is that "thymol" has been credited with being responsible for much of thyme's medicinal action, including the herb's ability to quell a cold, curb a cough, soothe sore joints and so much more. Read on and discover many more important uses for this "old-thymey" herb.

COLD & COUGH THYME

Thyme has been widely used for centuries as a remedy for the common cold. Today it is known that the fresh plant made into a tea or an alcohol tincture is the best and most active form to garner the medicinal benefits. Thyme fights the common cold by **causing the body to sweat out the toxins** which helps a person throw off those first symptoms of shivering, quivering and aching muscles that accompany the common cold. In addition, thyme acts as an **internal antiseptic against further infection**.

You can use thyme on its own. However, some herbalists believe that thyme is strengthened if it is combined with other cold and flu herbs. Echinacea is a great example. Research has shown that **due to the natural tannin content in thyme, it may accelerate the antibiotic action of echinacea**. Since echinacea is most effective when both water and alcohol are used to extract its principles, I always suggest purchasing a

308

tincture that has 70 percent alcohol and 30 percent water. Make a tea out of fresh or dried thyme by combining one teaspoon of the dried plant or two teaspoons of the fresh plant to eight ounces of boiling water. Cover and let the herb steep for 15 minutes. Strain the herb and add one teaspoon of the echinacea tincture to the tea. The hotter you drink the tea, the more likely you are to perspire so make sure you stay warm to prevent a chill. You can take up to six cups a day of this mixture. Often times, I have found that a hot bath helps start the "toxin-dumping" process and can speed up the healing process.

If you want to **cleanse the air of germs**, fill a glass spray bottle with four ounces of distilled water and add 50 drops of thyme essential oil. Shake the bottle vigorously each time before spraying since the essential oil tends to quickly separate from the water.

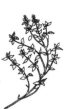

Thyme tea or the fresh plant tincture is also a **classic remedy for respiratory complaints** that include **whooping cough, tuberculosis, sinus ailments, asthma** and **sore throats**. "Thymol" once again comes into play by helping to soothe a cough as well as **bring up mucus, especially when it is deeply-seated, thick and yellow in color**. The tea should be taken as hot as possible and can be drunk four to six times a day. If you prefer the fresh plant tincture, add one-half teaspoon of it to eight ounces of hot water and drink it as hot as you can stand it. This can also be repeated up to six times a day. **When it comes to respiratory relief, it is sometimes necessary to use more frequent doses of thyme tea or tincture**. However, if at any time you feel nauseous or feel the frequent doses are giving you an upset stomach, either reduce the dose or discontinue.

For *topical* respiratory relief, I've had great success blending three to five drops of thyme essential oil into a tablespoon of either apricot kernel oil or castor oil and massaging the mixture on my chest. It creates a noticeable heat that can be a great comfort when you are battling lung-related ailments. (If you would like to make an even stronger respiratory rub, check out the box on page 310 and the formula for my "Breathe-Free Chest Balm.") **Thyme essential oil is extremely concentrated and should never be applied to the skin undiluted. The essential oil is also not recommended for children's tender skin since it can burn and sometimes cause a blister**.

*BREATHE-FREE CHEST BALM**

This is a very popular and effective chest balm that I created and students love to make. It works very well to relieve all kinds of respiratory problems, from the common cough to pneumonia.

The following formula will make one ounce.

Depending upon the consistency you prefer, you may want to adjust the amount of beeswax in the formula to make the balm thicker or smoother.

Place one teaspoon of melted yellow beeswax into a one ounce glass jar. (Baby food glass jars are excellent for this purpose). Add three teaspoons of room temperature castor oil. Heat the jar either in a shallow pan of boiling water or in the oven at 180° or less. Stir occasionally to blend the oil and beeswax. Once the base oil is completely dissolved with the beeswax, remove from the water bath or oven and start stirring the mixture *quickly* with a toothpick or slender wooden stick. *Do not use plastic since it will melt.*

When the mixture is lukewarm to cool—which can take anywhere from 10 to 20 minutes—start adding the essential oils. *Do not add the essential oils before the oil and beeswax have a chance to cool since the active principles within the oils will evaporate and you will lose their healing benefit.* Add one essential oil at a time, stirring well between each addition. The number in the "( )" is the exact amount of drops for that specific pure essential oil. DO NOT EXCEED THE RECOMMENDED DROPS. Essential oils are VERY CONCENTRATED AND EXTREMELY STRONG. Too much of any oil can cause more harm than good–especially when you are placing the balm directly upon your skin.

Thyme (14) Expectorant, colds, cough, stimulates immune system, antibacterial.

Eucalyptus (6) Strong antiseptic qualities, antiviral, antibacterial, expectorant action, bronchitis, coughs, sinusitis.

Camphor (6) Strong decongestant, coughs, sinusitis.

Wintergreen (6) Sinusitis, decongestant, stimulating.

Peppermint (6) Decongestant, sinusitis, uplifting to the senses, bronchitis, anti-inflammatory.

Lavender (3) Bacterial infections, sinus infection, sore throat, congestion, nervousness during illness, insomnia, strengthens the immune system.

Pine (3) Sinusitis, bronchitis, strong expectorant & decongestant, increases circulation to local area.

Clove (3) Bronchitis, asthma, warming.

Tea Tree (3) Bacterial infections, anti-viral, antifungal.

***DO NOT USE DURING PREGNANCY OR IF
TAKING HOMEOPATHIC REMEDIES.**

BATH THYME

A thyme bath has long been considered the perfect remedy for everything from **nervous exhaustion** to **soothing respiratory problems**. To make the bath, you're going to need a lot of thyme–about two cups of the dried herb or four cups of the fresh plant. Bring a large pasta-sized pot full of water to a boil and turn off the heat. Add the thyme, cover and steep for 10 to 20 minutes. While that's steeping, pour a hot bath. When the herb is ready, carefully strain the dark liquid into the hot bath water. Soak in the bath for up to 30 minutes, breathing in the fragrant vapors. The oils trapped within the herb tend to release very quickly whenever hot water touches them. The oils are absorbed into every pore of the body, causing the body to perspire profusely. Don't be alarmed if this happens–this is simply your body's way of throwing off any toxic material. This is a classic herb bath to take at the first sign of a cold or flu. Breathing in the aromatic fumes is also beneficial for those suffering from any kind of bronchial problems. **Bronchitis**, **whooping cough**, **painful barking coughs** and even **mild cases of asthma** can all be eased with a thyme bath. After getting out of the bath, it's very important to bundle up and get into bed since your body will continue to perspire for up to an hour afterwards.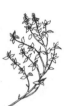

If you wish to "juice up" the aromatic oil content of this bath, place 10 drops of thyme pure essential oil into a tablespoon of either castor oil or apricot kernel oil and swish the mixture into the water just before you get into the tub. The only people who should not add the oil are those who have sensitive or fair skin since thyme essential oil has been known to burn and blister.

MOUTH & THROAT THYME

One of the most popular ways to use thyme is as **a gargle to disinfect and ease the discomfort of a sore throat**. It also does a bang-up job on **sore gums** when swished in the mouth for several minutes. An added bonus is that thyme **freshens the breath while killing those germs**. Another product on the market that makes that claim is Listerine, which just happens to include "thymol" at the top of its list of "active ingredients." To make your own gargle, sore gum rinse or mouth wash from thyme, use a double strength tea concoction (i.e., two heaping teaspoons of dried plant or four heaping teaspoons of the fresh plant steeped in eight ounces of hot water) or opt for the fresh plant tincture, adding 25 drops to several ounces of warm water.

OH, IT'S CRAMPING THYME

Whether the stomach starts cramping because of **nerves**, **stress**, **a disagreeable meal** or **menstrual difficulties**, thyme tea can work to **soothe and relieve tension**. In addition, thyme's **mild sedative** qualities also come into play without making you feel dopey. As you slowly sip an eight ounce cup of hot thyme tea, sit quietly or, better yet, lie down.

Thyme tea has also been used to **quell the painful griping of gastritis** as well as **increase the appetite**. To encourage the latter, drink an eight ounce cup of the tea 15 to 30 minutes before eating. Thyme can also be employed as an excellent after dinner, **digestive tea** if you're feeling bloated after a meal.

THE JOINTS OF THYME

Add ten to fifteen drops of thyme essential oil to a tablespoon of a light, penetrating base oil (such as apricot kernel oil) or use thyme *extracted* oil or thyme tincture and you have an excellent healing rub for **inflamed joints**, **sprains** and **shingles**.

For inflamed joints and sprains, you could use either of the oils or the tincture. However, **for shingles, I would not use the pure essential oil or tincture since it could burn and aggravate the condition**. Instead, use the *extracted* oil. To make this, simply pack a widemouthed jar tightly to the brim with fresh or dried flowers and stems. Cover the herb with equal parts of olive oil and wheat germ oil. (You can substitute peanut or sesame oil for the olive oil). If you are using the fresh plant, place a piece of muslin over the top held in place by a rubber band. If you are using the dried plant, use the lid. Place the jar in a sunny window for four to six weeks. After that period, strain the oil through a muslin cloth, wringing out every last drop from the oil-soaked herbs. To give the oil added preservative power, add one drop of benzoin tincture for every liquid ounce of oil. You now have a dandy oil which will keep fresh for up to six months if kept in a cool, dark place.

WOUND THYME

Thyme's strong antiseptic abilities make it a number one remedy for **infected wounds**, **insect bites** and **fungal problems such as athlete's foot**. The tea is a little weak for this purpose, so I suggest using the fresh plant tincture or *diluted* essential oil. For the tincture, soak a cotton pad with the liquid and place it over the area to be treated. For the essential oil, either blend 10 drops in a tablespoon of apricot kernel oil or add 10 drops to four ounces of cold water and use as a wash. If all you have is the plant, that will work. Take a small handful of the *fresh* plant, chew it into a wet poultice and press it into your skin. Hold it in place with a handkerchief, a string or piece of tape and check it frequently.

WORM THYME

Thyme is very effective to rid the body of **hookworms**. Even though the herb is strong, it is safe for children to use. I would use a double-strength tea made from the *fresh* plant *or* opt for the ease and convenience of the fresh plant tincture. You can take up to three cups a day of the double-strength tea. For the tincture, add 25 to 30 drops to two or three ounces of hot water. Repeat this every two to three hours.

In addition to using thyme, include one or two handfuls of freshly ground pumpkin seeds into your diet each day along with two to six cloves of *fresh* garlic. The diet in general should be fairly bland and should not include any dairy, meat, sugar, wheat or alcohol since this gives the hookworms something to feast upon. Drink plenty of distilled water and eat lots of leafy greens and fresh fruit. Before bedtime, drink one cup of senna *pod* (*not* leaf) tea, made by pouring eight ounces of hot water over one tablespoon of senna pods and steeping them in a covered container for two hours or longer. (The longer you steep the pods, the better). By morning, this should promote a gentle bowel movement. Eat no food the following morning until you have had a bowel movement. Senna *leaves* should not be used since they are both addictive and create horrible bowel cramps. Since hookworms can be very hard to get rid of, diligence with this or any other natural healing program is mandatory.

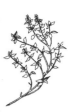

THYME TO PURIFY THAT WATER

Author John Heinerman claims that fresh thyme can be used to **purify water** when traveling in countries where purity is an issue. He suggests using one good handful of fresh thyme for every quart of suspicious water. Cover the vessel and simmer the herb in the water for 20 minutes. Strain the herb and, according to Heinerman, you now have "safe drinking water that won't give you any more diarrhea and fever." What you also have is a quart of strong thyme tea.

THYME TO GET RID OF THOSE BUGS

Hang dried thyme in closets or place the plant in muslin drawstring bags to **deter moths** from infesting woolen coats and sweaters.

Bugged by bothersome flies? No problem. Simply fill a glass spray bottle with four ounces of distilled water and add 50 drops of thyme pure essential oil. Shake vigorously each time before you spray the air since the essential oil has a tendency to separate from the water.

THYME TO STIMULATE THE BRAIN

Place eight to ten drops of thyme essential oil into a lamp ring and feel your **energy surge**. You may also get a temporary **boost to your brain power** which can be good for students who need a little aromatic motivation. The aroma of thyme essential oil is also considered good for **depression** as well as **debilitating conditions** brought on by a prolonged illness.

SOME CAUTIONS TO BE AWARE OF

Since thyme herb and essential oil are uterine stimulants, **do not use the herb during pregnancy**. Seasoning your food with *small amounts* of the dried herb is okay. **Excessive use of thyme for days or weeks at a time may stimulate the thyroid gland too much. Ingesting too much of this herb can lead to symptoms of poisoning**. While you do need large doses of the herb tea when using it for respiratory complaints, the secret is to use thyme for short periods, with a week or so off in between. As mentioned previously, **thyme essential oil can be very hot and cause blisters on those with sensitive or fair skin if it is used undiluted**.

You can now see why this thyme-ly herb does far more than simply add punch to your poultry. In my opinion, it's about thyme people took this herb more seriously.

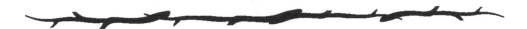

THE "DIRT" ON... THYME

Botanical ~	*Thymus vulgaris* (garden thyme or English thyme) and *Thymus serpyllum* (wild thyme or mother of thyme) are two of the common medicinal species.
Growth cycle ~	Perennial.
Medicinal uses~	Expectorant, anti-bacterial, anti viral, antiparasitic, anti-spasmodic, antifungal, antiseptic, antioxidant, carminative, diaphoretic, mild sedative.
Part(s) used for medicine ~	Leaves.
Vitamins/Minerals ~	Not applicable.
Region ~	Thyme is a native plant to the western Mediterranean. Can be grown from sea level to 8,000 feet. However, the higher the altitude, the more likely thyme will need to be an inside plant due to low temperature sensitivity. Thyme is hardy to temperatures as low as 30°F and as high as 110°F.
Wild or Domestic ~	Wild thyme/mother of thyme (*Thymus serpyllum*) is both wild and domestic whereas garden thyme and the hundreds of other species are more typically domesticated.
Poisonous look-alikes in the wild ~	No.
Hardy or Delicate ~	Hardy.

Height of mature plant ~   Six to eighteen inches.

Easy or hard to grow ~   Easy from either seed or root cuttings. Novice gardeners may have more trouble with stem cuttings.

Cultivation ~   Seed, root cutting, established plants, stem cuttings. Seed must have warm soil and warm temperatures that hover around 70°F or hotter in order to germinate. Place seed in 1/4" drills and barely cover with soil. Do not scatter seed too thickly.

Plant spacing ~   Six inches to one foot.

Pre-soak seeds ~   No.

Pre-chill seeds ~   No.

Indoor seed starting ~   Yes. If you live in climates that have late frosts, starting the seed indoors allows the plant to get a head start. Use either seed cells or flats.

Light/dark seed requirements ~   Light.

Days to germinate ~   If soil and air temperature are warm, seed can germinate within eight days. Typical germination takes 14 to 21 days. If soil is not kept warm, germination can sometimes be as low as 50 percent.

Days to full maturity ~   Approximately 90 days if kept consistently warm.

Soil type ~   Light, warm, sandy soil with a moderate amount of compost.

Water requirements ~   Moderate watering. Do not allow the soil to become bone dry or the plant will suffer.

Sun or shade ~   Full sun.

Propagation ~   Seed and underground roots.

Easy/hard to transplant ~   Easy. Wait until they reach four to five inches tall. Seedlings require regular watering, without drowning, until they become firmly established.

Pests or diseases ~   Virtually pest and disease-free. Thyme actually helps repel both whiteflies and cabbageworms.

Landscape uses ~   Classic ground cover and aromatic crevice plant. Can also work as an attractive border if it is kept clipped.

Gathering ~   Harvest the plant just before it blooms. Cut it several inches above the base.

Best fresh or dried ~   The volatile oils, including thymol, are most active in the fresh plant. However, if thyme is dried and stored correctly, it can work very well.

Drying methods ~   Thyme has a tendency to clump together when you harvest it. If this happens, pull the plant apart as much as possible and lay on a drying screen or clean piece of cloth out of direct sunlight. Thyme should be dried in a warm, dry area and checked daily. Don't over dry thyme since you will lose some of the oils that make it such a valuable remedy. Once ready, immediately strip the leaves from the stems and store them in an airtight glass jar.

Amount needed ~ Moderate use: 5 plants; Regular use: 15+.

Seed collection ~ Allow a number of plants to fully flower. In late summer, occasionally tap the flower heads into the palm of your hand to check for seed development. Once you are able to tap several seeds into your hand, clip that stem and place it head first into a paper bag. Set it in a dry, warm area away from direct sunlight. Shake the stem occasionally inside the bag to release more seeds.

Companion planting ~ Thyme is thought to enhance the growth of tomatoes, potatoes and eggplant. It also helps repel whiteflies and cabbageworms. Planting stinging nettle nearby is said to increase the volatile oil content of thyme.

Container planting ~ Yes. Thyme makes an excellent container plant for indoor or outdoor use. It is especially recommended to start thyme in pots if your outdoor winter temperatures dip below 30°F since a hard freeze will kill plants and compromise spring germination. Also, make sure the pot is well-drained since thyme doesn't like to stand in water.

Common mistakes ~ Some people believe that since thyme does not need much water, it is okay to allow the soil to become bone dry. Unfortunately, if this pattern continues, you will wake up one morning with a dying plant that will be difficult, if not impossible, to bring back to life. Water whenever the soil starts looking parched and spray the plant with a fine mist of water if you live in areas that are especially dry and hot.

Interesting facts/tips ~ Six pounds of seeds will sow one acre. To ensure years of healthy growth, propagate a few new plants each year to replace those that may be lost to age or are damaged by weather. There are well over 100 species of thyme. Some say there are as many as 400. All share similar medicinal properties. However, some of the more scented varieties such as pinewood thyme and nutmeg thyme don't agree with everyone when used for medicine. Save those for culinary use. If you have any plants that die back or dry out in the garden, gather them together and place them on barbecue coals to add a lovely smoky flavor to meat.

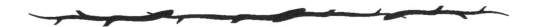

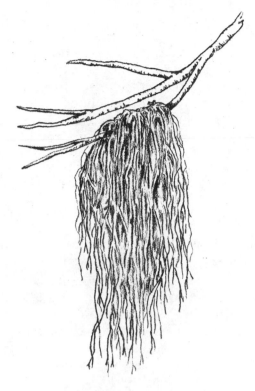

Chapter 35

Usnea

~

You'll Really, Really Lichen This Fungus For Infection

Usnea barbata / Usnea longissima
Usnea ceratina / Usnea dasypoga
Usnea birta / Usnea florida
Usnea Californica
Hardy perennial

Medicinal Uses: *Anti-bacterial, antifungal, anti-viral, antibiotic, immune-supporting, vulnerary, pectoral, diuretic*
Medicinal parts of plant: *Whole plant*
Forms: *Fresh plant tincture, fresh and dried plant, extracted oil, salve*

WHAT IS ITS CHARACTER?

I've always looked on this fabulous forest find as the elder statesman of the woods. Perhaps it's because it takes months and months of the right conditions within a thicket of timber for usnea to fully develop. Or maybe it's because it resembles a ragged beard as it hangs stiffly from tree branches. Whatever the reason, I have a feeling its long period of maturation has given it a chance to soak up the wisdom, energy and secrets of all the other trees and plants that surround it. To the untrained eye, usnea may look like an odd piece of "forest lint" clinging to the various tree branches. But if you only knew the stories it could tell….

WHERE DO I FIND IT?

Usnea–which has various medicinal varieties including *Usnea barbata, Usnea longissima, Usnea ceratina, Usnea dasypoga, Usnea hirta, Usnea florida and Usnea Californica*–is also known as "Larch moss," "Bear lichen, "Beard lichen" or, the most popular, "Old Man's Beard." The last reference refers to the fact that usnea often resembles an old man's beard as it hangs off the branches of pines, oaks, Douglas firs and apple trees. Typically, you'll find usnea on these trees *above* 3000 feet and preferably in areas of the forest that are shaded and densely populated with plant life. These trees can be standing, recently fallen or dead. Usnea does not care. I've found copious amounts of usnea on dead, downed oaks.

HOW DO I GROW IT?

You don't grow usnea. Rather, it appears *very slowly* hanging on the branches of trees that grow within a dense forest setting. It evolves after a fungus forms the base for chlorophyll-bearing algae to spread out and provide food sugars for both entities. Putting it more simply, usnea is a lichen, which is part fungus and part algae. When the two come together, they form a plant life that is unlike either the fungus or the algae, with chemicals that are unique only to usnea. Instead of cultivating usnea, cultivate the knowledge of where you can find this very useful lichen in the wild.

HOW DO I HARVEST IT?

Harvesting usnea is as easy as breathing. Simply pull it off the branch and place it in your gathering sack. It takes *a lot* of usnea to make a tincture or extracted oil since it's very light in weight and tends to compress down into a single mass when many pieces are pressed together. I have found the easiest way to harvest usnea is to find a downed tree that serves as a horizontal "catch basket" for this lovable lichen. **One impor-**

tant note: usnea tends to accumulate heavy metals from the air. Keep this in mind when you are wildcrafting this lichen. In other words, do not harvest in areas that have obvious high amounts of airborne pollution. Do not harvest around old or working mines or in areas that are dumping grounds and landfills for waste products of known or unknown origin. Also, pick usnea at least 200 feet from heavily travelled roads due to the potential contamination from car fumes.

HOW DO I USE IT?

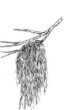

Years ago, a friend of mine begged me to take a class with her called "Communing with Nature—A Guided Journey Through the Wilderness Portals." Just the title made me nervous. I enjoy a nature hike, but something about this class worried me.

Our guide through nature's portals was named Lark—a woman who was so thin and pale that a mild breeze would have easily sent her soaring into the next zip code. Her skin was paper thin with a road map of soft blue veins that ran underneath in variegated patterns. Lark didn't exactly talk; it was more like whispering, which made our guided journey difficult at best since the group spent a great deal of time muttering "What did she say?" and "Huh?"

Lark loved plants. Lark loved trees. Lark loved dirt. Lark did *not* like people. I say this because every time someone asked her a question, she'd cut them off with a quick "Shhh!" and then tell us the plants were communing with her and she had to pay attention.

Lark also did not like humor. That was a pity because when she lead us into a dark crevice of the forest, shaded with layers of dense pine trees and thick stands of oaks, she introduced the group to a curious little gray-green growth that hung like icicles from the tree branches. She approached it with reference, softly caressed it's rough exterior and spoke in her trademark whisper. "This is usnea," she uttered. "It's very special. It's a lichen. A lichen is not really a plant. It's two organisms living together as one. And through their relationship, they join, forming an eternal partnership in the ecosystem we call nature." At this point, Lark choked up and a tiny tear rolled down her cheek.

I came closer to the tree and examined the usnea and said, "It's a fungus, Lark. Calm down." While the class enjoyed this little bit of levity, Lark did not. She ignored me for the rest of the class. I would never forget my guided journey through that wilderness portal and I would always remember that funny plant called usnea. The only problem was that there was not a whole lot of available information on this lovable lichen. I set out to learn more about usnea and discovered that it was truly a fabulous fungus when it comes to **infection** and **respiratory ailments**.

319

PULL APART THE "OLD MAN'S BEARD"

If you come upon this plant life affectionately known as "Old Man's Beard," take a single piece of the gray-green stem and gently pull it apart. Hidden inside, you should find a resilient white cord that is stiff when the plant is dry and similar to a crude piece of elastic when it is wet. If you cannot find this inner white thread, you are not looking at usnea. The outer part of the plant (i.e., the gray-green rough "tendrils") contains the strong antibiotic properties. The inner core, including the white thread, contains the immune-stimulating *polysaccharides*.

The active ingredient in all the usnea varieties are lichen acids—especially something called *usnic acid*. **Usnic acid is considered "poorly water soluble" which means that teas are only mildly effective. However, teas can still be used in a pinch**. The best ways to use usnea are chewing it right off the tree, tincturing it in a grain alcohol/distilled water solution and, for *external use*, making a heat extracted oil from handfuls of the stuff or crushing it into a powder to sprinkle on wounds as a disinfectant.

How to Make A Homemade Usnea Tincture

You will need a wide mouth, quart glass jar (canning jars are good for this purpose), grain alcohol (which is sold under the brand name "Everclear"), distilled water and of course, *fresh* usnea. As you collect the usnea, work it into a ball to condense it as much as possible. You should harvest enough to have two or three good sized handfuls. Once you determine the weight in ounces of the usnea, multiply that by three. That will give you the amount of alcohol and distilled water that is needed. For example, if three good handfuls weigh six ounces, six multiplied by three equals 18 ounces. Of that 18 ounces, 70 percent must be grain alcohol and 30 percent is distilled water. Seventy percent of 18 comes out to 12.6. I would round that up to 13. Thus, for six ounces by weight of fresh usnea, you would add 13 ounces of grain alcohol and five ounces of distilled water. Stuff the usnea tightly in the glass jar and pour the grain alcohol and distilled water over it. If the usnea absorbs a lot of it, you haven't condensed the plant enough in the glass jar. Store the jar in a cool, dry, dark place for a minimum of 60 days. Many herbalists believe that fresh tinctures, such as this one, are best after a full year of soaking. When you are ready, strain the herb from the alcohol/water solution through a muslin cloth, squeezing every last drop of the liquid from the herb. Keep the tincture in dark amber bottles and in a cool, dry location. It should keep for five years or longer.

What is usnea good for, you ask? How about this laundry list of physical problems which have been *proven* to react positively to usnea.

- **Streptococcus**
- **Staphylococcus (especially impetigo)**
- **Trichomonas**

- **Candida albicans**
- **Vaginal chlamydia infection**
- **Infected wounds**
- **Tuberculosis, pleurisy, pneumonia**
- **Infected gums**
- **Any fungus infection (including athlete's foot)**
- **Ringworm**
- **Colds & Flu**
- **Bronchitis**
- **Sinus infection**
- **Urinary tract infection**

What's even more amazing about usnea is that the active principle, *usnic acid,* is considered **"more effective" than penicillin against some bacterial strains, including human tuberculosis, staphylococcus, streptococcus and pneumonococcus**. What's more, while drugs destroy intestinal flora, usnea does not. This allows the body to retain more of its natural defenses to fight the condition.

THE STREP BUSTER!

For **strep** conditions, the recommended dose is 20 to 35 drops of the tincture every two hours during waking hours. Place the drops into two ounces of warm, distilled water, gargle as long as you can and swallow. (This also works for your run-of-the mill **sore throat**). I would personally combine equal amounts of echinacea tincture to the strep blend to supercharge the infection-fighting potential. Understand that with strep *you must be tenacious in your approach if you choose a natural versus antibiotic healing route.* If you do not feel you can keep plugging away every two hours, it might be best to use the antibiotic approach.

SOOTHES IMPETIGO

Impetigo—a skin disease brought on by a bacterial infection that creates pus-filled lesions on the skin—is typically associated with young children. Staph or strep is considered the root of impetigo. Like strep, you must be diligent when using plant medicinals for impetigo since, left untreated or treated without persistence, impetigo can lead to severe kidney infections. Lymph and blood cleansing teas such as burdock root, cleavers, yellow dock and red clover should be considered as part of the protocol in addition to echinacea tincture and fresh garlic to fight the infection. Combining equal parts of usnea with the echinacea tincture will help potentiate echinacea's action as well as serve as another heavy duty antibacterial agent. The impetigo pustules must not be allowed to spread up into the nose. To dry them up, saturate a cotton ball with usnea tincture (do *not* dilute with water) and hold it against the lesions several times a day. Do not wash the tincture off in between.

THE TRICHOMONAS EFFECT

Usnea is also considered "superior" to the drug Flagyl (metronidazole) which is commonly prescribed for women who have **trichomonas**. Trichomonas is a parasite infection of the uterine cervix. Flagyl has been found to cause cancer in some women and can be found in the bloodstream, cerebrospinal fluid and breast milk of nursing mothers. Nursing mothers are warned to avoid the use of Flagyl for this reason. However, usnea is safe in proper dose amounts. For trichomonas, the recommended dose at the onset of the condition is 10 to 30 drops of usnea tincture taken in two ounces of warm, distilled water every two hours (during waking hours) for one week. After the first week, maintain a dosage of 20 to 30 drops of the tincture, three times a day until the infection is completely out of the system. For those whose immune systems are not charging at full throttle, it might take consistent daily doses of the tincture for three or more months. My most conservative advice to anyone who sees *no* results after 10 days of continual usnea use *or* who feels the infection worsening, is to discontinue the herbal remedy and seek antibiotic treatment.

THIS LICHEN WILL LOVE YOUR WOUND

If you fall down in the woods while you are collecting usnea (or any other plant) and scrape your skin, you can apply a saliva-moistened ball of this lichen to the **wound** to halt infection and speed healing. Usnea also works as an **antimicrobial compress to stop bleeding in the wound**. If you don't want to depend upon "happening upon" usnea when and if you cut yourself, you can always carry a small bottle of the powdered herb in your pack and sprinkle it onto the wound or use the tincture, applying it full-strength or diluted half and half with water. Other options include the oil and salve.

THE ALL-AROUND ANTI-INFECTION REMEDY

As mentioned previously, usnea combines *exceptionally* well with echinacea whenever one needs a reliable **internal and external anti-infection remedy**. This could be everything from an **infected boil, carbuncle** or **cut** to the **common cold** and **bronchitis**. However, if you add echinacea, do not use the combination *internally* for more than 14 days since echinacea loses effectiveness after that point.

KEEP YOUR RESPIRATORY TRACT HEALTHY

Naturopathic doctor Alfred Vogel writes enthusiastically in his classic herbal tome *The Nature Doctor* about picking usnea off low lying branches and chewing it during winter ski trips. He comments that he had to "fight with the deer for this **great natural antibiotic**." Dr. Vogel says that continued use of usnea throughout the winter months helped clear up **respiratory tract infections that produced plenty of yellow, thick phlegm** as well as **acted as a natural preventative against the condition**. If you live in wet and/or cold climates and are prone to seasonal respiratory conditions with lots of catarrh (inflammation of the mucous membrane of the nose and/or throat), usnea could be your remedy. A good maintenance dose is 15 to 20 drops of the tincture diluted in several ounces of warm distilled water taken upon rising.

How to Make A Healing Usnea Oil & Salve

Take several condensed handfuls of fresh usnea and stuff it very tightly into a 16 ounce wide mouth glass jar. Once you cannot get anymore usnea in the jar, cover the plant with extra virgin olive oil. Instead of placing the lid on the jar, cover it with a piece of muslin cloth, held in place by a rubber band. Put the jar in a south-facing window or directly in bright sunshine. The hotter the bottle becomes, the better the extraction will be. If you can find wide mouth amber or cobalt blue jars, you will be able to generate even more heat. Large vitamin bottles and Ovaltine jars are great for this purpose. Keep the jar in the sunshine for a minimum of three months. Check it periodically to make sure it hasn't turned rancid due to water or bacteria getting inside the jar. After three or more months, decant what you need, leaving the plant matter and remaining oil in the jar to continue "cooking." To make a salve from the oil, pour the oil into a glass jar and gently heat it in a 200°F oven. Add just enough yellow beeswax to give it a smooth texture. When the wax has completely melted into the oil, stir the salve with a wooden stick (a toothpick works well for this purpose) to make sure the oil completely blends with the beeswax. Set it aside to cool. To "juice up" the infection fighting potential of this salve, remove the jar from the oven and continue stirring until the jar feels lukewarm to the touch. At that point, for every ounce of salve, add 15 drops of tea tree oil essential oil. Stir rapidly to make sure the essential oil completely dissolves and is not floating on top.

GREAT GUM HERB

For **infected gums**, place one dropperful (approximately 20 to 25 drops) into two or three ounces of warm water and swish it around your mouth for three minutes. You can do this up to six times per day. To increase the effect, add one dropperful *each* of myrrh tincture and echinacea tincture to the water.

DOSE DECISIONS

Dose requirements can vary with usnea depending upon the ailment you are treating. For example, for most **acute bacterial infections**, one dropperful taken three times a day is sufficient. However, for whatever reasons, your body may require more or less of the herb. Usnea is often considered to be most effective for chronic conditions when two to seven dropperfuls are taken three times a day for three to six months. *However, this can always be modified based upon your individual chemistry.* I encourage anyone who is not sure about proper dosage to work in tandem with a qualified herbalist or naturopathic physician who can guide you toward the best dose for your ailment. In addition, they can also suggest other natural treatments that are directed at treating your whole body.

SOME CAUTIONS YOU SHOULD KNOW

Cautions for usnea are as follows: **Since the alcohol tincture can sometimes be irritating when used internally, it is best to dilute it in a little bit of water instead of using it full strength. If you decide you want to drink usnea in tea form, don't overdo it thinking that "more is better" because you could experience gastrointestinal upset.** The typical herb to water ratio is one heaping tablespoon of a tightly packed clump of the dried herb steeped in eight ounces of boiling distilled water for 20 minutes. However, usnea tea should only be a last ditch effort since the active principles are barely active in water. **Pregnant women can take usnea in small amounts after their first trimester. In rare cases, contact dermatitis has occurred in some people who harvest quantities of usnea. The same skin condition has occurred with a few people who apply it to their skin to treat a wound.** If this happens to you and a rash develops, discontinue use of usnea, *both internally and externally.* Finally, **if you want to pick it in the forests, stay away from any brightly colored yellow or orange species since they are poisonous.** My best advice if you are unsure about what to pick is to take somebody with you who knows the area and can identify usnea.

Every time I pick usnea in the summer, I remember Lark and her bony body and wispy voice. If I ever run into her on some back road that leads into the densely shaded places of the forest, I'll speak softly and tell her that I talked to the usnea and it sends her its regards.

THE "DIRT" ON...USNEA

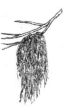

Botanical ~ *Usnea barbata, Usnea longissima, Usnea ceratina, Usnea dasypoga, Usnea hirta, Usnea florida* and *Usnea Californica*

Growth cycle ~ Perennial.

Medicinal uses~ Anti-bacterial, antifungal, anti-viral, antibiotic, immune-supporting, vulnerary, pectoral, diuretic.

Part(s) used for medicine ~ Entire plant.

Vitamins/Minerals ~ Not applicable.

Region ~ Usnea is also known as "Larch moss," "Bear lichen, "Beard lichen" or, the most popular, "Old Man's Beard." The last reference refers to the fact that usnea often resembles an old man's beard as it hangs off the branches of pines, oaks, Douglas firs and apple trees. Typically, you'll find usnea on these trees above 3000 feet and preferably in areas of the forest that are shaded and densely populated with plant life. These trees can be standing, recently fallen or dead. Usnea does not care. I've found the most copious amounts of usnea on dead, downed oaks.

Wild or Domestic ~ Wild.

Poisonous look-alikes in the wild ~ There are no poisonous look-alikes that are gray-green in color. However, if you happen upon lichens that are brightly colored yellow or orange, stay away since those are indeed poisonous. My best advice if you are unsure about what to pick is to take somebody with you who knows the area and can positively identify usnea.

Hardy or Delicate ~ Hardy.

Height of mature plant ~ One to seven inches.

Easy or hard to grow ~ Easy when the forest environment is just perfect.

Cultivation ~ You don't grow usnea. Rather, it appears very slowly hanging on the branches of trees that grow within a dense forest setting. It evolves after a fungus forms the base for chlorophyll-bearing algae to spread out and provide food sugars for both entities. Putting it more simply, usnea is a lichen, which is part fungus and part algae. When the two come together, they form a plant life that is unlike either the fungus or the algae, with chemicals that are unique only to usnea. Instead of cultivating usnea, cultivate the knowledge of where you can find this very useful lichen in the wild.

325

Plant spacing ~   Not applicable.

Pre-soak seeds ~   Not applicable.

Pre-chill seeds ~   Not applicable.

Indoor seed starting ~   Not applicable.

Light/dark seed requirements ~   Not applicable.

Days to germinate ~   Not applicable.

Days to full maturity ~   Not applicable.

Soil type ~   Not applicable.

Water requirements ~   Not applicable.

Sun or shade ~   Shade with filtered sunlight.

Propagation ~   When the algae meets the fungus, usnea happens.

Easy/hard to transplant ~   Not applicable.

Pests or diseases ~   Pest and disease-free.

Landscape uses ~   Not applicable.

Gathering ~   Harvesting usnea is as easy as breathing. Simply pull it off the branch and place it in your gathering sack. It takes a lot of usnea to make a tincture or oil since it's very light in weight and tends to compress down into a single mass when many pieces are pressed together. I have found the easiest way to harvest usnea is to find a downed tree that serves as a horizontal "catch basket" for this lovable lichen. **One important note:** usnea tends to accumulate heavy metals from the air. Keep this in mind when you are wildcrafting this lichen. In other words, do not harvest in areas that have obvious high amounts of airborne pollution. Do not harvest around old or working mines or in areas that are dumping grounds and landfills for waste products of known or unknown origin. Also, pick usnea at least 200 feet from heavily travelled roads due to the potential contamination from car fumes.

Best fresh or dried ~   Best fresh but dried is fine.

Drying methods ~   Often, usnea is already technically dried when you collect it. However, when it is taken out of its secluded, moist forest setting and brought home, it does tend to dry out more readily. I place small two to three inch clumps of the lichen in an air dryer and leave it for one week. After that, I store it in airtight, glass containers. Instead of powdering it ahead of time, I like to keep it intact until I need it.

Amount needed ~   Moderate use: 35 clumps of harvested usnea; Regular use: 100+

Seed collection ~   Not applicable.

Companion planting ~   You don't plant usnea. But it does have an affinity in the wild for oak and conifer trees.

Container planting ~   Not applicable.

Common mistakes ~   Confusing common moss with usnea. Whenever in doubt, do the "usnea test." Take a single piece of the gray-green stem and gently pull it apart. Hidden inside, you should find a resilient white cord that is stiff when the plant is dry and similar to a crude piece of elastic when it is wet. If you cannot find this inner white thread, you are not looking at usnea.

Interesting facts/tips ~   Usnea is one of those plant forms that grows in groupings of trees. In other words, you could walk for a mile through the forest and see none, then happen upon a tree that is chock full of the lichen. It's an herb that I tend to always be on the lookout for when I'm out harvesting other medicinal plants since setting off to "gather usnea" exclusively could leave you empty handed at the end of the day.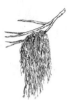

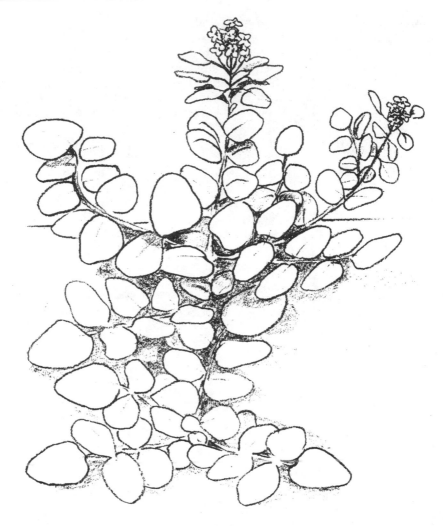

Chapter 36

DIVE INTO WATERCRESS

Nasturtium officinale
("W.F.")
Hardy perennial

Medicinal Uses: *Mineral-rich tonic, diuretic, expectorant, blood builder, hypoglycemic*

Medicinal parts of plant: *Leaves*

Forms: *Fresh plant, tea*

WHAT IS ITS CHARACTER?

Other herbs might rule the prairies, meadows and deserts—watercress rules the streams and ponds of the world. Sure, there might be a few reeds or cattails hanging around those waterways, enjoying the constant H_2O, but watercress is the "big fish," "the main man," "The Godfather." It sinks its roots into the soggy soil and intertwines those long stems to form a thicket of growth that says "I own the place. Watch it!" Not content to own just a part of a stream, it sends emissaries (i.e., seeds) in the down current to populate distant riverbanks and take over yet another corner of the river market. I have this strange feeling that all the other plants that grow nearby are only there because watercress gave them the "okay." They know not to grow too close though or watercress will choke them out. Yes, it's not easy growing upstream. But somebody's got to be in charge.

WHERE DO I FIND IT?

Watercress is native to the Mediterranean region and Europe. In the United States, it is usually found growing in or on the banks of streams, ponds and swamps, from sea level to 8,000 feet.

HOW DO I GROW IT?

Broadcast the seed into a water-soaked mound of rich, fertile soil or in a flat area that has a constant source of moisture. Press seed into dirt, barely covering. *I cannot stress it enough that if watercress is not given a steady soaking of water on a daily basis, it will not thrive.* Seedlings usually start popping out of the ground within 15 days. If you have a stream or pond on your property that has a clean, non-polluted source, this is the perfect place to plant watercress. Watercress naturally grows in dense patches that need to be thinned to avoid overcrowding. Once it takes hold in a stream or pond, seed will be carried several inches or several hundred feet depending upon the force of the current. Seeds can be started indoors in dirt flats or individual cells as long as you follow the same growing instructions for outside and keep the plant constantly moist, if not soaking. Watercress usually matures within 60 days.

HOW DO I HARVEST IT?

It can be harvested year-round, even in areas that experience freezes. In those locations, you need only to break through the ice to uncover the dark green plant. The active medicinal principles in the leaves are highest when watercress is in flower–usually during spring and summer. However, I have gathered generous handfuls of watercress from streams in southern California in late December and found it to be very potent. **Important note**: it is important that you gather watercress from streams and ponds that have a non-polluted source. If you have the slightest doubt as to the purity of the water, *do not harvest watercress.* Microorganisms such as giardia (a painful intestinal ailment that can cause long-term debility and systemic weakness) is one of the organisms that can live on the leaves and stems of watercress. Watercress is best used fresh in order to obtain the greatest vitamin and mineral benefit. However, it can be used dried and powdered for culinary purposes. To do this, thoroughly rinse or soak the plant for 20 to 30 minutes in pure water, remove and pat dry with a towel. Lay the stems on a dry towel out of direct sunlight. Do not stack watercress on top of each other since mold can form due to the innate water content. When you can easily crumble a leaf into a powder, strip the leaves from the stems and store them in an airtight glass jar. Powder the leaves as needed.

HOW DO I USE IT?

My first introduction to watercress was not staring down at it in a shallow mountain pond. Rather, this herb was staring up at me from a small triangular shaped piece of bread.

When I was a youngster, my mother did everything she could to make a "nice young lady" out of me. I had other plans, but that didn't stop her. She'd curl my hair, put a pretty dress on me, slip my feet into patent leather Mary Janes and cover my hands in little white gloves. We would then go to a place called "The Tea Room" where blue-haired ladies met from 3:00 to 4:00 pm to speak in hushed tones, drink tea and eat small triangular shaped thinly sliced bread, covered in cream cheese and watercress. Meanwhile, I'd be drawing pictures on my pad of paper. Pictures of me at the beach, me at the park, me just about anywhere else but that stuffy tea room.

"Eat the sandwich, Laurel," my mother said to me. "The watercress will make you smart." I was having trouble learning subtraction at the time, so I figured I'd give the leaf a try. I bit into the perky green plant and was immediately overwhelmed by the most bitter, mustard-like taste. I reached into my mouth, trying valiantly to extract the watercress from the bread and cream cheese. Needless to say, we left "The Tea Room" soon after that, bursting my mother's bubble of me ever becoming a "nice young lady."

Fast forward about 20 years and I am standing at a clear mountain pond in Northern California. Beneath me lay that same bitter leaf, enjoying life in its natural habitat. Perhaps it was maturity, perhaps it was the herbalist in me or perhaps it was because I was hungry that I gladly snapped off a few leaves and ate them without causing a scene. They were still as pungent tasting as ever, but this time I knew exactly what the herb was doing for me. No, it wasn't making me smarter. But it was flooding my body with more minerals and vitamins than your average drug store multi-vitamin.

LOVE THAT VITAMIN-RICH "SCURVY GRASS"

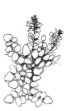

Watercress was called "scurvy grass" by early settlers who brought the plant to America in hopes of preventing that dreaded disease which debilitates the body due to a lack of vitamin C. They hadn't read any scientific lab studies on why it worked — they just knew it did. The fact is, watercress is loaded with lots of essential dietary fiber, vitamins A, B_2, B_9 (folic acid), C, D and E and charged with minerals such as copper, manganese, iron, iodine, phosphorus and calcium. Every cup of watercress has 53 mg. of calcium, 19 mg. of phosphorus, 0.6 mg. of iron, 18 mg. of sodium, 99 mg. of potassium, 1,729 I.U. of vitamin A, 28 mg. of vitamin C and 6.5 mg. of magnesium. In addition, one-third of watercress is pure sulphur. One source states that watercress contains four times more vitamin C, weight for weight, than lettuce and more calcium than whole milk!

The great thing about this plant is that it grows almost anywhere in the world. Since it requires continual water, it is usually found in shallow mountain ponds or stream beds. The plant can be gathered and eaten throughout the year. However, the active medicinal principles in the leaves are highest when watercress is in flower–usually during spring and summer.

So what can watercress do for you? Besides being an **incredible natural "multi-vitamin,"** this pungent plant achieves much of its healing success from its **blood purifying abilities**. Because of this, watercress can work as a **preventative to illness**, a **rehabilitation tonic** and a **treatment for skin ailments**. In addition, watercress is also *very* effective as an **expectorant for respiratory ailments such as bronchitis, asthma and even tuberculosis**.

GET FRESH WITH WATERCRESS

Before delving into each one of these, I must say that the best way to get the most medicinal benefit from watercress is to eat it *fresh*. Some herbal reference guides include the herb in its dried form in a few tea formulas. But many herbalists and nutritionists believe that only the *fresh* plant has the high vitamin and mineral count. Thus, either find a non-polluted mountain pond, create a makeshift "pond" in your backyard and grow it yourself or find a good health store that sells fresh organic watercress.

A REHABILITATION TONIC

Let's start off with watercress' preventative abilities. This, of course, goes back to the belief that watercress could prevent diseases such as scurvy. With all the innate vitamins and minerals within the leaves, this idea is not exactly a quantum leap of logic. For centuries, watercress was used as part of a "**Spring Tonic" to rid the body of leftover winter colds**. The idea was that if you flooded your body with a healthy dose of fresh, leafy, spring greens (such as watercress, nettle, dandelion leaves and alfalfa), you could literally blast any stubborn winter ailment from your body. Likewise, it would prevent any further illnesses from roosting in your body.

This brings us to watercress' **rehabilitation uses**. There's no need to be sickly, weak and anemic when you have herbs such as watercress to get you walking vertically again. When folks are getting over a **debilitating illness**, it never ceases to amaze me how they often eat so poorly and do nothing to fortify their body. When you are in this condition, your body needs nutritious foods and a hefty dose of vitamins and minerals. And believe me, the more natural the source, the better for your body. Watercress **tones the liver** as it **cleanses the blood of "the crud" that may be hanging on during an illness. Watercress can be eaten fresh or taken in tea form while you are fighting the effects of the common cold—especially if one of the symptoms is a runny nose**.

As a **maintenance or preventative tonic**, eat one handful of watercress a day, either fresh or lightly steamed for several minutes. If you would like to enjoy this potent plant in liquid form, consider the following mineral tea to boost your body's immunity. Combine two heaping tablespoons *each* of *fresh* watercress leaves, *fresh* dandelion leaves, *fresh* parsley, *fresh* nettle leaves and fresh peppermint leaves. Add one heaping teaspoon of the following *dried* herbs: horsetail, red raspberry leaves, alfalfa, rose hips and red clover blossoms. Place the herbs into a gallon-sized ceramic or glass container that has a cover. Pour one gallon (16 cups) of boiling *distilled* water over the herbs. Stir briskly with a wooden spoon, cover and allow to steep for 20 minutes. Do not strain the herbs. This allows the plant matter to continue steeping and become stronger. Decant the mineral tea as needed, serving it cold or hot in eight ounce cupfuls. Store whatever you don't use in the refrigerator. It should keep for several days. **During periods of rehabilitation from long term illnesses, there is no way you can overdose on this tea mixture. The** only exception to that rule would be if you were pregnant since watercress, parsley, dandelion and peppermint have been known to stimulate the uterus and bring on a menstrual cycle.

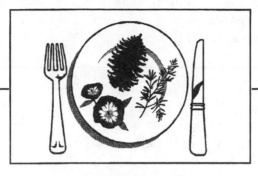

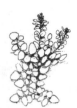

Wild Food Facts

Watercress is one of the wild food forager's favorite cuisine. It perks up salads, adds a tang to sandwiches and gives the day hiker a much-needed burst of energy, thanks to the many vitamins and minerals within the plant.

Stir a small handful of the finely cut leaves into scrambled eggs a few minutes before serving and you will have a tasty breakfast treat. Toss a few handfuls into a boiling hot steamer and steam this water-loving herb for no longer than two minutes. Serve it as you would spinach, as a side dish. I love placing a handful of chopped watercress into soups and stews minutes before serving them. This allows the watercress to slightly warm up and soften but it doesn't drain the plant of its vitamins and minerals.

A healthy, very "wild" salad can be made by combining a handful of fresh watercress, a handful of fresh chickweed, a handful of chopped fresh blue violet leaves and a handful of fresh, young dandelion leaves into a bowl. Mix them together and sprinkle a tablespoon each of fresh lemon juice and extra virgin olive oil over the greens. If you wish, add a chopped, hard-boiled egg. This is a great salad but I wouldn't overdo it until your system gets used to the taste (and the energy) of wild food since too much can lead to frequent trips to the bathroom.

If you are looking for a tasty salt-substitute, crush the dried watercress leaves into a semi-fine powder and use it straight or mix it with equal parts dried basil or dried nettle.

GET GREAT SKIN WITH WATERCRESS

Any herb such as watercress which is known as an "A-1" blood purifier, is also going to be a great aid for **skin ailments**. Everything from **acne** and **rashes** to **eczema**, **psoriasis** and **ringworm**. Use the herb both internally as a tea and externally as a face toner. To make a skin cleansing tea and skin toner, take three ounces (by weight) of *fresh* watercress. Pour 12 ounces of boiling distilled water over the plant, stir rapidly with a wooden spoon and then cover. Steep for 20 minutes, strain and drink eight ounces of the tea. Use the remaining four ounces as a skin wash. If you are treating acne, wash your face first with a good soap and then apply the watercress wash with a cotton ball. If you are using the wash for eczema, psoriasis or a rash, dip a clean, cotton flannel cloth into the mixture, wring it out and then wrap the herb-soaked cloth around the affected area.

If you have a **wart**, juice a handful of fresh watercress leaves (stems included) and saturate a cotton ball with the liquid. Hold the cotton ball in place over the wart with a piece of masking tape, changing it only when the juice dries up. Eating a handful of fresh watercress daily as well as drinking one cup of tea will help to purify your blood and speed up the disappearance of the wart.

EXPECT SOME EXPECTORANT ACTION

As an **expectorant for respiratory conditions**, many herbalists feel you can't beat watercress' "mucus-moving" capabilities. The best way to use the herb is through juicing it in a blender. According to author Dr. John Heinerman, one fantastic formula that actually "cured" a Vietnam vet's drug-resistant **tuberculosis** included watercress, a turnip and a dash of Kyolic liquid fermented garlic. To make it, place one large handful of fresh watercress into a blender and add eight ounces of cold water. Juice the mixture then add a medium-sized cubed turnip. Continue blending until everything is liquified. Divide the mixture into two equal portions and drink one portion eight hours apart *with meals.*

THE KIDNEY & BLADDER ENCOURAGER

Watercress is a natural **diuretic**. Because of this, it is great for **minor kidney and bladder problems** that occasionally arise. Since it eliminates excess water from the body, those who suffer from **PMS** could benefit from including it in their diet two weeks out of the month to reduce bloating and add a needed dose of minerals and vitamins.

THINGS YOU SHOULD KNOW

For all its leafy goodness, there are some things you have to remember about watercress.

If you are gathering watercress in the wild, make sure you are picking watercress and not the deadly water hemlock.

Make sure the water is not polluted or near any kind of wild animals. The fecal matter from these animals carries a deadly parasite, the liver fluke. This was once and still is a common source of typhoid.

Some naturalists say that if you boil the plant in water for 15 to 20 minutes, you can kill the parasite. Unfortunately, boiling the plant that long kills most of the medicinal benefits. My advice is to either cultivate it yourself (it grows *very* easily from seed) in a makeshift "pond," or purchase it from the store. Stored in airtight bags, it will keep in the refrigerator up to three days.

Watercress is contraindicated for those with gastric or duodenal ulcers and inflammatory kidney disorders.

While this is one great plant, don't get excessive with it. Too much of it can lead to kidney and bladder irritation due to its diuretic ability. Overdosing can also irritate the mucus lining of your intestines. One or two handfuls are enough to gain a healing benefit. **If you decide to juice watercress, I suggest diluting it with a little water or mix it with other juices since undiluted watercress juice can cause inflammation of the throat and stomach**.

Finally, **medicinal doses of watercress can stimulate the uterus. Because of this, pregnant women are advised not to take the herb. However, a few leaves on a piece of bread are okay**.

And if that slice of bread happens to be triangular and covered with cream cheese, take a bite to see if you like it. But if you don't care for it, remember to remove your white gloves before picking it out of your teeth.

THE "DIRT" ON... WATERCRESS

Botanical ~	*Nasturtium officinale*
Growth cycle ~	Perennial.
Medicinal uses~	Mineral-rich tonic, diuretic, expectorant, blood builder, hypoglycemic.
Part(s) used for medicine ~	Leaves.
Vitamins/Minerals ~	Vitamins A, B_2, B_9 (folic acid), C, D and E and charged with minerals including copper, manganese, iron, iodine, phosphorus and calcium. Every cup of watercress has 53 mg. of calcium, 19 mg. of phosphorus, 0.6 mg. of iron, 18 mg. of sodium, 99 mg. of potassium, 1,729 I.U. of vitamin A, 28 mg. of vitamin C and 6.5 mg. of magnesium. In addition, one-third of watercress is pure sulphur.
Region ~	Native to the Mediterranean and Europe. In the United States, it is usually found growing in or on the banks of streams, ponds and swamps, from sea level to 8,000 feet.
Wild or Domestic ~	Both.

Poisonous look-alikes in the wild ~

Yes. Some people apparently have mistaken young water hemlock for early spring watercress. Water hemlock (*Cicuta douglasii*)—considered to be "the most toxic plant in North America"—attacks the nervous, circulatory and respiratory system. One mouthful can be fatal. Upon closer examination, the new growth of water hemlock is very different than young watercress. However, the fatal mistake might have been made if the wild forager was under the impression that "all plants that grow in or along stream beds are related to watercress." While that deduction might sound far-fetched, I have actually heard someone make that statement. Scary, eh?

Hardy or Delicate ~

Hardy.

Height of mature plant ~

The floating stems can be up to three feet in length. However, typically the top six to eight inches is all that can be seen above the water.

Easy or hard to grow ~

Easy.

Cultivation ~

Broadcast seed into a water-soaked mound of rich soil or in a flat area that has a constant source of moisture. Press seed into dirt, barely covering.

Plant spacing ~

Watercress will naturally grow in dense patches. Trying to control this is futile.

Pre-soak seeds ~

No.

Pre-chill seeds ~

No.

Indoor seed starting ~

Yes, seeds can be started indoors in dirt flats or individual cells as long as you follow the same growing instructions for outside and keep the plant constantly moist, if not soaking.

Light/dark seed requirements ~

Light.

Days to germinate ~

10 to 15 days.

Days to full maturity ~

Approximately 60 days.

Soil type ~

Rich, fertile and, preferably, *under* water.

Water requirements ~

Watercress doesn't just want to be watered, it wants to be *in* water. In order to thrive, watercress must always be either drowning in water or water-soaked.

Sun or shade ~

Full sun.

Propagation ~

Seed and underground roots.

Easy/hard to transplant ~

Fairly easy but I prefer to direct seed watercress.

Pests or diseases ~

Virtually pest and disease-free.

Landscape uses ~

If you have a moving pond, stream or natural spring on your property that has a clean, non-infectious source, you have the ideal location for growing watercress.

Gathering ~

Can be harvested year 'round, even in areas that experience freezes. In such a case, you need only to break through the ice to uncover the dark green plant. The active medicinal principles in the leaves are highest when watercress is in flower–usually during spring and summer. However, I have gathered generous handfuls of watercress from streams in southern California in late December and found it to be quite effective. **Important note:** it is important that you gather watercress from streams and ponds that have a non-polluted source. If you have the slightest doubt as to the purity of the water, do not harvest watercress. Microorganisms such as giardia (a painful intestinal ailment that can cause long-term debility and systemic weakness) is one of the organisms that can live on the leaves and stems of watercress.

Best fresh or dried ~

Fresh. It can be used dried and powdered for culinary purposes.

Drying methods ~

Thoroughly rinse or soak the plant for 20 to 30 minutes in pure water, remove and pat dry with a towel. Lay the stems on a dry towel out of direct sunlight. Do not stack watercress on top of each other since mold can form due to the innate water content. When you can easily crumble a leaf into a powder, strip the leaves from the stems and store them in an airtight glass jar. Powder the leaves as needed.

Amount needed ~

Moderate use: 20 plants; Regular use: 35+++

Seed collection ~

I have found it difficult to successfully harvest the seed from watercress since I plant it under water. Let nature take its course and you should have an abundant supply of watercress without having to worry about collecting seed.

Companion planting ~

In the wild, I've seen watercress growing at the foot of cottonwoods and aspens that are in or nearby a moving stream. Aside from that, there aren't many herbs that require as much water as watercress.

Container planting ~

Others have successfully seeded watercress into containers and enjoyed a year 'round bounty of this mineral-rich plant. I've tried it just so I could say I did it, but I spent the better part of my day constantly keeping that darn pot consistently wet so it wasn't worth it.

Common mistakes ~

It isn't called watercress because it likes the desert. The most common mistake is simply not supplying watercress with enough water.

Interesting facts/tips ~

Turkish peasants rely on watercress to temporarily relieve the pain of cancer.

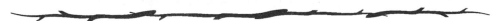

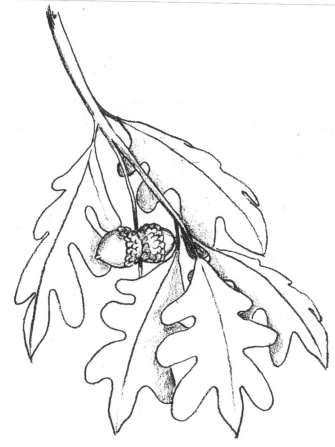

Chapter 37

WHITE OAK BARK

~

A MIGHTY FINE HERB

Quercus alba
("W.F.")

Hardy perennial

Medicinal Uses: *Highly astringent, antiseptic, mild stimulant, tonic, hemostatic, antivenomous*

Medicinal parts of plant: *Inner bark of branch or trunk (preferably, young branches only), leaves and freshly fallen acorns*

Forms: *Tea, tincture, capsules, fomentation*

WHAT IS ITS CHARACTER?

Throughout the centuries, there are herbs that have been referred to as "Grandfather" plants. While the title can shift, I'd have to say the oak tree has genuinely earned that reputation. This old, often gnarled, but always magnificent tree has a majesty, stability and character shared by no other plant or tree. It grows slowly and deliberately. As it matures, it acts like a sponge, imprinting every experience, every word and every thought of every century in which it has lived. I've often stood in front of an old, regal oak and wondered how many stories it could tell. Once I learn to talk "oak," I might find out. There's a wonderful story about what the oaks do at night when no one is looking or listening. The mature oaks are said to speak in whispers with each other, while the young, more energetic oaks pull up their shallow roots and dance thunderously in the full moon. A warning goes out to all who heed this story: beware where you lay your camp if you are in an oak forest and be careful under whose boughs you whisper secrets or hatch infernal plans. You never know who may be listening....and who they might tell.

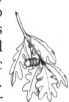

WHERE DO I FIND IT?

Depending upon who you talk to, there are between 85 and 200 species of oak trees. From the five foot tall "scrub oak" to the over 100 foot black oak, many species have naturally hybridized in the wild. For this reason, you can find this venerable tree in just about any region. All oaks share similar medicinal properties. However, many vary in the amount of tannic acid. For medicinal purposes, the white oak is most commonly used, since it has a lower tannin content. Thus, the information in this chapter regarding the oak's cultivation and medicinal use will focus on the white oak tree.

White oak (also known by the name "Tanner's oak") is found in the United States throughout the eastern states, parts of the upper midwest and in some portions of east Texas. It might be scattered in other areas not mentioned. However, it will have a better chance of sustaining life for decades (if not centuries) if it is cultivated in areas where it is native. It does best in rich, moist, clay-like soil that has superior drainage and full sun.

HOW DO I GROW IT?

You can cultivate white oak (or any oak) two ways: from established two-year-old or older saplings or from seeds (acorns). If you want to get a head start and fear your thumb is not as green as you'd wish, I suggest opting for the sapling. Plan to plant the sapling within days of purchasing it. The best weather for planting trees (especially bareroot trees) is a damp, chilly one. Hot, dry weather is hard on young trees. Allow the soil to determine how often watering should occur. Never allow the sapling to experience bone-dry conditions. White oak can be a slow grower in some regions — in others, it has been known to grow up to three feet each year. The better the soil, the more it will flourish.

If you'd like to try your hand at planting acorns, it is always best to plant them when they are brown but before they fall from the tree. White oak acorns are known to often sprout while still on the tree. If you have a choice, pick those acorns first to use as seeds since they have established a desire to reproduce. Dig a small hole with your finger one inch to one and one-half inch deep. Drop the acorn in the hole and firmly cover it with soil. It doesn't hurt to add a little compost to the hole to encourage a healthy start. Give it enough water without drowning it. Expect slow but steady growth over the two years that follow. If you cannot plant the acorns immediately, they can be stored at 34°F in a high humidity environment. To accomplish this, they could be placed in flats filled with sphagnum moss or straw and stored in the refrigerator. This should only be for short-term purposes since the longer they are left in storage, the less likely they are to successfully sprout.

HOW DO I HARVEST IT?

The following information applies to *all* species of oaks. The inner bark of the young branches or trunk should be collected in either early spring or late fall when the tannin content is the highest. Of the two seasons, I think early spring is by far your best choice. Because all oaks take so long to grow, I never harvest from the trunk of the tree unless it has recently fallen. In general, I don't harvest the inner bark from *any* tree since it scars them and could potentially kill them if too much bark is taken. Besides, the young branches are ten times easier to harvest due to the innate suppleness which makes the inner bark a cinch to peel back. Dry the strips of inner bark in a cool, dry, dark place. They are ready to store when you can easily snap a section in half. Collect oak leaves in early fall, before the first freeze. Leaves need to be dried quickly. This means the room should be hot but not humid or the leaves will mold. Collect acorns when they have turned from green to brown, either on the tree or after they have recently fallen. One old trick for collecting those recently fallen acorns is to spread four or five old sheets under the tree and pick them up every day or so as they fall. Acorns should be used *fresh*.

Note: *The acorns from the white oaks mature in one growing season. Acorns from red oaks do not mature until the end of their second growing season. The way to tell the difference between a white oak and a red oak is by the leaf. White oaks have smooth, round edges; red oaks have bristly terminal points.* (For more information on how to use acorns as a nutritious food, check out the "Wild Foods Facts" box on page 348 and 349.)

HOW DO I USE IT?

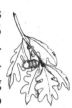

I didn't want to go to my first summer camp—especially one that was called "Get To Know Nature Summer Camp." But go, I did, along with 65 other little 10-year-old girls from that wilderness capital, Los Angeles, California. Our idea of the wilderness was camping in the backyard and turning off the porch light. We hardly had time to throw down our sleeping bags on our cabin cots when the sound of a shrill whistle beckoned us to the camp fire pit. Three female camp counselors were waiting there to greet us. I may have only been 10, but I remember thinking that they seemed a little spacey. They wore tie-dye shirts and painted bell-bottom jeans with huge yellow daisies, peace symbols and the words "Flower Power" painted up and down the pant legs. "We want to get you all started on this groovy adventure," one of the counselors yelled out. "We're asking each one of you to hike up into the woods and find a rock or a tree or a flower and introduce yourself. Become friends with whatever you find. If at anytime during your stay here at 'Get To Know Nature Summer Camp' you feel the slightest bit lonely, homesick or if you're just not groovin', I want you to remember that rock, or tree or flower is your new buddy. Now go find that special friend!"

All 65 of us spread out faster than Kentucky bootleggers. I think some girls were running in the direction of Los Angeles, hoping they could make it back home before sunset. Warily, I climbed up into the thicket of trees and overgrowth and stopped when my little legs finally gave out. I sat down on a large rock to catch my breath. I considered calling that rock my "new friend" just to get the whole thing over with but the idea of having a rock for a buddy seemed somewhat pitiful.

While I came to grips with the realization that I would be spending the next seven days in this "Flower Power" nightmare, I looked down and found the forest floor littered with tiny bowl-shaped "cups" that were about the size of a penny. Some of them had tan protrusions growing out of them. I popped the protrusion out of the cup and, in a moment of carefree bliss, tossed it on the ground and stomped on it as hard as I could. It broke open to reveal a soft, meaty center. I smelled this curious thing and, being in an adventurous mood, I bit into it. It was horribly bitter but it had an odd taste that sort of grew on me.

In the distance, the shrill sound of that awful whistle echoed throughout the camp, summoning our return. I quickly gathered several handfuls of this strange, wonderful nature find, stuffing my pockets with it. Before leaving, I patted the trunk of this oversized tree and said, "You're my new friend." I had no idea what it was called or the reason for those odd little cupped balls. But somewhere, deep down, I fell in love with that tree.

LOCATION, LOCATION, LOCATION!

It wasn't long before someone kindly informed me that I had been in the presence of an oak tree and those "cups" with "tan protrusions" were acorns. With the ability to positively identify one tree in this entire world, I felt a great sense of accomplishment. This was strengthened by the fact that nearly everywhere you turn in this country, there is one or more of the 200+ oaks located nearby.

To coin a phrase, the mighty oak has three things going for it: location, location and location. From Italy to Japan—from British Columbia to South Africa—the oak tree stands as a symbol of strength.

And it is one powerful healing herb to boot. To some herbalists, oak is on their top ten list. The active ingredients that make the healing possible are *tannin* and *quercin*. Quercin has almost the same effect as salicin which is found in white willow bark. The leaves, acorns, and inner bark are all equally valuable, with the inner bark being the most active of the bunch.

WHITE OAK—THE OAK MOST FAVORED

As I indicated earlier, *all* oaks have similar healing properties. The only difference is that some are higher in tannic acid than others. Traditionally, white oak is the "designated oak" that is used for medicinal purposes. One reason for this is that the inner bark, leaves and acorns are *lower* in tannic acid which makes it milder on the system than, say, red oak which has extremely high tannin levels.

All oaks are traditionally **very astringent**. White oak is no exception to the rule. You can thank the natural abundance of tannic acid in the herb for that astringent ability. When you need to stop runny things from running and tighten loose things so they stop flapping, you want to reach for white oak.

DIARRHEA DILEMMA

The inner bark or the dried leaves of the white oak tree can help bring an end to **acute diarrhea** or **bleeding diarrhea**. Use one heaping teaspoon of the dried leaves or one teaspoon of the inner bark to every eight ounces of water. If you use the leaves, make an *infusion* (i.e., steep the leaves in hot water). For the bark, simmer it in the water for 10 minutes before straining and sipping the tea. Take no more than three cups each day for no longer than three days since the tannic acid in the bark and leaves can be irritating to your system.

If you think that the diarrhea may be caused by a bacterial infection in your intestines (due to bad food or contaminated water), I would consider using several cloves of fresh garlic and taking a teaspoon of echinacea tincture every two hours in an attempt to rid your system of the bacteria. However, if it is a particularly stubborn bacterial infection—such as those that can be caught in foreign countries—white oak, garlic and echinacea may not be enough to kill it. If the bacterial infection becomes more serious after two days, please discontinue the use of the herbs and seek medical attention. In a case such as this, an antibiotic may be the best route.

White oak really goes to town when the ailment stems from **gastroenteritis**–a debilitating inflammation of the stomach and intestines. For gastroenteritis, use only the *leaves* of the oak tree. Place one-half ounce of oak leaves and one-half ounce of raspberry leaves (another astringent herb) into a pan and pour one pint of boiling hot water over the leaves. Do not boil them—rather, let the herbs steep in the water until cool. When cool, strain and sip three or four ounces of the tea throughout the day. You can also warm up this oak/raspberry combination and use it as an enema. If your condition worsens or fails to show any improvement after one week, discontinue use of the herbs. If the gastroenteritis is chronic, I would seek the advice of a trained holistic practitioner who can suggest additional herbs as well as dietary advice that could help.

VARICOSE VEINS

Whenever someone asks me what I suggest for **varicose veins**, I always tell them about white oak bark. The track record is very impressive and can work even when the problem is considered "hopeless." Fortunately, pregnant women can take the herb and obtain relief. For minor problems, take two capsules of white oak bark three times a day with meals. For more advanced conditions, take the capsules as indicated *and* use the following *fomentation* externally.

To make the fomentation, you will need to brew a very concentrated bark tea. Place four tablespoons of white oak bark into two pints of *cold* distilled water. Bring the mixture to a boil. Continue to boil the tea until it is reduced to *one pint*. At that point, dip a clean, cotton white sock or a large piece of clean, cotton flannel into the tea and securely cover the entire leg area. One trick with the sock is to cut off the toe end of the sock so that you can pull it up higher on your leg. Cover the flannel or sock with plastic wrap which will help hold in the heat. Leave this fomentation on overnight. For cases that are considered "serious," in addition to the six capsules, drink one to two cups of white oak bark tea each day with a pinch of cayenne pepper added. Continue this process, doing it six days on and one day off, until you see marked relief.

HEMORRHOID HELPER

Since white oak bark can support the veins and is known as a remedy for sagging tissue, it can help give relief to **hemorrhoid** sufferers. At the first sign of the hemorrhoid, drink one cup of white oak bark tea up to three times a day for up to three days. Instead of the tea, you can take two or three of the capsules three times a day with meals for several days.

FOR THOSE "SAGGING" FEMALE CONCERNS

Remember, white oak dries it up and tightens it up. For this reason, a cup or two of the bark tea each day during your period can help reduce an excessive **menstrual flow**.

If **leucorrhea** discharge is troubling you, try a white oak bark douche. Place one-quarter cup of white oak bark in four cups of water and bring it to a boil. Simmer covered for 30 minutes and then allow the tea to cool before straining and using as a douche.

White oak bark can be used **during pregnancy for uterine pro-lapse**, **varicose veins** and **hemorrhoids**. Take one capsule of white oak bark powder two times a day.

THE ULTIMATE HERB FOR GUMS & TEETH

White oak bark should be the first herb on the list for gum and teeth problems.

If **gum diseases such as pyorrhea** are troubling you, oak bark can help. There have been cases where patients were due to have their teeth removed due to severe gum disease. Using only white oak bark as inter-vention, these patients have reversed their gum deterioration and saved their teeth. How did they do it? They made a pliable paste out of oak bark powder and water and pressed it into their gums, making sure to pack it up and into the gum lining whenever possible. (Make sure not to add too much water or the paste will not adhere to the gums. If you do end up with the paste becoming too soggy, simply add a little more of the pow-dered bark until the paste is firm). The pack should be placed on the gums every evening and left on until morning. Yes, you will resemble a traveling hobo and your "significant other" may look at you rather strangely. However, it has been shown that if this pack is used every night, within 14 days, there should be improvement with tighter teeth and firmer gums.

During the day, swish oak bark tea in your mouth several times. If you don't want to make the tea, place 25 drops of the tincture in several ounces of warm water and use that instead. This mouthwash can also be used as a maintenance treatment for those who want to keep their gums in tip-top shape between visits to their dentist. To "juice up" the mouthwash, I combine one ounce *each* of white oak bark tincture, myrrh tincture and prickly ash bark tincture into a three ounce glass bottle. Shake the tinctures together and place 25 drops of this combination in several ounces of warm water and swish that in your mouth.

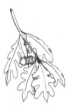

Besides protecting and tightening the gum tissue, this mouthwash (either with or without the added herbal tinctures) has been known to **recalcify the teeth** as well as **help to prevent cavities**. The bark tea can also be used if you don't want to use the tinctures. When I first heard that oak bark could prevent cavities, I was a bit wary. But, I started using it in tincture form every night as a mouthwash after brushing my teeth. I can honestly say that my teeth *and* gums are in better shape because of it.

Speaking of brushing your teeth, here's a good **herbal tooth powder** that cleans, soothes sensitive gums and helps prevent cavities. Combine one ounce *each* of baking soda, white oak bark *powder* and prickly ash bark *powder*. Purchase the herbs in powder form since you cannot grind them into the finely powdered consistency that is needed with the typical home grinder.

A concentrated cup of white oak bark tea (made by rapidly boiling two cups of water and one tablespoon of white oak bark for 20 minutes) has been used to treat **thrush** in babies and young children. Thrush, a yeast infection of the mouth which can eventually invade the entire body, is noted by white spots on the side of the mouth and an extremely coated white tongue. There is also a pervasive, toxic stench to thrush which can sometimes be smelled across a room. The first step is to give the baby acidophilus which will help bring back balance to the system. If you are still nursing the child, take acidophilus as well. Give the child several ounces of the white oak bark concentrate tea three or four times a day, making sure to swab the inside of the mouth with the tea. There have been cases when the child rebounded from thrush after only one day of consistent applications of the tea concentrate.

THROAT INFECTIONS

Consider using white oak bark tea as a gargle to relieve a **sore throat**, **swollen tonsils** or the pain of **bronchitis**. Boil a tablespoon of the bark in 12 ounces of distilled water for 20 minutes. Strain and gargle the tea several times a day. Repeat every 30 minutes if needed.

WOUNDS, LEG ULCERS & MINOR BURNS

Sprinkling the powdered bark into **wounds** will help tighten tissues and speed healing. If the wound is bleeding profusely, first place a pinch of cayenne into the cut. Bleeding should stop within seconds.

For **leg ulcers**, a paste can be made by mixing the powdered bark with a little water. Place the bark poultice over the ulcer, cover it with a piece of gauze and hold it in place with tape. Check the poultice every few hours. This poultice often helps drain and dry up old leg ulcers that are slow to heal.

For **minor burns**, make a strong tea from the bark and let it cool. Soak a piece of cotton flannel into the tea and cover the burned area with it. If the cloth becomes warm on the skin, place it back in the cool tea and reapply.

NIP THAT NOSEBLEED

Use the finely powdered bark as a snuff during a **nosebleed**. This can quickly constrict and cut off the flow of blood. Make sure you don't try to sniff too much up your nose or it can get awfully uncomfortable.

POISON IVY RASH

Soaking in a cool, white oak bark bath can reduce the itching and pain of a **poison ivy rash**. Make the bath by boiling a handful of white oak bark in several quarts of water for 30 minutes. Allow the mixture to cool and then strain it into a lukewarm to cool bath. Soak in the bath for as long as needed.

POISONOUS AND VENOMOUS BITES

Moving from poison ivy rashes to **snake bites**, every hiker should take along a baggie filled with powdered white oak bark...just in case. Making a paste out of the oak powder and water, apply it quickly over any poisonous or venomous bite. If you don't have water, have the person who suffered the bite spit into the oak bark powder to make the poultice. The astringent action of the herb has been shown to draw out the poison. In addition, drinking white oak bark tea can also leech out the poison. In a case such as this, *any oak species will do*. If you are stuck in the woods without your trusty supply in your pack, take the leaves off an oak tree and chew them into a wet pulp, then apply the wet leaves over the area. This should in no way be a substitute for getting medical attention. Rather, use the oak bark *en route* to the hospital.

LYMPH EDEMA AID

Herbalist and author Matthew Wood considers white oak bark a "specific" remedy for **edema resulting from the removal of lymphatic glands or the spleen**. Wood suggests taking either one cup of the bark tea, two capsules, or three drops of the bark tincture three times a day each day until relief is felt. In addition, this remedy works well for **women who have had lymphatic glands removed near the breasts and are suffering from edema down the arm or nearby**. Try applying the tincture externally as well to the area for further relief.

COULD OAK REDUCE THE DESIRE FOR ALCOHOL?

There is some evidence to support the idea that **daily use of white oak in small doses may reduce the desire for drinking alcohol**. For some people, white oak tends to gradually give alcohol an unpleasant taste, thereby squelching their desire for it.

From the research I've been able to uncover, it seems that white oak is not necessarily suited for those who would fall under the heading of "hopeless alcoholics." Rather, it works better for those who drink out of loneliness or lack of companionship. Dorothy Shepherd, British homeopathic doctor and author of the book *A Physician's Posy,* wrote that white oak is specific for "sherry tippers who are never really drunk, but are never free from the influence." In other words, the difference is between someone who is able to "manage" their liquor intake and someone who cannot. The former could possibly benefit from white oak. I should emphasize that using white oak to reduce or eliminate alcohol cravings without seeking help as to *why* you like or feel you need to drink is not going to solve anything. Studies have shown that once white oak is no longer taken, the desire for alcohol can eventually return.

The inner bark can be used in tincture form, at a dose of 10 drops in several ounces of warm water morning and night. However, studies that date back to the late 1800's describe the use of an "acorn brandy tincture" to be the most effective way to curb the alcoholic tendency. In the study, English oak or European oak (*Quercus robur*) was used, which has similar medicinal action to white oak. However, the standard white oak (*Quercus alba*) can be used if you cannot obtain English oak. Fill a glass jar with the *unshelled fresh acorns* and pour a good brandy over them until they are covered. Place the lid on the jar and set it in a dark, cool cupboard for 14 days. Shake the bottle vigorously twice a day. At the end of 14 days, strain the acorns and place the remaining brandy tincture in a dark glass jar. Take 10 drops of the brandy tincture in several ounces of warm water morning and night. The "anti-alcohol" effects of either the inner bark or acorn tincture have been felt in as little as 10 days — for others, it takes longer. It all depends upon your individual body chemistry, your genetic history, how long you have been drinking and the emotional reasons why you drink.

THINGS YOU SHOULD KNOW

White oak—as well as all the other oak species—should not be overused due to their high tannic acid content. Too much tannic acid in the body can be slightly poisonous. The great thing about oak is that it takes very little of the herb to experience the astringent effect.

Due to the strong astringency of those tannins, **drugs may have reduced absorption in the body**. For this reason, if you depend upon a certain medication, I would not take any oak species since it might be absorbed by the herb.

I may not have known the name of the oak tree when I first spotted it during my summer camp initiation. But I can assure you, it has been a favorite and a friend ever since.

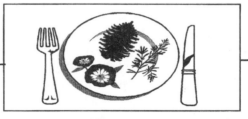

Wild Food Facts

When it comes to wild food, turn to the oak's plentiful acorns. The shelled acorns of white oak can be eaten raw since they have less tannic acid. Still, after about one or two, you will feel your tongue start to dry up thanks to the inherent astringent action of the herb. Some wild food foragers say that the shelled acorns of the white oak are less bitter than other species. I disagree. The first one or two taste like a fine hazelnut coffee to me. After that, it's just bitter, bitter, bitter.

Thus, with white oak or any oak species, you must leech the tannins out of the acorns before consuming them. Remove the acorn "cups" if they haven't already fallen off and break open the outer shell with a wooden mallet to reveal the soft, meaty center. Peel off the thin brown "skin." If you cannot get all of it off, the remainder should break free once you place the meaty pits in boiling water. Fortunately, it doesn't take much pressure to break the acorn's outer shell. It does, however, take time. So, collect a whole lot of acorns and then invite some friends over for a "shelling party." By the way, certain species of oaks produce larger acorns. Two of the western oaks that grow nice big acorns are the California or "live" oak (*Quercus agrifolia*) and the canyon oak (*Quercus chrysolepis*). If you have access to these species, it makes more sense to use them since you will get more acorn for your trouble.

Once you have a sufficient amount of shelled acorns, there are two ways to leech the tannins. The first and most common way is to bring a large pot of water to a boil and toss in the shelled acorns. When the water turns brown, strain the acorns and repeat the process. Continue until the water shows little sign of color. This means the tannic acid has been leeched out. By the fourth or fifth change of water, it is normal for the acorns to darken. To speed up the leeching process, have two pots of water going at one time—one serves as the leeching pot and the other is heating up for the next batch. Depending upon the species of oak, it can take anywhere from four to ten changes of hot water to complete this process. Red oak species have a higher tannic acid content and will take a longer time to leech. As previously mentioned, the water color is a good indication of the acorns' readiness. However, another test is to taste the acorns. When they no longer have a bitter taste, they are ready.

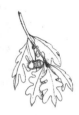

The second way to leech acorns is to fill a large glass gallon jug with the shelled acorns and cover them completely with hot water. Cap the jug and let them sit for 24 hours. The next day, pour the water off and replace it with more hot water. Continue this process for four or five days or until the acorns lose their bitter taste. *If you have the time, this is the preferred way to leech the tannins since the acorns retain more of their flavor and oils.*

When the acorn centers are fully leeched, strain the water and grind them immediately. If you wait until they dry, you will end up breaking blades since they become very hard. A meat grinder is your best bet for the initial grinding which should be on the coarse side. Lay the coarsely ground acorns on a cookie sheet and dry them in a 180°F oven. Once they are completely dry, they can be ground into a finer consistency using a hand mill, stone grinder or heavy duty blender. This flour may be used to give a wonderfully nutty flavor to breads (when used half and half with regular flour), muffins and pancakes. It can also be added to soups and stews to provide a thicker consistency as well as offer an added boost of nutty and nutritious flavor. Take some of the coarsely ground acorns and slowly roast them in your oven at 250°F and you have a nutty-tasting coffee substitute.

Here's a great recipe for acorn bread compliments of author and wild food expert Christopher Nyerges.

Combine one cup acorn flour, 3/4 cup whole wheat flour, 1/4 cup carob flour, three teaspoons baking powder, one teaspoon sea salt, three tablespoons honey, one egg, one cup milk and three tablespoons cooking oil. Mix well and pour into a greased pan. Bake for about 45 minutes (or longer if necessary) at 250°F.

Note: Nyerges says that he uses the same recipe for making pancakes by simply adding a little more milk or water until he gets the proper pancake batter consistency.

THE "DIRT" ON... WHITE OAK

Botanical ~ *Quercus albus*

Growth cycle ~ Perennial.

Medicinal uses~ Highly astringent, antiseptic, mild stimulant, tonic, hemo-static, antivenomous.

Part(s) used for medicine ~ Inner bark of branch or trunk (preferably, young branches only), leaves and freshly fallen acorns.

Vitamins/Minerals ~ Calcium, manganese, phosphorus, potassium, sodium, magnesium, iron, copper, iodine, selenium, sulfur and vitamin B_{12}. Acorns have between four to eight percent protein and are a high carbohydrate food.

Region ~ There are between 85 and 200 species of oak trees. From the five foot tall "scrub oak" to the over 100 foot black oak, many species have naturally hybridized in the wild. For this reason, you can find this venerable tree in just about any region. All oaks share similar medicinal properties. However, many vary in the amount of tannic acid. For medicinal purposes, the white oak is most commonly used, since it has a lower tannin content. White oak (also known by the name "Tanner's oak") is found in the United States throughout the eastern states, parts of the upper midwest and in some portions of east Texas. It might be scattered in other areas not mentioned. However, it will have a better chance of sustaining life for decades (if not centuries) if it is cultivated in areas where it is native. It does best in rich, moist, clay-like soil that has superior drainage and full sun.

Wild or Domestic ~ Both.

Poisonous look-alikes in the wild ~ No.

Hardy or Delicate ~ Very hardy.

Height of mature plant ~ A mature white oak tree is between 60 and 120 feet.

Easy or hard to grow ~ Easy from seed (acorn) as long as you have lots of patience and time. If you would rather forego the initial slow development, buy saplings that are two years old or older.

Cultivation ~ You can cultivate white oak (or any oak) two ways: from established two-year-old or older saplings or from seeds (acorns). If you want to get a head start and fear your thumb is not as green as you'd wish, I suggest opting for the sapling. Plan to plant the sapling within days of purchasing it. The best weather for planting trees (especially bareroot trees) is a damp, chilly one. Hot, dry weather is hard on young trees. Allow the soil to determine how often watering should occur. Never allow the sapling to experience bone-dry conditions. White oak can be a slow grower in some regions—in others, it has been known to grow up to three feet each year. The better the soil, the more it will flourish.

If you'd like to try your hand at planting acorns, it is always best to plant them when they are brown but before they fall from the tree. White oak acorns are known to often sprout while still on the tree. If you have a choice, pick those acorns first to use as seeds since they have established a desire to reproduce. Dig a small hole with your finger one inch to one and one-half inch deep. Drop the acorn in the hole and firmly cover it with soil. It doesn't hurt to add a little compost to the hole to encourage a healthy start. Give it enough water without drowning it. Expect slow but steady growth over the two years that follow. If you cannot plant the acorns immediately, they can stored at 34° F in a high humidity environment. To accomplish this, they could be placed in flats filled with sphagnum moss or straw and stored in the refrigerator. This should only be for short-term purposes since the longer they are left in storage, the less likely they are to successfully sprout.

Plant spacing ~ White oaks should be spaced a good 25 feet or more apart.

Pre-soak seeds ~ No.

Pre-chill seeds ~ No. However, as noted above under "Cultivation," this would apply if you are storing the seeds to plant at a later date.

Indoor seed starting ~ No.

Light/dark seed requirements ~ Dark.

Days to germinate ~ Some acorns are already sprouting while still on the tree. Germination in the ground varies from region to region and depends upon the soil composition.

Days to full maturity ~ You can't measure the maturity of a white oak in days. Try years. One grower told me that "you should know if the tree is going to make it after 10 or 15 years!"

Soil type ~ Rich, moderately composted, moist and well-drained.

Water requirements ~ Keep the area around the trunk slightly damp but never expose the tree to constant moisture.

Sun or shade ~ Full sun.

Propagation ~ Seed (acorn).

Easy/hard to transplant ~ Easy from sapling.

Pests or diseases ~ Over watering or allowing the tree to stand in puddles of water leads to root rot.

Landscape uses ~ Excellent windbreak and shade tree.

Gathering ~ The following information applies to *all* species of oaks. The inner bark of the young branches or trunk should be collected in either early spring or late fall when the tannin content is the highest. Of the two seasons, I think early spring is by far your best choice. Because all oaks take so long to grow, I never harvest from the trunk of the tree unless it has recently fallen. In general, I don't harvest the inner bark from any tree since it scars them and could potentially kill them if too much bark is taken. Besides, the young branches are ten times easier to harvest due to the innate suppleness which makes the inner bark a cinch to peel back. Collect oak leaves in early fall, before the first freeze. Collect acorns when they have turned from green to brown, either on the tree or after they have recently fallen. One old trick for collecting those "recently fallen" acorns is to spread four or five old sheets under the tree and pick up the fruits every day or so as they fall. Acorns should be used fresh. Note: The acorns from the white oaks mature in one growing season. Acorns from red oaks do not mature until the end of their second growing season. The way to tell the difference between a white oak and a red oak is by the leaf. White oaks have smooth, round edges; red oaks have bristly terminal points.

Best fresh or dried ~ **Inner Bark**: dried; **leaves**: fresh or dried; **acorns**: fresh.

Drying methods ~ **Inner bark**: Dry the strips of inner bark in a cool, dry, dark place. They are ready to store when you can easily snap a section in half. **Leaves**: These need to be dried quickly. This means the room should be hot but not humid or the leaves will mold. **Acorns**: must be used fresh.

Amount needed ~ One tree.

Seed collection ~ Simply collect the acorns off the tree or when they fall to the ground.

Companion planting ~ I've seen chickweed, blue violet and skullcap growing under the shade of the mighty oak.

Container planting ~ No!

Common mistakes ~ Planting a white oak out of its native region. It will not flourish in a hot desert climate. Find out what native species of oaks grow in your area and plant those varieties to ensure success.

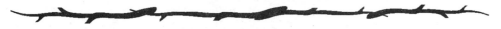

Interesting facts/tips ~ If you want to add a natural dose of calcium to your seed flats, line the bottom of the flat with a layer of fresh oak leaves and clean, broken egg shells. Acorns are a high energy, nutritious food crop that have been a staple for many cultures. Southern California Indians are said to have gathered as much as 500 pounds of acorns for each family, which lasted one year.

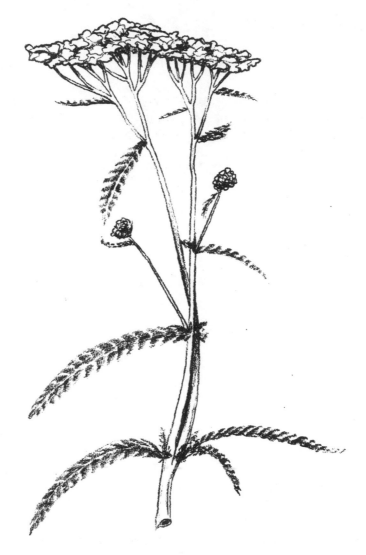

Chapter 38

GET A YEN FOR YARROW

Achillia millifolium

Hardy perennial

Medicinal Uses: *Diaphoretic, tonic, alterative, stimulant, hemostatic, vulnerary, anti-inflammatory, antispasmodic, diuretic, urinary antiseptic, emmenagogue*

Medicinal parts of plant: *Flower heads, leaves, root*

Forms: *Tea, tincture, fresh flowers and leaves*

WHAT IS ITS CHARACTER?

People may refer to yarrow as a weed. Herb books might give it the same label. But I don't think yarrow sees itself as a "weed." Whenever I come upon it in meadows or along road sides, yarrow always carries itself with a certain refinement. Its feathery leaves drape across the long stem like an elegant scarf swept to the side. Yarrow holds its flower head high, always rigid and looking above the tall grass in search of people who will notice and admire it. The other plants may think yarrow is putting on airs, but it stays resolute in its desire to be a little more educated than the other plants and perhaps rise above its "weed" standing. Yes, if yarrow were a person, I have a feeling it would listen to Vivaldi, crave appetizers such as hearts of palm and asparagus tips and read only the classics.

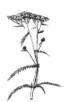

WHERE DO I FIND IT?

Yarrow is native to Europe and Asia. In the United States and Canada, it is typically found in the wild from 2,400 to 10,000 feet along roads, walking paths, trails and sunny meadows.

HOW DO I GROW IT?

Yarrow is grown from seed, rootstock or established plants. Choose a sunny location and broadcast seed into moderately rich, well-drained soil in early spring once there is no longer any danger of frost. Press seed into the soil and keep moist without drowning. It takes anywhere from 12 to 14 days for the seed to germinate. Once it becomes established, thin the seedlings to 12 or 18 inches apart. Yarrow can be started indoor in seed seed cells. Transplant outside when the seedlings are three inches tall. Yarrow doesn't like to stay in the same soil year after year. Because of this, toward late summer, divide clumps of established plants and move them to various locations throughout your garden.

Yarrow is a great plant for the garden since it attracts beneficial insects such as ladybugs and parasitic wasps that eat aphids, scale and whiteflies. This wonderful plant also repels ants, flies, Japanese beetles and termites. Some people plant yarrow near building foundations to deter termites. The only disease that might affect yarrow is powdery mildew but this only occurs if the herb is over watered or is standing in soil that is not well-drained.

HOW DO I HARVEST IT?

Harvest as yarrow begins to flower, usually in early to mid-summer. In high altitude regions (above 6,000 feet), yarrow may not flower until early to mid-September. Cut the stem about one foot below the flower head.

Unless you want to use the fresh root, do not attempt to gather yarrow by pulling on its stem in an attempt to break it. This often results in removing the whole plant, root and all. If necessary, use clippers to cut the stems. Pay attention to the flower heads when harvesting. If they are lacking in moisture or partially dry, do not gather that plant. It has passed its prime.

As for the roots, pull them up after the flower heads are well developed. They are usually easy to gather but you will need a lot of them since they can be small. Only gather roots if you know you will use them because you are killing the plant to do so.

To dry yarrow flowers, strip the leaves completely off the stems, gather together eight to ten, foot-long stems with attached flower heads and secure them on the stem end with a rubber band or string. Hang them flower end down in a dust-free, dry, warm area. I say "dust-free" because yarrow seems to attract dust as it dries and it is difficult to blow or shake it loose. Once dry, snap off the flower heads and crumble them into an airtight, glass jar. Store in a dark, cool, dry place.

As for the roots, clean them thoroughly with a quick water bath, pat them dry and place them on a cloth or in an air dryer away from direct sunlight. If exposed to continual warmth, they should be ready to store within one week.

HOW DO I USE IT?

When I was in my early 20's, I visited a local German woman who had a knack for choosing the perfect plant for whatever was ailing you. I had been feeling a bit sluggish and thought maybe she could give me some herbal relief. She was a tiny woman, no more than four and a half feet tall, with a shock of beautiful white hair that she rolled into a loose bun. Rumor had it she was in her 90's but for years she always looked as though she was perpetually in her sixties. Her physical energy was phenomenal and her mind was sharper than mine. Sometimes it was hard to understand her thick German accent, but if you caught every other word, the whole conversation tended to make sense.

"How you doing?" she asked me with urgency.

"I'm alright, I guess. Just not feeling, you know, perky." I said.

"What's this 'perky?'"

"Perky. You know...energetic."

"Ah...Perky...Yes..." She stood back and looked me over, up and down, one hand cupped under her chin. For a moment, I felt as though I was being sized up for market. Then she spoke. Her voice was decisive and abrupt. "You are stopped up right *here!*" With that, she pointed her finger toward my "female region."

"No," I said, "Everything is okay down there."

"It's not okay!" she exclaimed, her voice rising several octaves. "There is no flow! *No flow!* You hear me?!?" she said, pounding her little fist on a nearby table.

"But...I'm..."

"I give you what will make you flow and you will feel this 'perky' feeling once again." She scooped her hand into a huge, wide mouthed glass jar filled with tiny, dusty white flowers and emptied several handfuls into a large plastic bag. "*Take this!*"

"What is it?" I asked.

"Just take it! When you get up, first thing you do is put one handful of these flowers into a bottle and pour two quarts of hot water over them. Let the whole thing cool down. When it's cool, strain the flowers and drink the whole two quarts in half an hour. Do that for four days and you will feel this 'perky' feeling again."

With that, she literally pushed me out the door and sent me on my way. The next morning, I did exactly as she said. I had no idea what I was taking but I trusted her. As the mysterious herb steeped, the odor was less than wonderful. It didn't improve as the tea cooled. I strained the flowers and stared at those two quarts of liquid that would be trickling inside of me within the next 30 minutes. I drank and I drank and I drank until I thought I couldn't drink another drop. Then I drank some more. Besides the fact that the taste of this tea was bordering on horrible, I felt as if I were bloated like a beached whale. I got the entire amount down in about 29 minutes and sat down to rest. I didn't sit long, though. Nature called and soon most of what I had just drunk was coming out the other end. For the next two hours, I wore a trail in the carpet that led to the bathroom. I began to feel like "Betsy Wetsy," that children's doll that wets two seconds after you give her a bottle.

As much as I didn't care for the experience, I continued this "drink and drain" routine for the required three remaining days. On the third day, I awoke feeling less sluggish and actually had less trouble downing those two quarts of tea. By the fourth and final day, I was feeling...well...perky. I couldn't wait to tell the old woman. I rushed down to her house and met her in the garden.

"It did the trick," I said enthusiastically.

"Of course, it did!" she said. "What? You think I'm stupid?!? You are flowing now, right?"

"Oh, yeah, I'm flowing all over the place," I said. "Will you tell me the name of the herb?"

She leaned down and cut the stem of a weedy-looking flower. Handing it to me, she said, "You figure it out."

I didn't need a botanist's help with this plant—I knew it very well. It was yarrow. I had used it many times to bring down a fever and stop a cold, but I couldn't figure out what yarrow had to do with knocking out that sluggish feeling.

Years later, as I got more interested in learning about the whole body effects of herbs, the pieces started to come together. Yarrow works as a **tonic** and **alterative** on the system. This means that it cleanses and tones the body wherever it needs it, moving energy into places that are stagnant and lacking that all-important "flow." When energy is not flowing or circulating in a certain area of the body, it is very easy for that part of the body to slow down and eventually shut down. It's the same as if you didn't use your legs for several weeks. They would become like jello and it would be difficult to move, let alone walk.

Yarrow gets things moving in ways that can be dramatic in their effect. It's one of those herbs that, if taken correctly, can deliver the healing outcome you need within days...and sometimes, hours.

THE COLD-BUSTING, FEVER-DOWNING HERB

Yarrow has been used for centuries to **reduce high fevers** and nip **colds and flu** in the bud. Throughout history, it has been used to treat **typhoid**, **smallpox**, **malaria** and **pneumonia**. Yarrow works by promoting a heavy perspiration that, in turn, releases trapped toxins through the pores of the skin. Yarrow also stimulates the liver to throw off toxic waste and revs up the kidneys to eliminate their accumulated waste products via the urinary tract. While yarrow is doing all this, it's also increasing circulation which forces the lymph glands to dump built-up congestion that often contributes to sore joints and overall aches and pains during an illness.

The secret with using yarrow effectively during a cold, flu or fever is to *drink at least one quart of the tea as hot as possible and as quickly as possible.* In other words, you want to get as much of that tea inside of you in the shortest amount of time. The optimum cold and flu dose is *two quarts* but one quart will suffice. The herb to water ratio is one teaspoon of dried yarrow flowers (or two teaspoons of fresh yarrow flowers) for every eight ounces of *very* hot distilled water. Increase the amount of herb accordingly when making the quart sizes. Allow the herb to steep covered for 10 to 15 minutes, before straining and drinking as hot as possible.

To get the most herbal bang for your buck, I suggest soaking in a yarrow bath while you drink the tea. This helps to speed release of the toxic waste via the pores.

To make the bath, bring two quarts of tap water to a rolling boil. Turn off the heat and add one cup of yarrow flowers. Cover and let the yarrow steep for 20 minutes. Meanwhile, pour a hot bath and make sure the bathroom is very warm so you do not get a chill. When the tea is ready, strain it into the bathtub. Soak for 20 to 30 minutes, drinking one quart or more of the prepared yarrow tea while in the bathtub. The first question people usually have at this point is, "Won't I be getting up to go to the bathroom if I'm drinking all that tea?" Well, maybe. But more likely, you will be losing so much water through perspiration that the quart or more of yarrow tea will only serve to rehydrate your body.

After soaking in the tub, dry off and bundle up in warm pajamas. Get straight into a cozy bed and stay there. The last thing you want is to get a chill. If you follow this procedure the minute you feel a cold or flu coming on, you can often lick it overnight and feel back on top of the world the next morning. However, the tea and/or the bath can also work if you have been sick with a cold or flu for days or weeks at a time. The important part to remember is that the tea must be taken as hot as you can stand it so that your body is free to release toxins via perspiration.

CONSIDERED A "FEMININE" HERB

Yarrow has been called a "feminine" herb at times throughout history because it tends to have an affinity with the female organs. This doesn't mean that men cannot benefit from the herb. For example, yarrow is known to **clear congestion in the pelvic region**. This could relate either to females or males. "Congestion" translates into any ailment where there is a lack of "flow." Yes, we're back to what that little German herbalist kept saying to me. "Flow" has nothing to do with a menstrual cycle. "Flow" pertains to how energy is moving or not moving through a particular region. When it comes to the pelvis, in a woman it could mean backed up energy that relates to her menstrual cycle. In other words, she might experience painful cramping before or during her period. She may not even have a period for months at a time. These all trace back to lack of energetic flow in the pelvis. Drinking two or three hot cups of yarrow tea each day from ovulation until menstruation begins can help release much of this pelvic tension and be an aid in regulating the period as well as soothing or eliminating the associated cramping.

During **menopause**, yarrow comes to a woman's aid once again as it nourishes the female reproductive system. One to two cups of lukewarm to cool yarrow tea a day helps to **reduce hot flashes** and, according to some sources, **may speed up the entire menopause experience**.

Drinking one to two quarts of cold yarrow tea each day for five to seven days in a row has been shown to **dissolve and eliminate cysts on the ovaries**. During this time you will probably lose a little weight due to the diuretic action of yarrow.

Both **men and women can benefit from yarrow's natural antiseptic ability to cleanse the urinary tract**. The herb is very effective for **cystitis**, an inflammation of the bladder. In this type of case, two quarts of cool yarrow tea should be consumed each day. The cool temperature helps to quell the "fire" from the inflammation. The large amount of tea is required to adequately clear out the built up uric acid in the urine. Stay off all coffee, caffeine and soda pop during the urinary cleanse since they only serve to antagonize the condition.

INSECT BITE & WOUND MENDER

Externally, yarrow works as a strong **natural antibiotic and antiseptic** for **insect bites** or minor **scrapes and wounds**. Make a poultice by mashing the fresh or dried flowers in the palm of your hand and then moistening them with enough of your own saliva or clean water to form a paste. Place it over the insect bite or wound.

If you are out in the wild and need a wilderness remedy to **stop bleeding from a cut or a nosebleed**, grab a few fresh yarrow leaves and chew them into a wet poultice. Press the wet leaves over the wound and the bleeding will stop within seconds. That same poultice can be carefully inserted up the nostrils to stop a nosebleed. In one of nature's oddest little twists, this fresh leaf poultice can also *promote a nosebleed*. When I first heard this phenomenon, my first question was "Why would someone intentionally want to make their nose bleed?" Well, aside from the sheer shock value, it could come in handy when one is in the middle of a **sinus headache**. Apparently the process of making the nose bleed, relieves pressure in the sinus cavity, thereby easing the headache. We're back to that "flow" thing again. A sinus headache is another classic example of stopped up energy. Once you get the energy moving, the pressure is released and the pain slowly fades. However, the idea of making your nose bleed to stop pressure in the head is a double edged sword. I'm not fond of blood in general, especially when it's pouring out of me. But if that's what it took to relieve the head pain, I would do it.

As an experiment I wadded up a fresh yarrow leaf and put it into one of my nostrils just to see if I could make my nose bleed on cue. After 15 minutes and no sign of blood, I removed the yarrow leaf. I suppose my body knew I was just testing the theory and that I didn't really need to release any pressure in my head at the time.

TOOTHACHE ANESTHESIA?

The *fresh* leaf or *fresh* root mashed into a wet poultice can be applied to **sore gums** or **toothaches to give temporary relief**. The poultice has a slight anesthetic quality to it which is especially active in the fresh root. There are stories of backwoods doctors using fresh yarrow roots, macerated in whiskey, and pressing them against the skin to numb the area before cutting. While I wouldn't rely on whiskey-soaked yarrow roots to effectively numb my skin prior to surgery, I have used the fresh root and leaf on my teeth and gums to relieve minor dental pain.

BLOOD SUGAR

Yarrow tea can also come in handy when you need to **raise your blood sugar**. One of the many symptoms of low blood sugar is feeling sluggish and dopey upon waking even when you have had a full night's sleep. If that sounds like you, try a hot cup of yarrow tea right before you go to bed. Essentially, what the tea does is maintain a higher level of blood sugar during the night so that when you wake, you're not starting from ground zero.

WONDERFUL SKIN WASH

Yarrow tea makes a good astringent wash for **skin problems such as acne and rashes**. Place one heaping teaspoon of the dried *root* in 12 ounces of water. Boil for 10 minutes and let stand until cool, then strain and apply with a cotton ball to the affected area several times a day. If the skin eruptions are chronic, look to your diet and consider a whole body cleanse to release the toxic waste. Burdock root is a classic remedy for chronic skin problems. (For more information on burdock, turn to Chapter 14).

NO MORE GRAY? NO MORE BALDNESS???

There have been claims that yarrow tea taken internally as well as in a hair rinse can **prevent baldness due to chemotherapy treatments**. I've also heard stories that **rinsing your hair with three cups of yarrow tea three times a week may restore its original color**! Since I have never seen this with my own herbal eyes, I cannot attest to its effectiveness. But, hey, it's worth a shot to see if the brew can beat the bottled hair color.

A FEW CAUTIONS

As I mentioned earlier, yarrow is not a "happy tasting" herb. This is not a tea you drink and say, "Ah, pour me another cup. I can't get enough." For this reason, I always add a teaspoon or more of raw honey to the tea which helps take the edge off. **Never use sugar of any kind when**

sweetening herb tea since sugar will alter the herb's healing value. If you find that the honey still makes you pucker, try adding a pinch of peppermint or ginger (one or the other, not both) to the cup and that should improve the taste. If you still don't like the taste and you're determined to get this herb into your system, I suggest using yarrow tincture at a rate of 30 drops for every eight ounces of water. **If you use the tincture instead of the tea, you will need to get large amounts of liquid into your system to promote that all-important "flow" of energy.** So, if the ailment calls for one or two quarts of tea, use the 30 drops of tincture per cup ratio. (For every quart of water, you would add 120 drops of yarrow tincture).

Some people simply cannot handle the odor of yarrow and find they are **allergic to it or become nauseated when they drink the tea. This is particularly common among people suffering from asthma or hay fever**. Those who have an allergy to arnica, calendula or chamomile, may also have an allergy to yarrow. If this is the case, it's best to consider another herb and leave yarrow on the hillside.

Because yarrow has such strong effects on the uterine muscles, **pregnant women should never use the herb**.

Finally, the large doses of yarrow that are often required sometimes cause slight headaches. This could be due to the accelerated dumping of trapped toxic waste from the liver. If this happens and becomes too painful, reduce your intake of yarrow or discontinue using the herb.

Yes, yarrow can sometimes be a bitter pill to swallow. But if you can hold your nose, think lovely thoughts and gulp it down fast, you may just get back in the "flow."

THE "DIRT" ON... YARROW

Botanical ~	*Achillea millefolium*
Growth cycle ~	Hardy perennial.
Medicinal uses~	Diaphoretic, tonic, alterative, stimulant, hemostatic, vulnerary, anti-inflammatory, antispasmodic, diuretic, urinary antiseptic, emmenagogue.
Part(s) used for medicine ~	Flower heads, leaves, root.
Vitamins/Minerals ~	B-complex vitamins (choline & inositol), potassium, phosphorus, magnesium, manganese, selenium, silicon.
Region ~	Native to Europe and Asia. Typically found in the wild from 2,400 to 10,000 feet along roads, walking paths, trails and sunny meadows.
Wild or Domestic ~	Both.

Poisonous look-alikes in the wild ~	No. However, the somewhat toxic tansy (*Chrysanthemum vulgare*) has a similar leaf to yarrow when it is young.
Hardy or Delicate ~	Hardy.
Height of mature plant ~	Three feet.
Easy or hard to grow ~	Easy.
Cultivation ~	Seed, rootstock and established plants. Broadcast seed into soil in early spring once there is no longer any danger of frost. Press seed into the soil and keep moist without drowning. Divide clumps of established plants at the end of each growing season.
Plant spacing ~	12 to 18 inches apart.
Pre-soak seeds ~	No.
Pre-chill seeds ~	No.
Indoor seed starting ~	Yes. Easiest to start in seed plugs.
Light/dark seed requirements ~	Light.
Days to germinate ~	Seven to fourteen days.
Days to full maturity ~	Approximately 90 days.
Soil type ~	Moderately rich, well-drained soil with moderate moisture.
Water requirements ~	Likes regular moisture without being drowned.
Sun or shade ~	Sun with filtered shade part of the day.
Propagation ~	Seed.
Easy/hard to transplant ~	Easy. Wait until the seedlings are three inches tall.
Pests or diseases ~	Virtually pest and disease-free. Yarrow, in fact, is one of the best plants for attracting beneficial insects such as ladybugs and parasitic wasps that eat aphids, scale and whiteflies. This wonderful plant also repels ants, flies, Japanese beetles and termites. Some people plant yarrow near building foundations to deter termites. The only disease that might affect yarrow is powdery mildew but this only occurs if the herb is over watered or is standing in soil that is not well-drained.
Landscape uses ~	Beautiful border and hardy filler.
Gathering ~	Harvest as yarrow begins to flower, usually in early to mid-summer. In high altitude regions (above 6,000 feet), yarrow may not flower until early to mid-September. Cut the stem about one foot below the flower head. Unless you want to use the fresh root, do not attempt to gather yarrow by pulling on its stem in an attempt to break it. This often results in removing the whole plant, root and all. If necessary, use clippers to cut the stems. Pay attention to the flower heads when harvesting. If they are lacking in moisture or partially dry, do not gather that plant. It has passed its prime. As for the roots, pull them up after

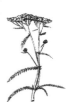

363

the flower heads are well developed. They are usually easy to gather but you will need a lot of them since they can be small. Only gather roots if you know you will use them because you are killing the plant to do so.

Best fresh or dried ~   **Flowers**: fresh or dried; **Leaves**: best fresh; **Root**: best fresh.

Drying methods ~   **Flowers**: strip the leaves completely off the stems, gather together eight to ten foot-long stems with attached flower heads and secure them on the stem end with a rubber band or string. Hang them flower end down in a dust-free, dry, warm area. I say "dust-free" because yarrow seems to attract dust as it dries and it is difficult to blow or shake it loose. Once dry, snap off the flower heads and crumble them into an airtight, glass jar. Store in a dark, cool, dry place. **Roots**: Clean them thoroughly with a quick water bath, pat them dry and place them on a cloth or in an air dryer away from direct sunlight. If exposed to continual warmth, they should be ready to store within one week.

Amount needed ~   Moderate use: 10 plants; Regular use: 25+.

Seed collection ~   Allow the flowers to dry on the plant. Tap or shake the flower heads into your hand before picking them to see if any seed is released. Bring a paper bag with you and immediately insert the plant, flower-head down, into the bag. Place it in a dark, cool, dry area to dry. Occasionally, rattle the flower heads against the paper bag to dislodge the seeds.

Companion planting ~   Plant yarrow around aromatic herbs such as spearmint, peppermint, lemon balm, horehound, thyme, rosemary and garden sage to increase their innate essential oil content.

Container planting ~   No. It can be done, but yarrow needs room to grow. Besides, you wouldn't be able to grow enough yarrow in the container to meet your needs.

Common mistakes ~   Thinking that the hybrid, decorative varieties of the yellow-flowered yarrow are the same as the medicinal species. Only use the yellow variety for the dried flower arrangements. While not a universal belief, I don't use the brightly colored pink yarrow species for medicine. Instead, I stick with the run-of-the-mill, classic off-white variety.

Interesting facts/tips ~   If you spoil yarrow with lots of compost, it will grow taller than usual. However, it will also produce less of the active volatile oils that make it so valuable. Also, yarrow should be moved to a new location every one to two years to ensure a strong medicinal crop. If you leave some plants in the same location, be sure to use the seeds from their flower heads to propagate new growth for the following year.

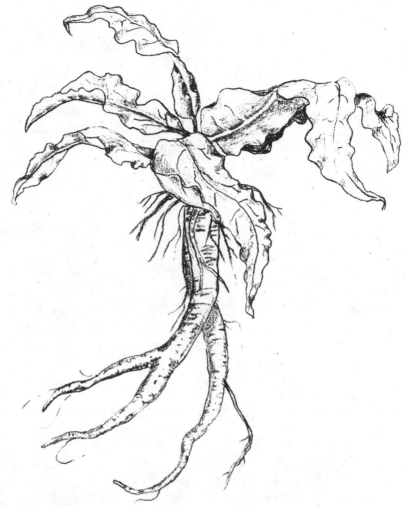

Chapter 39

JUST WHAT THE YELLOW DOCK ORDERED

Rumex crispus
("W.F.")
Hardy perennial

Medicinal Uses: *Alterative, bitter, general tonic, laxative, astringent, lymphatic cleanser, cholagogue*

Medicinal parts of plant: *Leaves, root*

Forms: *Tea, tincture, capsules, fomentation, skin wash*

WHAT IS ITS CHARACTER?

Yellow dock reminds me of an eccentric genius who is always disheveled and far from stylish in appearance. Yes, yellow dock is a bit of a slob–but a brilliant slob. This seedy, weedy, somewhat homely road side perennial spends every growing moment soaking up a mass of vitamins and minerals via its tenacious tap root. Under that slovenly cloak, lies a single-minded character that harnesses tremendous medicinal power and rugged toughness. Make fun of its appearance if you wish, yellow dock couldn't care less. It's too busy generating an awesome force that will course through its leaves in the spring and dive into the roots come fall. It's not really here to be your friend. Yellow dock is like the front line troops sent in to do battle and win the war. When you have yellow dock on your side, you suddenly realize that you can be a contender in the fight and even come out the winner.

WHERE DO I FIND IT?

Yellow dock (or "curly dock," as it is often called) is found in the wild from sea level to 10,000 feet in meadows, semi-moist fields, along road sides and streams and in ditches. In the wild, if left untouched and allowed to freely reproduce, yellow dock can grow in thick stands with plants spaced only inches apart.

HOW DO I GROW IT?

Yellow dock is easy to grow from seed. Broadcast seed thinly into moist, rich soil in an area that gets full sun. Press firmly and keep moist until germination which usually takes eight to ten days. Thin the seedlings about one to two feet apart if they appear to be crowding against each other. The herb can be grown in poor soil. However, it produces the best roots and leaves when it is grown in moderately rich, slightly composted, semi-damp dirt that has excellent drainage. If yellow dock is allowed to stand in areas that collect water, the roots will lack the distinctive yellow streak in the inner core that is an indicator of medicinal strength.

All docks dramatically change color from green in the spring to a deep coffee-rust in late summer. Keep this in mind if you are designing your garden around a particular color scheme. Dock makes a very large centerpiece, albeit one that can be rather weedy looking and unkempt. If not controlled, dock could easily take over your garden. While it adds wonderful nutrients to your soil, it can become invasive within several years.

HOW DO I HARVEST IT?

Harvest the leaves for "rubbing out" the pain of a nettle sting whenever they are needed. Dig the eight to twelve inch roots in October or November once the herb has turned from green to rust and has an abundance of seeds clinging to a dry stalk. Many herbalists believe that the later you can wait the better for digging roots. Mid to late November or even early December in some areas is preferred. Clean the long tap roots of dirt and slice them as you would a carrot in one inch pieces. Look at the center of the root; you should see the yellow/orange inner core which is where the "yellow" in yellow dock originates. The darker the yellow inner core, the stronger and more powerful the medicinal value. Lay the roots inside an air dryer that allows for circulation on all sides of the root. When they are completely dry, store them in an airtight glass jar in a cool, dark, dry space.

HOW DO I USE IT?

A few years ago, I was sitting around with some friends bemoaning the fact that no matter how many lottery tickets we bought, we never won the big prize.

"If you really want to make lots of money," one of my friends piped up, "you've gotta invent something that everybody needs or wants…"

"Or something that makes life easier…" another added.

"But it's got to be simple," I insisted. "Easy and cheap to make. Like that little piece of rubber that someone added to the dust pan so you don't scratch the floor. Now, that was genius."

"How about those plastic reflectors that divide lanes on the freeway?" someone said. "That's easy, simple and so obvious I can't believe I didn't think of it. I heard that guy gets a quarter of a penny for every one of those. Do you have any idea how much money that adds up to?!"

"You know what I wished I'd invented?" said one friend. "Geritol."

"Geritol?" I questioned.

"Yeah! All that 'liquid iron' in a bottle. It's like an anemic's best friend! That's a great seller. Everybody loves it."

"Well, you know…" I started to say.

"Oh, gawd, you're not going to try to tell us there's an herb that can beat Geritol, are you?" my friend said.

"Well, yes" I said. "And this herb beats it by a mile!"

You can call it yellow dock or just plain ol' "dock." There are those who refer to it as that '#!%$!' out of the yard.

Yellow dock gets no respect and that's too bad. It's actually a good thing if yellow dock happens to pop up in your garden. Wherever it grows, it is an indicator that there is naturally-occurring iron in the soil. We're talking 40% iron compounds in its little root! Research has shown that yellow dock has more organic iron than any other known plant.

Because of the rich iron content (along with the high amounts of calcium, phosphorus, and vitamin A and C), yellow dock is considered to be one of the top ten **blood purifiers**. That means yellow dock has the ability to cut through the crud in your body, **detoxify your system** and **stimulate your organs to operate at maximum efficiency**.

GOT NO GET UP AND GO?

Since yellow dock is so high in iron, it makes sense that it works for those who are **iron-deficient**. Because yellow dock is a plant, your body recognizes the organic iron and is better able to process and assimilate it into the system wherever and whenever it is needed. This differs greatly from "iron fortified" pills and liquids which are made from inorganic compounds that the body often does not recognize, and therefore, does not metabolize.

One old herbal book claims yellow dock "soothes thy womyn during her weakness." Translated, that simply means that when a woman's get up and go has got up and left due to a lack of iron in the body, yellow dock can come to the rescue. This can happen during **menstruation** or any other time in a female's life when, due to age, **menopause**, diet, **chronic anemia** or **illness**, the body becomes depleted of iron.

If you suffer from **anemia**, you might see a vast improvement as yellow dock's blood purification properties help to release built up toxins and then fortify the blood with easily assimilated iron. Of course, anemia can be a sign of a poor diet, lack of vitamins and stress. Yellow dock can certainly help add iron to your bloodstream, but if you continue with poor dietary habits and/or don't get enough sleep, it will be similar to putting a band aid on an ax wound.

Yellow dock is a wonderful herb for a woman during **pregnancy** since it replenishes whatever iron is lost and helps give the mother both energy and stamina. Either the tea, tincture or capsules can be used. One cup of the root tea each day is sufficient. I would drink it six days on and one day off for several weeks and then take a week or so off to give your body a chance to assimilate what it needs and release what it doesn't want. As for the tincture, use one-half to one full teaspoon diluted in several ounces of warm water upon rising and before bedtime. If you prefer the capsules, the recommended dose is one or two capsules with meals.

LIVER LOVER

Yellow dock has the ability to **stimulate and clear congestion in the liver**. In doing so, it **increases the bile flow** and the dumping of poisons that may have collected within the liver. A warm cup of yellow dock root one or two hours after a meal can work as a **mild laxative**. In addition, if you eat an exceptionally heavy meal full of fatty meat and dairy products, a warm cup of yellow dock root tea taken after the meal **helps break down the fat and make digestion easier**. If you're still feeling sluggish the following day, a cup of yellow dock tea in the morning and one in the afternoon taken between meals can help improve overall digestion.

THE EMPHATIC LYMPHATIC

While it's detoxifying the liver, yellow dock is also **draining and clearing the lymph glands**—another place pockets of pesky poisons love to set up camp. Lymphatic cleansing herbs are important when you feel congestion building up along the lymph channels. Those areas include the neck (specifically from underneath your ear lobes and extending down toward the center of your throat), the armpits and the groin. Sometimes when there is congestion in these areas, you can feel painful bumps or swellings. This simply means that there is a blockage of energy in that area that needs to be cleared. Yellow dock, along with several other lymphatic and blood cleansing herbs, just might be able to do the trick.

Here's a good formula: combine one teaspoon each of yellow dock root and burdock root in a saucepan. Add two cups of cold distilled water and bring the mixture to a boil. Simmer on low heat for 15 minutes. Strain the roots and add two droppersful (approximately 50 drops) of cleavers tincture made from the *fresh* plant. You can repeat this process up to three times a day. In order to really get that lymph moving, make sure you drink plenty of water during the day to cleanse the entire system.

If the lymphatic swelling is causing you exceptional discomfort, cover the area with a yellow dock fomentation. To do this, make a strong decoction (boiling the herb rather than steeping it) from yellow dock root, dip a clean cotton cloth in the hot tea, wring out the excess liquid and apply it as hot as can be tolerated to the affected areas. When the fomentation cools down, dip the cloth back into the hot tea and repeat the process. Continue for as long as needed.

THE SKIN "DETOXIFIER"

With all this toxic elimination taking place, it's no wonder that yellow dock is also famous for treating **topical "eruptive" skin problems**. This can be everything from **acne** and **psoriasis** to **poison ivy rashes** and common **skin rashes**. Used both internally as a tea and externally as a hot, astringent fomentation, skin wash or bath, yellow dock tends to not only soothe but reduce the discomfort.

Yellow dock tea alone works well but there are specific application methods and combinations that work for each skin ailment. For **poison ivy/oak rashes**, the root should be boiled in vinegar (one ounce of the root to one and one-half pints of vinegar), left to simmer for 30 minutes, strained and then either applied directly to the rash or poured into a bath.

369

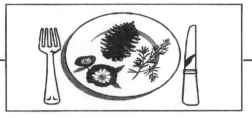

Wild Food Facts

Yellow dock leaves are best gathered in early spring when they are still tender. They have a tart vinegar taste that becomes progressively bitter as the plant matures. Try eating them raw or added to a salad to give it a "wild" bite. I like to steam the spring leaves as you would cook spinach or add them to a pot of boiling water. Cook them until tender and eat them with dash of lemon and butter or as is. Wild food forager and author Christopher Nyerges has a great recipe for spring dock leaves. In a cast iron skillet that has a layer of oil added, place equal portions of chopped yellow dock leaves, diced tomatoes and diced brown onions. Cover the skillet and gently sauté until tender. The dish needs no seasoning, says Nyerges, due to the sour (dock), sweet (cooked onion) and salty (tomato) combination.

There is a slight warning on overdosing with yellow dock leaves. Like spinach, sorrel and rhubarb, dock can have varying amounts of oxalic acid depending upon its growing location. Compared to rhubarb, which can have "toxic" levels of oxalates, dock is a minor player. Still, you don't want to overdo on consumption. Oxalic acid leeches calcium from the body and can cause severe digestive tract irritation. However, you would have to consume large portions to accomplish this. The first symptoms of oxalic acid poisoning are mild nausea and stomach cramps. However, the sour taste of yellow dock has always prevented me from overdosing on the cooked leaf.

A wild flour can be made from the seeds, although it takes a lot of plants to accumulate enough seed to make flour. If you want to try this, use only one-third yellow dock flour with two-thirds regular flour. Any more than that and the resulting bread can become too mushy.

This also works for stinging nettle rashes. In fact, yellow dock is the "classic" remedy for nettle stings. There's the old saying, "Nettle in, dock out." For the most immediate relief, use a fresh yellow dock leaf chewed into a wet poultice. Apply this to the skin and you will feel an instant cooling sensation. Within minutes, the stinging should subside along with any pain. You might ask how you are going to "happen to find" a yellow dock leaf when you are stung by nettle. Well, of all the natural antidotes that grow near nettle in the wild (which include plantain, mullein, blue violet, jewelweed and hounds tongue), yellow dock tends to be the most prevalent.

When it comes to **acne—especially teenage acne which is accompanied by oily skin and eruptions on the face, neck and back—**it is best to combine one-half heaping teaspoon of yellow dock root with one-half heaping teaspoon of burdock root. Pour 16 ounces of *boiling* distilled water over the herbs and continue to simmer the concoction for 20 to 30 minutes. At this point, the tea should have boiled down to half its original volume. Drink one cup of this tea combination three times a day for two weeks, take one week off and then repeat the process. During this time, drink one ounce of pure water for every pound of weight. In other words, a 128 pound person should drink one gallon of water each day. You need this amount of fluid to cleanse and hydrate the cells so that they can release every bit of toxic debris. Understand that the acne may become worse when you begin the procedure due to the toxic dumping. For this reason, you can also incorporate a hot yellow dock root bath into the schedule twice a week since the heat from the bath quickens the release of the toxins via the pores. To make the bath, combine one ounce of yellow dock root to two quarts of boiling water. Simmer for 30 minutes, strain and add to a hot bath.

HEAVY METAL REMOVER

I once told a woman that yellow dock helped to **remove heavy metal poisoning**. She misunderstood and took my comment to mean that this herb would remove the effects of "heavy metal" rock music. Go figure. As for the *real* heavy metals—such as lead, copper and even small amounts of arsenic—herbalist Dr. John R. Christopher has a tested formula which many have used successfully for years.In a pint sized jar, combine three ounces of yellow dock root with three ounces of bugleweed herb and one ounce of lobelia. Stir the dried herbs together well so they are completely mixed. Take one ounce of this herbal mixture and pour one pint of hot water over the herbs. Cover and allow to steep for 15 minutes. Strain and drink two to three cups of the tea every day. Dr. Christopher also suggested taking three chaparral capsules or tablets *with the tea*. Chaparral works as an effective liver detoxifier, especially when there are serious poisons in the body. Continue the tea and chaparral capsules/tablets for six days in a row with one day off for three consecutive weeks.

After three weeks, the external process of heavy metal detoxification can begin. To do this, place one to three pounds of Epsom salts in a hot bath. Soak for 30 minutes, three times a week on alternate days. Continue this procedure for three weeks. Rest from the bath for one week and then continue after that if needed. During this time, you are still taking the tea formula as mentioned. What I have found is that the bathroom will often take on a peculiar, metallic odor. In addition, the bathtub may show signs of dark or grey rings around the sides. This is actually a good sign and shows that the body is efficiently dumping the toxic metals.

THINGS YOU SHOULD KNOW

Those with a delicate stomach should only drink one to one and a half cups a day of yellow dock since it really can stimulate the body and release trapped debris from the liver and colon. Yellow dock contains a high amount of tannins that give it astringent properties. **Those with a history of kidney stones are asked to use this herb "cautiously" since the tannins could exacerbate the condition. While you are using yellow dock, you must eliminate coffee, Chinese or black tea and any other beverages that have caffeine. Mixing caffeinated beverages with iron-rich herbs such as yellow dock can produce highly toxic results.**

Yellow dock may not be the prettiest plant in the yard. But when you need what it can offer, it might be the best dock on the block.

THE "DIRT" ON... YELLOW DOCK

Botanical ~	*Rumex crispus*
Growth cycle ~	Hardy perennial.
Medicinal uses~	Alterative, bitter, general tonic, laxative, astringent, lymphatic cleanser, cholagogue.
Part(s) used for medicine ~	Leaves, root.
Vitamins/Minerals ~	Massive amounts of iron (yellow dock is thought to have more organic iron than any other known plant), vitamins A & C (with four more times beta carotene than carrots and more vitamin C than oranges), manganese, B-complex, magnesium, protein, phosphorus, selenium, calcium, potassium, niacin.
Region ~	Yellow dock (or "curly dock," as it is often called) is found in the wild from sea level to 10,000 feet in meadows, semi-moist fields, along road sides and streams and in ditches. In the wild, if left untouched and allowed to freely reproduce, yellow dock can grow in thick stands with plants spaced only inches apart.
Wild or Domestic ~	Both.
Poisonous look-alikes in the wild ~	No. However, yellow dock has a handful of "kissing cousin" plants that are collectively referred to as "dock." The two most commonly confused "docks" are red dock (*Rumex aquaticus*) and water dock (*Rumex britannica*). Fortunately, both share similar medicinal qualities with yellow dock, The greatest differences are that red dock is the largest of the "docks," reaching heights of six or seven feet tall and water dock is a much more astringent medi-

cine than yellow dock. When young, yellow dock's leaves can also be mistaken for rhubarb.

Hardy or Delicate ~ Very hardy.

Height of mature plant ~ Three to five feet tall.

Easy or hard to grow ~ Easy.

Cultivation ~ Seed. Broadcast seed thinly into moist, rich soil. Press firmly and keep moist until germination. Thin seedlings if they appear to be crowding against each other. If yellow dock is allowed to stand in areas that collect water, the roots will lack the distinctive yellow streak in the inner core that is an indicator of medicinal strength.

Plant spacing ~ One to two feet.

Pre-soak seeds ~ No.

Pre-chill seeds ~ No.

Indoor seed starting ~ No.

Light/dark seed requirements ~ Light.

Days to germinate ~ Eight to ten days.

Days to full maturity ~ Approximately 90 to 120 days.

Soil type ~ Can be grown in poor soil. However, it produces the best roots and leaves when it is grown in moderately rich, slightly composted, moist dirt that has excellent drainage.

Water requirements ~ Likes regular moisture but never allow it to stand in water.

Sun or shade ~ Full sun.

Propagation ~ Seed.

Easy/hard to transplant ~ Hard. Yellow dock transplants poorly due to its tap root. Direct seeding is your best bet.

Pests or diseases ~ Virtually pest and disease-free.

Landscape uses ~ Dock dramatically changes color from green in the spring to a deep coffee-rust in late summer. Keep this in mind if you are designing your garden around a particular color scheme. Dock makes a very large centerpiece, albeit one that can be rather weedy looking and unkempt. If not controlled, dock could easily take over your garden. While it adds wonderful nutrients to your soil, it can become invasive within several years.

Gathering ~ Harvest the leaves for "rubbing out" the pain of a nettle sting whenever they are needed. Dig the eight to twelve inch roots in October or November once the herb has turned from green to rust and has an abundance of seeds clinging to a dry stalk. Many herbalists believe that the later you can wait the better for digging roots. Mid to late November or even early December in some areas is preferred.

Best fresh or dried ~ **Leaves**: fresh; **Root**: dried.

Drying methods ~ Clean the long tap roots of dirt and slice them as you would a carrot in one inch pieces. Look at the center of the root; you should see the yellow/orange inner core which is where the "yellow" in yellow dock originates. The darker the yellow inner core, the stronger and more powerful the medicinal value. Lay the roots inside an air dryer that allows for circulation on all sides of the root. Once they are completely dry, store them in an airtight glass jar in a cool, dark, dry space.

Amount needed ~ Moderate use: 5 plants; Regular use: 15+.

Seed collection ~ Allow yellow dock to naturally go to seed. This usually takes place in late summer to early fall, depending upon your geographic region, when the plant has turned from green to rust. The stalk should be fairly dry and may even be easily breakable. Strip the multitude of seed heads off the stalk in small handfuls. Gently rub your hands together to release the coffee-colored seed from the heart-shaped "wings" that hold the seed. It is nearly impossible to sift out all the chaff from the seed so don't worry about it. When it comes time to plant seed, toss the chaff along with it. As always, fresh seeds are more potent than dried. For this reason, as you collect seed for saving, scatter a handful around the area. When it comes to collecting seed, one plant is more than enough to accommodate you.

Companion planting ~ Since dock is the classic remedy for "rubbing out" the sting of nettle, you may want to plant it within an arm's reach of nettle. Some gardeners plant garden sorrel (*Rumex acetosa*) or sheep sorrel (*Rumex acetosella*) which are also in the "dock" family but referred to as "sour dock" due to their sour tasting leaves. If you do this, give the sorrel and dock plenty of space (four or more feet) so they don't get tangled up and easily confused when it comes time to harvest the sorrel leaves.

Container planting ~ No.

Common mistakes ~ Treating yellow dock like a king and doting on it. In the wild, dock thrives in moderate to poor soil and only gets watered when it rains. If you give it too much attention, the roots can often be small and the leaves underdeveloped.

Interesting facts/tips ~ Yellow dock can be used as a cover crop to enrich poor soil. However, it is extremely invasive and could choke out other plants if left unchecked.

Chapter 40

How To Make Herbal Stuff

Here are detailed descriptions on how to make the various preparations described in the herbal chapters.

IMPORTANT NOTE!!!

When you are making any herbal preparations, please DO NOT USE ALUMINUM OR CAST IRON POTS.

Aluminum and cast iron can alter the ability of the herb to work as a medicinal agent. Use either a good grade of stainless steel (one that is not made partly with aluminum) or Pyrex. Enamel pans are fine. However, make sure there are no chips or cracks.

In addition, while it is not imperative, it is always best to use *distilled* water when making medicinal herb teas. When distilled water comes in contact with the plant matter, it has a tendency to extract more of the healing nutrients out of the herb than spring water which still has minerals in it.

THE FOLLOWING HERBAL PREPARATIONS ARE FOR *INTERNAL USE*

INFUSION

The most common way to make an herbal tea. The medicinal properties are extracted in water by a more gentle process. An infusion is generally used for the more delicate parts of a plant (i.e., the flowers and leaves). Hot (**NOT** boiling) water is poured over the herb. The mixture is then allowed to steep for 10-20 minutes.

A cold infusion may also be indicated. This requires pouring cold water over the herbs and allowing the mixture to stand, covered, overnight.

The suggested tea to water ratio for an infusion is one heaping teaspoon of the *dried* herb or two heaping teaspoons of the *fresh* herb to eight ounces of distilled water.

The per cup dose for infusions varies depending upon the ailment you are treating.

DECOCTION

A decoction is called for when using the "tougher" plant parts (i.e., roots, barks, berries, leaf buds, nuts). Boiling water is necessary to extract the medicinal essence from the core. The herb is usually first placed into cold water and brought to a boil. The mixture is then allowed to simmer for 10 to 20 minutes (or longer if indicated). The harder the plant material, the longer it will take for the medicinal elements to be released.

The tea to water ratio varies from herb to herb and formula to formula. One typical tea to water ratio for a decoction is one heaping teaspoon of the dried herb to 12 ounces of cold distilled water. *Note: Once the herb has simmered for 10 to 20 minutes, you will end up with less water than you started with due to evaporation.*

The per cup dose for decoctions varies depending upon the condition being treated.

CAPSULES

Whether it is for convenience or those times when an ailment calls for using a large dose of an herb, capsules can sometimes be a good way to take plant medicine. Many people prefer to make their own capsules since they can create herb combinations that are not always available in pre-packaged bottles. Unless you own a high tech grinder that can pulverize herbs into a ultra-fine powder, you will need to purchase any roots, barks, leaves or flowers in a finely ground powdered form. The finer the powder, the more you can pack into the capsule.

Capsules come in different sizes: #000, #00 and #0. Respectively, this translates to triple aught, double aught and single aught. Triple aught capsules are the largest of the three. It is difficult to determine how many milligrams each size capsule will hold since that is dependent upon how firmly you pack the capsules and how fine the herb powders have been ground.

Packing capsules with herb powders is a very "zen" procedure. In other words, it is time consuming and allows your mind to wander. Try to pack each end of the capsule with as much herb powder as possible before slipping the two sections together. Store capsules in recycled, amber colored glass vitamin bottles. When making your own capsules, always remember to label the bottle since after awhile, all herb capsules start to look the same.

There are times when capsules are not the best way to ingest an herb. When an herbal remedy calls for a diaphoretic (perspiration-inducing) action, for example, you need the hot herb tea to generate that effect. Some herbs hold most of their medicinal activity when they are used fresh in teas or in tinctures. For those herbs, the capsules with their dried powder would not be effective. Another problem I have had with capsules is that they often do not break open and release their herb(s) until they hit the colon. In some cases, capsules *never* break open, traveling through the entire body completely intact and offering no healing assistance along the way. If you want to see how fast a homemade capsule might break open, fill one up with your herbs and drop it in a glass of warm water. Watch the clock and see how long it takes for the gelatin to dissolve and disperse the herbs. If after two hours, nothing has happened, you may want to reconsider using those particular capsules.

Capsule doses vary depending upon the ailment you are treating. However, a typical dose is usually two capsules taken three times a day with meals.

TINCTURE

A tincture is another convenient and very effective way to take herbal medicine. Tinctures are especially helpful when a specific herb is recommended to be taken *fresh*. You may not always have access to a fresh plant. But by preserving that fresh plant in an alcohol solution, you can secure that freshness and have it available throughout the year. Herbal tinctures can be made with brandy, 80 proof vodka or 190 proof alcohol (known as "grain alcohol" and sold under the name "Everclear"). Alcohol tinctures are very potent. Ten to fifteen drops placed under the tongue or diluted into eight ounces of hot water are equivalent to about one cup of tea.

Some tinctures are made from vegetable glycerine. There are herbalists who feel that glycerine tinctures are best for internal use—especially for children under the age of 12 and those adults with alcohol sensitivities or addictions. Glycerine tinctures are also preferred by those whose religious faith does not allow the use of alcohol. Unfortunately, vegetable glycerine tinctures have some disadvantages. First, they usually lack the potency of alcohol tinctures, thereby requiring *double or triple* the required dose in order to get the desired medicinal effect. Secondly, vegetable glycerine is incompatible with resinous herbs—such as myrrh—which demand an alcohol solvent to coax out the hard-to-release medicinal core. Many parents choose vegetable glycerine tinctures for their children since they don't want to give them alcohol. However, the tincture dosage for children is measured in *drops*, thereby making the alcohol content fairly negligible. I will say that alcohol-based tinctures that are made with 100 percent *grain* alcohol and no water concern me. These are *very* strong and can cause serious physical reactions with both children and adults. One way to significantly reduce the alcohol content in *any* alcohol-based tincture is to place the tincture into eight ounces of *boiling* water that has been removed from the heat. The heat burns off most of the alcohol while still retaining the medicinal value of the plant. Whatever alcohol remains is very minor.

377

The only time I always reach for a glycerine tincture is when my "patient" is an animal. An animal's system is overly-sensitive to alcohol. Depending upon the weight and general health of the animal, the alcohol could quickly be absorbed into their system and worsen their condition or cause a fatal effect.

Making effective homemade *glycerine* tinctures is an art. You must know exact ratios and whether the herb is even suitable for extraction via glycerine. I've made my fair share of glycerine tinctures and never been quite happy with the result. If I need a glycerine tincture, I buy it at my local herb store or through a trusted herb company. Glycerine tinctures have a shorter shelf life than straight alcohol-based tinctures—ranging anywhere from three to five years.

It is very easy to make a standard homemade alcohol tincture. (Please do not attempt to substitute vegetable glycerine in place of the alcohol for the following formula. *It will not work).*

The herb to alcohol ratio is as follows: For *fresh* herbs, the herb to alcohol ratio is either 1:1 or 1:2. The first number represents *weight;* the second number represents *volume.* Thus, a 1:1 ratio means that for every one ounce by *weight* of **herb**, you would add one ounce by *volume* of **alcohol**. With *fresh* herbs, I have found the simplest way to achieve this is to tightly pack a wide-mouth, glass jar with the fresh herb. Pour either brandy, 80 proof vodka or grain alcohol over the plant matter until it is completely covered. *If using grain alcohol, I usually fill the bottle three-quarters with the alcohol and one-quarter with cold distilled water. This reduces any chance of alcohol poisoning if you give the grain alcohol-based tincture to someone with any sensitivity to this "high octane" liquor.* Store the bottle in a dark, dry, cool space for at least 60 days. Many seasoned herbalists believe that *fresh* plant tinctures are not really "ready" until they have soaked for one full year. The choice is completely up to you. Every day, vigorously shake the bottle and let the alcohol move around the packed herb. When you are ready to process the tincture, strain the alcohol from the herb through a clean muslin or cotton cloth, pressing every last drop of liquid from the plant material. If I only need a small amount of the volume, I simply pour whatever I want out of the bottle without straining the plant material.

Now, onto making tinctures from *dried* plants.

The herb to alcohol ratio is typically 1:4. (For every one ounce by *weight* of the herb you will need four ounces by *volume* of the alcohol solvent). Thus, if you had four ounces by weight of *dried* herb you would need 16 ounces by *volume* of alcohol. Combine the dried herbs and alcohol into a wide mouthed, glass bottle. For this method, always allow enough room in the bottle so that the herbs and alcohol are not packed right to the top. Place the lid on tightly and shake the contents vigorously. Put the bottle in a cool, dark place for 14 days. Three times each day, shake the bottle so that the contents have a chance to move around. On the 14th day, strain the liquid through a clean muslin cloth. Once all the liquid has been emptied, twist the muslin cloth tightly to force out the remaining tincture.

Both fresh and dried tinctures should be stored in dark bottles and kept in a dark, cool cupboard. They can last as long as 10 years depending upon how well they are stored and how often they are used.

Important note: When using homemade grain alcohol tinctures, I think it is always best to dilute the tincture in hot water first and allow the mixture to cool to lukewarm before ingesting. This should prevent any negative physical reaction from the alcohol.

As always, doses vary depending upon the condition you are treating. A typical tincture dose is one dropperful (which is approximately 25 to 30 drops) placed under the tongue or diluted in several ounces of warm water. Placing the tincture in warm water helps speed its delivery into the bloodstream. This dose is taken a minimum of two times a day.

FLUID (LIQUID) EXTRACT

A fluid or liquid extract is the most concentrated way in which an herbal medicine can be prepared. Extracts are far stronger than a tincture. One ounce of a fluid extract is equal to ingesting one ounce of the original herbal plant. What is confusing for many people is that the term "extract" is often used when referring to "tinctures." The confusion is easy to understand since almost all fluid extracts are made with alcohol. The most common ways to make extracts are through cold percolation (passing a percentage of alcohol and water through a measured amount of dry herb), evaporation of the liquid via heat or extracting the plant essence through massive pressure.

While opinions differ, some herbal practitioners are recommending tinctures over extracts because they feel that the process needed to make the extract removes too much of the volatile compounds in the plant. Extracts can be tricky for the beginning herbal student to make. Many herbs require very specific alcohol to water ratios in order to extract the greatest healing benefit from the plant. For this reason, if you are a beginning herbal student, it might be best to purchase the extract from a trusted herb company.

The suggested dose for an extract is one-half to one teaspoon of the extract taken straight or diluted in several ounces of warm, distilled water. The latter is considered a better and faster way to deliver the herb into your bloodstream.

SYRUP

Homemade herbal cough syrups are as old as time and easy to make. First, you will need to make either an infusion or decoction, depending upon whether the herb you are using falls into the flower/leaf category or the root/bark/berry/nuts category. Use two cups of distilled water and follow the same herb to water measurements (i.e., one heaping teaspoon of the *dried* herb or two heaping teaspoons of the *fresh* herb to eight ounces of distilled water. For the syrup, simply double the measurements to meet the two cup criteria). Allow the infusion or decoction to cook down to half its original volume (i.e., one cup of liquid should remain). This usually takes about 30 to 45 minutes. Take the liquid off the heat, strain out the herbs, return the tea to the pot and gradually stir in two cups of raw honey. Bring the mixture to a slight boil and take it off the heat again. Add one or two "thumb-size" chunks of fresh ginger root to the syrup. This helps preserve it as well as catalyze the herb(s). Let the mixture slightly cool before placing it into a dark, corked bottle for storage. **NOTE:** *the bottle must be corked since screw-capped bottles may explode if any fermentation takes place.* Store the syrup in the refrigerator. It should keep for several months.

For Figuring Children's Doses, Remember "Clark's Rule"

Clark's Rule bases the herbal dose upon the child's weight. According to Clark's Rule, an "adult" is considered 150 pounds. Thus, all factoring is based upon 150 pounds. The child's weight is then divided into 150 to determine what approximate fraction of the "adult" dose to give. For example, if the child weighs 50 pounds, the fraction would be 50/150 or 1/3 of the recommended adult dose. If the child weighs 30 pounds, the fraction would be 30/150 or 1/5 the recommended adult dose. If the child is at an in-between weight, always factor down rather than up to make sure you don't give the child too much of a dose.

When using tinctures, figure out the child's dose by dividing the child's weight in half. That number is how many **drops** you need to administer (i.e., a 60 pound child would require 30 drops of the tincture for each dose). For extracts, which are much stronger than tinctures, figure the child's weight, cut that in half and then cut *that* number in half. Thus, a 60 pound child would require 15 drops of the extract for each dose.

Children under the age of two years old require extra-special care. Some herbs are gentle while others are considered too strong for their delicate bodies. Any mother who wishes to use herbal medicine should read as much possible about herbal care directed specifically for children.

THE FOLLOWING HERBAL PREPARATIONS ARE FOR EXTERNAL USE ONLY.

LINIMENT

Herbal liniments are great when you need to add a burst of external circulation to sore muscles and aching joints. An herbal liniment can be made two ways. The first way is to combine one and one-half cups of the dried herb to two cups of inexpensive vodka or pure apple cider vinegar. Put the herbs and vodka/cider vinegar in a large dark glass bottle and shake vigorously. Keep the mixture in a cool, dark cupboard for one to two weeks, shaking the mixture at least twice a day. After that period, strain the herbs and add one to two tablespoons of olive oil. The olive oil helps to make the liniment spread more easily. Before using, always shake the bottle to distribute the olive oil.

The second way to make a liniment involves the use of pure essential oils. This version requires no "incubation" period as mentioned above. Simply fill a bottle with eight ounces of inexpensive vodka and add 40 to 50 drops of whatever essential oil you wish to use. Don't substitute apple cider vinegar this time because the vinegar will not blend well with the aromatic essential oils. It is best to use the essential oil blend within several days of making it since the essential oils lose their aromatic "punch."

For both types of liniments, use gentle but persistent friction against the skin. The liniment should be rubbed into the skin with a brisk motion so that all of it is absorbed.

FOMENTATION

Not to be confused with *fer*mentation. A fomentation is a fancy term for saying "a cotton cloth soaked in hot or cold liquid." One would use a fomentation on someone who has pain or inflammation. To make a fomentation, you will need a clean, cotton cloth (flannel is best). An herbal tea is brewed up to three times the normal strength. The cloth is then soaked in the tea liquid, wrung out and—once the burning heat disperses—is placed across or around the affected area to be treated. Retaining the heat is important with fomentations since it is the moist heat which contributes to the healing process. For this reason, placing plastic wrap over the hot, herb-soaked cotton cloth is recommended along with a heavy towel. Once the cloth becomes cool, remove and repeat the process. **NOTE:** If the area to be treated is swollen due to a sprain or break, USE COLD, NOT HOT fomentations.

POULTICE

This is one of the most effective forms of external herbal relief. A poultice can be made many different ways, but here are two of the more common approaches.

When using **fresh herbs**, you can either lightly heat the indicated plant's flowers or leaves in a sieve until moist or bruise (rub the leaves or flowers between your palms) or macerate (lightly chew until moist) and apply the plant directly to the area that needs to be treated. Hold the fresh herbal poultice on the area with your palm or hold it in place with a piece of masking tape. Check the poultice every half hour or so and replace it if it becomes dried out.

The second way to make a poultice is using *dried herbs.* Grind the dried herbs into a granulated or fine powder form. The amount of herbs needed will depend upon the size of the area you want to treat. For an average size poultice (3" x 3") combine two to four tablespoons of the dried, powdered herb with enough hot water to make a thick paste. To give the dried herb poultice extra drawing action, I sometimes mix in a tablespoon of castor oil. Stir the contents briskly until the mixture is smooth and uniform. (You might want to flip it between your palms, as you would a meat patty, in order to knead the contents together). Immediately apply this mixture to the affected area and cover with plastic wrap to hold it in place. If heat is required, a hot water bottle is preferred. However, a regular electric heating pad will do. Usually, a dried herb poultice is left on two to eight hours depending upon what you are treating. When it is removed, throw it away. It should *never* be reused.

Generally, poultices are used to draw out infections and poisons (such as insect bites) or reduce inflammations.

SALVE /OINTMENT

Some call them salves; some call them ointments. Either way, you're talking about the same thing. I prefer to say salve. Salves are used for their emollient, protective and healing effects. It can be a messy job to make a salve but, often times, the specific herbal salve you need is either unavailable on the commercial market or difficult to find. Thus, making it yourself is the only way. Here's how:

Use a Pyrex or stainless steel saucepan. Buy inexpensive wooden spoons for stirring. *Plastic will not work because they melt with the heat.* You will need a one quart glass mason jar for straining the ointment into and smaller glass containers for storing the ointment. Once again, plastic jars will not work since the hot oil will melt the sides. Finally, a muslin cloth cut approximately 16" x 16" will be necessary to fit over the one quart glass jelly jar for use in straining and separating the herb particles from the oil. (A muslin drawstring "jelly bag" used for canning is actually your best bet, but they are often hard to find).

To make approximately 12 to 14 ounces of a salve, you will need 16 ounces of extra virgin olive oil, two ounces of beeswax, two ounces of the *dried* herbs **OR** four ounces of the finely cut *fresh* herb and one-half teaspoon of benzoin tincture as a preservative. In a pinch, you can use regular olive oil (i.e., not extra virgin) but the first pressing is always considered the best.

Combine the herb(s) and olive oil in a saucepan and heat the mixture on low on top of the stove. Keep covered so the herbal oils do not escape into the air. Every 10 minutes or so, stir and "pumice" the herbs with a wooden spoon to make sure the herbs are saturated with the olive oil and breaking down into the oil. Continue for two hours, making certain the mixture *never* gets so hot that it starts to burn.

The idea is to gently pull the medicinal qualities out of the plants. If you cook the mixture too fast, the healing volatile oils are extracted too quickly and are often "burned out" of the mixture. Your final salve will smell like burnt grass and it will not have the highest medicinal benefit. You don't want to overcook any herb, but *you have to really watch it with flowers and leaves* (such as red clover) since they are very delicate. What I like to do with more delicate plant material is bring the mixture *just* to a boil and then turn off the heat, letting the oil sit covered for 20 minutes. Then, turn the burner on low again and repeat the process. You don't have to stare at the stuff the whole time, but please *don't leave it unattended since these mixtures have been known to pop, explode and even voluntarily catch on fire when they get too hot and are not stirred.*

After two hours of cooking, the plants may look darker. Turn off the heat and cover the pot. Allow the mixture to sit covered for up to eight hours. Before straining the herb from the oil, gently melt two ounces of yellow beeswax in the one quart glass mason jar. You can use a double boiler to melt the beeswax or place the mason jar in a 180° F oven.

Once the beeswax has melted, secure the 16" x 16" muslin cloth around the neck of the jar with a rubber band and slowly strain the herbal oil through the cloth. To make sure all the oil has been extracted from the herbs, carefully remove the muslin cloth and squeeze it tightly until the last drop is forced through the herbs. Return the strained herbal oil to the pan and gently bring it back up to a boil before pouring it into the hot, melted beeswax. Using a wooden spoon, quickly stir the oil and beeswax for three or four minutes to make sure they are completely blended together. Continue stirring and add one teaspoon of benzoin tincture as a natural preservative. If you wish, you can now pour the liquid salve into separate glass jars for storage. However, you will need to do it quickly because the salve will start to harden within minutes. When the salve cools, tightly secure the jars and store them in a dark cupboard or in the refrigerator. If kept out of the refrigerator, the salve will usually last up to two years. If refrigerated, it can last as long as five years.

HERBAL OIL EXTRACTION

This is not to be confused with the *pure essential* herbal oils which are steam distilled. (See next entry). *This* herbal oil is used more as an external rub (similar to a liniment). The healing essence of the herb is extracted from the herb using heat. An herbal oil extraction can be made two ways.

The first method is when you need the oil right away and can't wait for it to "mature." For *dried* herbs, combine one ounce of plant matter by *weight* to eight parts of olive oil *by volume*. In other words, one ounce (by weight) of the dried herb to eight ounces (by volume) of the oil. If you are using *fresh* herbs, the herb to oil ratio is one part *fresh* herbs *by weight* to four ounces *by volume* of the oil. Stir the oil and herb together in a stainless steel or Pyrex saucepan. Heat the mixture on a very low temperature, stirring constantly. DO NOT heat the oil too fast because you can burn the herbs. Allow the oil and herbs to gently simmer for 30 minutes, then turn off the heat. Cover and allow it to sit for about 30 minutes. Then, reheat the liquid, stirring constantly, until it starts to simmer again. Let it simmer for 15 to 20 minutes on low heat before turning off the burner and covering the pan. You can repeat this two or three times more, depending upon how strong you want the oil extraction. Obviously, the more you let the hot oil blend with the herbs, the better. I've kept this going for up to 12 hours with great results. However, the more the liquid is simmered, the more it will evaporate. When you're finished, strain out the herbal sediment through a muslin cloth and pour the hot herbal oil into a dark, amber glass jar. Although it is optional, stirring in one-half teaspoon of benzoin tincture will make the oil last longer and prevent rancidity. Let the mixture cool at room temperature. Store the herbal oil extract in a dark, cool cupboard. It should last up to two years.

You'll need both patience and time to make an herbal oil extract the old fashioned way. But if you don't need it right away, I think the following process produces a much better oil with fuller herbal powers. The ratio of herbs to oil (*weight to volume*) is the same as mentioned above. *Include an additional three tablespoons of wheat germ oil for extra "preservative" powers.* Pack a wide mouthed glass canning jar three-quarters of the way full with the fresh or dried herbs and pour the required amount of oil over them. Make sure the canning jar has a wide enough opening so the herbs can come out easily once the oil is ready to "harvest." Tightly close the lid. Shake the bottle so that the contents are thoroughly mixed together, then place the canning jar directly in the sun or on a windowsill so that the sun shines directly on it for at least five hours each day. Every day, shake this mixture at least once to circulate the herbs and oil. Occasionally, check the odor of the oil to make sure it hasn't "turned" (i.e., gone rancid). If that happens, you have to throw it out and start all over.

One very important note: prior to placing the **fresh** herbs into the glass jar, put them into a large bowl and sprinkle a very light coating of cheap vodka or grain alcohol over the plant. Toss the plant matter between your hands to make sure the alcohol is evenly distributed. You don't soak the plant in alcohol, by the way. A simple light drizzle will do. Set the bowl aside for three to six hours and then pack the moist herb into the glass jar and pour the oil over it. Instead of using the jar's lid, place a layer of muslin cloth over the canning jar, securing it with a rubber band. The reason for the muslin is that if you place an airtight lid over fresh herbs and oil, the natural water from within the plant can breed bacteria. The alcohol pre-soak helps alleviate part of this problem as well but the muslin allows for water evaporation. Before I figured this out, I ruined lots of fresh herbal oils due to spoilage. You can tell if a fresh herbal oil is spoiled when you open the lid and need to step back several feet due to the awful odor. Even with the alcohol pre-soak and muslin cover, these herbal oils can still turn rancid due to invading bacteria. If that happens, you will need to discard the oil and start over. By the way, since you will only have a muslin cloth over the top, you will not be able to vigorously shake the bottle of fresh herbs as you would the bottle that contains dried herbs and has a lid.

Keep the jar in the sunshine for at least four weeks. However, the longer you can keep the jar in the sun the better. One herbal supplier I know states that all of his "sun extracted oils" spend 1000 hours in the heat. That comes out to a little under six weeks. I've had jars in a south-facing window for *four years* and the resulting oil is very strong. When you finally harvest the oil, strain the herbs through a clean, muslin cloth. Press every last drop of the oil from the cloth. (Remember, the strainer should be plastic or stainless steel—*NOT* aluminum). Adding a half teaspoon of benzoin tincture helps the oil last longer. Place the strained oil into an amber glass jar and store it in a dark, cool spot. This oil can last anywhere from one to four years.

PURE ESSENTIAL OILS

Pure essential oils *cannot* be made at home. These are highly concentrated, steam-distilled preparations that require sophisticated equipment and expert handling in order to produce a safe, effective product. Contrary to some literature—much of which is published in Europe—essential oils should *never* be ingested. Due to the exceptionally high concentration of plant matter, essential oils can be extremely toxic if swallowed. Some essential oils—such as wintergreen, mugwort and pennyroyal, to name a few—are fatal in doses as small as one-half teaspoon.

Used properly externally, essential oils have many medicinal and aromatic properties. Here are some of the most popular ways to enjoy these aromatic oils.

Steam Inhalation

An herbal inhalation is a great way to clear congestion from the bronchial tubes and lungs and help soothe sore throats. Fresh herbs, dried herbs or pure essential oils are used. However, I feel essential oils are the most effective way to benefit from this herbal treatment.

Fill a large pot (pasta pots work well) with tap water and bring it to a rolling boil. Set the pot aside. Situate yourself in a comfortable position in front of the covered pot and drape a towel over your head to form a "tent." Place eight to ten drops of the pure essential oil into the water. Inhale the herbal fumes deeply, taking care not to get so close to the steam that you burn your skin or interior nasal passages. Continue for 10 to 20 minutes. Essential oils will usually evaporate and lose their fragrance within five minutes since they are not water soluble. When this happens, simply add five to eight more drops into the hot water.

(Dried herbs can be used in steam inhalations as well. Place one large handful of the herbs into the pot, stir thoroughly and breathe deeply.)

Massage Oil

A massage oil can be used on stiff joints, sore muscles or rubbed on the chest to break up respiratory congestion. The essential oil is placed into a "base oil." The best base oils, in my opinion, are those that soak quickly into the skin and are not extra greasy. Two that meet this criteria are apricot kernel oil and grapeseed oil. For every ounce of the base oil, add 25 to 30 drops of the pure essential oil. Keep the bottle tightly capped to retain as much of the aromatic healing value as possible. These massage oils can last up to two years before losing their aromatic power.

Herbal Spray

Herbal sprays are easy and inexpensive to make. Fill an eight ounce glass or plastic spray bottle with seven ounces of cold *distilled* water. To this mixture, add 100 drops of any pure essential oil. Shake vigorously before using and spray freely around sick rooms to disinfect as well as create a pleasant aromatic environment. The herbal spray usually lasts up to one month before losing its therapeutic potency.

Lamp Ring diffusers/Electric or candle diffusers

These are used for diffusing a pure essential oil into the atmosphere to benefit from the physical as well as mental properties of the fragrance. Lamp rings are available in brass, glazed ceramic and unglazed ceramic. I don't think the unglazed ceramic is worth purchasing since most of the essential oil evaporates into the porous clay before it can be released into the environment. Use eight to ten drops of the pure, undiluted essential oil in the lamp ring. Place it on an *unlit* light bulb that does not exceed 75 watts. Any hotter than that and the essential oil will burn and smoke.

There are dozens of electric and candle diffusers on the market, some of which have restrictions on the kinds of essential oils that can be used in them. Comparison shop before buying to see which electric or candle diffuser works best for your needs.

~ Quick Reference Chart ~ General Planting Information ~

HERB	GROWTH CYCLE	HARDY/ DELICATE	HEIGHT	CULTIVA -TION	SOIL	WATER	SUN/SHADE
Alfalfa	Hardy perennial	Very hardy	1 to 3 feet	Seed	Well-drained, fertile	Moist	Full to partial sun
Anise	Annual (perennial if left to go to seed)	Hardy	Up to 2 feet	Seed	Rich soil with some compost	Light moisture	Full sun
Aspen	Perennial	Hardy	100 feet	Nursery stock	Rich, cool & aerated	Reg. moisture	Partial sun
Blue violet	Perennial	Hardy	3 to 6 inches	Seed	Rich with light compost	Moist	Shade
Burdock	Biennial	Hardy	6 to 7 feet	Seed	Deep & loose	Moist	Partial sun
Chickweed	Annual	Very hardy	3 to 7 inches	Seed	Undemanding	Moist	Shade & cool
Cleavers	Perennial	Hardy	2 to 7 feet	Seed	Rich, aerated & mulched	Moist	Shade & cool
Cornsilk	Annual	Hardy	5 to 10 feet	Seed	Needs rich nitrogen content	Moist	Full sun
Fennel	Tender perennial	Hardy	Up to 6 feet	Seed	Rich & well-drained	Moderate	Full sun
Fenugreek	Tender annual	Hardy	1 to 2 feet	Seed	Fertile & well-drained	Light watering	Full sun
Horehound	Hardy perennial	Hardy	1 to 2 feet	Seed, root division, cuttings	Sandy & well-drained	Moderate	Partial sun

HERB	GROWTH CYCLE	HARDY/ DELICATE	HEIGHT	CULTIVA -TION	SOIL	WATER	SUN/SHADE
Lemon balm	Hardy perennial	Hardy	1 to 3 feet	Seed, root division	Rich & moist	Reg. moisture	Partial shade
Marshmallow	Hardy perennial	Hardy	4 to 5 feet	Seed, root division, root cuttings	Fertile & well-drained	Reg. moisture	Partial sun
Mullein	Hardy biennial	Hardy	6 to 8 feet	Seed	Poor & well-drained	Light watering	Full sun
Mustard	Hardy annual	*Very* hardy	1 to 3 feet	Seed	Works in rich, but can tolerate sandy & dry	Light watering	Full sun
Onion	Biennial	Hardy	1 to 2 feet	Seeds or sets	Medium/sandy, well-drained	Moist	Full sun
Pine	Perennial	Very hardy	Up to 150 feet	Nursery stock	Fertile	Moderate	Full sun/partial shade
Red clover	Biennial	Hardy	1 to 3 feet	Seed	Fertile & rich	Moderate	Full sun /partial shade
Rose hips	Perennial	Hardy	2 to 18 feet	Seed, cuttings, buddings nursery stock	Either heavy & loamy or rich & composted	Light watering	Full sun/partial shade
Rosemary	Perennial	Hardy	3 feet	Seed, cuttings, est. plants	Light, sandy & well-drained	Very light water	Full sun
Sage	Hardy perennial	Hardy	1 to 2 feet	Seed	Light, sandy & well-drained	Very light water	Full sun

HERB	GROWTH CYCLE	HARDY/ DELICATE	HEIGHT	CULTIVA -TION	SOIL	WATER	SUN/SHADE
Skullcap	Hardy perennial	Delicate to hardy	12 to 18 inches	Seed, root cutting, root division	Rich & fertile	Constant moisture	Partial sun
Spearmint	Hardy perennial	Hardy	3 feet	Root division, stem cuttings seeds	Rich, moist, well-drained & slightly alkaline	Constant moisture	Partial sun
Stinging nettle	Hardy perennial	Very hardy	2 to 7 feet	Seed, cuttings, seedlings, root division	Rich & well-drained	Reg. moisture	Full sun/partial shade
Thyme	Perennial	Hardy	6 to 18 inches	Seed, root. cuttings, est plants	Light, sandy	Moderate	Full sun
Usnea	Perennial	Hardy	1 to 7 inches	Not applicable	Not applicable	Not applicable	Shade
Watercress	Perennial	Hardy	Up to 3 feet	Seed	Rich, fertile & under water	Best sitting in water	Full sun
White oak bark	Perennial	Very hardy	60 to 120 feet	Est. 2 year old saplings or seeds (acorns)	Rich, moderate compost & well-drained	Slightly damp	Full sun
Yarrow	Hardy perennial	Hardy	3 feet	Seed, rootstock est. plants	Rich & well-drained	Moderate	Partial sun
Yellow dock	Hardy perennial	*Very* hardy	3 to 5 feet	Seed	Moderately rich, well-drained	Moderate	Full sun

~ Herbal Remedies & Their Healing Uses ~

AILMENT	HERB(S)	FORM	ACTION
Acne	Burdock	Tea, skin wash	Cleanses and purifies the blood.
	Yarrow	Skin wash	Astringent action tightens pores.
	Yellow dock	Tea (combined with burdock), bath	Cleanses and purifies the liver and bloodstream.
Addiction	Alfalfa	Tea, capsules, sprouts, powder	Replenishes lost vitamins & minerals as it nourishes body.
	White oak	Tincture	Tends to curb desire for alcohol, giving it a disagreeable taste.
Allergies	Marshmallow	Capsules (add = parts astragalus)	Calms the immune system, making it less sensitive to itself.
	Red clover	Tea	Cleanses the liver, bloodstream and kidneys.
	Stinging nettle	Tea, capsules (500 mg.), root extract	Acts as a natural antihistamine.
Arthritis	Alfalfa	Tablets, tea	Helps release uric acid from joints.
	Burdock	Tea	Cleanses and purifies the blood.
	Cornsilk	Tea (made from fresh "silk")	Believed to break up uric acid in joints.
	White pine	Bath	Helps relieve joint discomfort.
	Rosemary	Massage oil, tea	Provides temporary relief by stimulating circulation.
	Stinging nettle	Tea, bath, urtication	Cleanses uric acid from joints. Stimulates circulation.
	Thyme (topical use)	Extracted oil, massage oil, tincture	Provides temporary relief by increasing stimulation.

AILMENT	HERB(S)	FORM	ACTION
Constipation	Chickweed	Tea	Gently stimulates the bowel.
	Fenugreek	Tea	Gently stimulates the bowel.
Cough	Anise (hard, dry cough)	Tea	Expels mucus.
	Blue violet	Tea, syrup	Calms and soothes the cough reflex.
	Fennel	Tea, syrup	Expels mucus.
	Fenugreek	Tea (combine with one part thyme)	Expels mucus.
	Horehound	Tea, syrup, lozenges	Relaxes bronchi and expels mucus.
	Marshmallow	Tea, added to cough syrups	Provides a soothe coating of cooling relief for inflamed tissues.
	Mullein	Tea, syrup, smoking	Calms and soothes tight, dry unproductive coughs.
	Mustard	Chest pack	Generates tremendous heat which pulls congestion from lungs.
	Onion	Chest pack, cough syrup	Sulphur compounds pull toxins and congestion from lungs.
	White pine	Bark or needle tea, cough syrup	Expels mucus once the feverish & infectious stage has passed.
	Red clover	Tea	Has gentle sedative and restorative abilities.
	Stinging nettle	Root extract, root or leaf tea	Nourishes entire body while strengthening respiratory system.
	Thyme	Tea, tincture, topical massage oil, bath	Acts as a natural antiseptic, expels mucus.
	Usnea	Fresh plant tincture	Strong natural antibiotic.
	Watercress	Fresh plant (juiced)	Generates expectorant action.

392

AILMENT	HERB(S)	FORM	ACTION
Cystitis	Aspen	Tea (blend with uva ursi)	Tones weak urinary organs.
	Cleavers	Tea, tincture (fresh plant)	Soothes as it acts as a natural diuretic.
	Cornsilk	Tea (blend with mineral-rich herbs)	Cools the "fire" in the kidneys. Acts as a natural diuretic.
	Marshmallow	Tea	Provides a soothe coating of cooling relief for inflamed tissues.
	White pine	Tea (blend with uva ursi & buchu)	Acts as a urinary antiseptic.
	Usnea	Fresh plant tincture	Strong natural antibiotic.
	Yarrow	Tea (cool)	Natural antiseptic abilities cleanses and tones pelvic region.
Diarrhea	Aspen	Tea (add equal parts bayberry bark)	Acts as gentle astringent as it tones intestines.
	Marshmallow	Tea	Soothes inflamed tissues and provides relief.
Digestion (Poor)	Anise	Tea	Warms digestive tract/prevents fermentation of food.
	Aspen	Tea	Tones stomach lining.
	Fennel	Tea, ground seeds	Warms digestive tract. Prevents bloating.
	Horehound	Tea	Bitter taste promotes better liver function.
	Lemon balm	Fresh leaf tea	Indicated for poor digestion due to nervous tension.
	Rosemary	Tea	Improves liver function by increasing bile flow.
	Skullcap	Tea, tincture (fresh plant)	Antispasmodic. Helps when worry brings on digestive problems.
	Spearmint	Tea (combine with chamomile)	Gentle antispasmodic ability calms and reduces cramping.

AILMENT	HERB(S)	FORM	ACTION
Diarrhea	Aspen	Tea (add equal parts bayberry bark)	Acts as gentle astringent as it tones intestines.
	White oak	Bark or leaf tea	*Extreme* astringent action. Recommended for bleeding diarrhea.
Fever	Aspen	Tea (drink cool)	Cools the "fire" and relieves minor muscle aches.
	Cleavers	Tea	Cools the body, releasing trapped heat.
	Mustard	Bath, foot bath	Stimulates body to release trapped toxins via perspiration.
	Yarrow	Tea, bath	Encourages profuse perspiration and release of toxins.
Gas	Lemon balm	Fresh leaf tea (add = parts peppermint)	Soothes general nervous tension.
Headache	Aspen	Tea (drink cool)	Has a mild "aspirin-like" effect on the body.
	Blue violet	Tea, tincture, compress	Acts as an anti-inflammatory.
	Mustard	Foot bath	Pulls pressure and blood congestion from the head.
	Rose hips (migraine)	Tablets that include 100 mg. vitamin C	Taken at the onset of headache, can reduce symptoms.
	Rosemary	Tea, essential oil in base oil	Relieves tense, nervous headaches brought on by stress.
High Blood Pressure	Alfalfa	Capsules, tea	Nourishes as it calms the body.
	Cornsilk	Tea	Acts as a natural diuretic, relieving pressure.
	Onion	Raw or cooked plant	Innate sulphur compounds are thought to be responsible for this.

AILMENT	HERB(S)	FORM	ACTION
Inflammation	Aspen/ Cottonwood	Salve, oil	Cools, relieves pain and reduces swelling.
	Chickweed	Tea, fresh poultice	Cools and reduces painful swelling.
	Marshmallow	Tea, fresh root or leaf poultice	Provides a soothe coating of cooling relief for inflamed tissues.
	Mullein	Flower oil (topical use only)	Cools and eases pain.
	Onion	Raw or cooked plant poultice	Pulls congestion and toxins from area.
	Stinging nettle	Urtication	Microinjections of formic acid disperse pain and congestion.
Insomnia	Anise	Tea (made with warm milk)	Warms the body while soothing the nervous system.
	Lemon balm	Fresh leaf tea	Gently soothes the nerves. Helps prevent nightmares.
	Skullcap	Tea, tincture (fresh plant)	Effective when insomnia is caused by pain.
Lymphatic swelling	Burdock	Tea, fresh leaf poultices	Encourages lymphatic drainage as it cleanses the blood.
	Cleavers	Tea, tincture (fresh plant)	Gently stimulates the lymph system to cleanse toxins.
	Mullein	Tea	Stimulates release of toxins as it reduces pain.
	Red clover	Tea	A "specific" for single, hard, swollen glands.
	Yellow dock	Tea	Encourages lymphatic drainage.
Measles	Burdock	Tea, salve (external use only)	Purges impurities from the bloodstream.

395

AILMENT	HERB(S)	FORM	ACTION
Menopausal Support	Alfalfa	Tea	Nourishes ovaries, adrenals and the pituitary gland.
	Red clover	Tea	Gently sedates and nourishes the whole body.
	Sage	Tea (drink tea lukewarm or cool)	Helps reduce night sweats.
	Yarrow	Tea (cool to lukewarm)	Helps reduce hot flashes and may speed up menopause.
	Yellow dock	Tea, tincture	Provides a rich source of iron and vitamins.
Nausea	Anise	Tea	Soothes the stomach lining.
	Spearmint	Tea (add ginger & cinnamon)	Aids in nausea caused by morning sickness.
Nursing	Alfalfa	Tea	Enriches milk.
	Anise	Tea	Produces more milk while reducing chance of colic in infant.
	Fennel	Tea	Produces more milk while reducing chance of colic in infant.
	Marshmallow	Tea	Increases and enriches the flow of mother's milk.
	Sage	Tea (drink cold)	*Reduces* the flow of milk. Good for weaning a baby.
	Stinging nettle	Tea	Increases breast milk. Adds a healthy dose of minerals to body.
PMS	Burdock	Tea	Detoxifies the liver of excess estrogen.
	Lemon balm	Fresh leaf tea	Calms and soothes the nerves.
	Stinging nettle	Tea	Cleanses the liver. Acts as a whole body tonic.
	Watercress	Fresh plant	Reduces bloating, replenishes lost minerals and vitamins.
Recovery from illness	Alfalfa	Tea	Supports the body with necessary vitamins and minerals.
	Stinging nettle	Tea	Nourishes the body with minerals and vitamins.
	Watercress	Tea, fresh plant	Acts as a "multi-vitamin" as it cleanses liver and bloodstream.
	Yellow dock	Tea, tincture	Provides a rich source of iron and vitamins.

396

AILMENT	HERB(S)	FORM	ACTION
Skin Rashes	Blue violet	Tea	Cleanses and purifies the blood.
	Burdock	Tea	Cleanses and purifies the blood.
	Chickweed	Salve, bath	Acts as an anti-inflammatory and anti-itch remedy.
	Cleavers	Tea, tincture (fresh plant)	Stimulates the lymph system and cleanses the bloodstream.
	Red clover	Tea	Cleanses the liver, bloodstream and kidneys.
	Watercress	Tea, skin wash	Cleanses the bloodstream, cleanses and tones the skin.
	White oak	Bath	Provides itch relief and is cooling to *poison ivy rashes*.
	Yarrow	Skin wash	Astringent action tightens pores.
	Yellow dock	Tea, skin wash, fresh leaf poultice	Blood purifier. Neutralizes *poison ivy/stinging nettle rashes*.
Sore Throat	Blue violet	Tea (gargle)	Soothes and reduces inflammation.
	White pine	Fresh or dried needle gargle, fresh sap	Acts as an antiseptic for the throat.
	Red clover	Tea (gargle)	Soothes and heals damaged tissue.
	Rosemary	Tea (gargle)	Natural antiseptic ability speeds healing.
	Sage	Tea	Strengthens the gums and mucous membranes as it kills bacteria.
	Thyme	Tea or tincture (gargle)	Strong antiseptic action helps kill infection.
	White oak	Bark tea	Astringent action tightens tissues and reduces pain.

397

AILMENT	HERB(S)	FORM	ACTION
Wounds	Aspen	Tea wash, fomentation	Soothes inflammation.
	Blue violet	Tea wash	Soothes and cools inflammation.
	Cleavers	Fresh plant poultice	Cools and soothes as it relieves pain.
	Lemon balm	Fresh leaf poultice	Acts as a slight anesthetic and anti-infection agent.
	Marshmallow	Root or fresh leaf poultice	Acts as a gentle drawing poultice to pull out any infection.
	Onion	Raw plant poultice	Pulls pain from area, prevents infection and speeds healing.
	White pine	Fresh sap	Acts as a "band-aid" to prevent infection.
	Rosemary	Dried powdered leaf	Sprinkled on wound, has antiseptic and antibacterial qualities.
	Sage	Fresh leaf poultice	Antiseptic abilities help to prevent infection.
	Thyme	Tincture, plant, diluted essential oil	Acts as a strong disinfectant.
	Usnea	Tincture, fresh poultice, salve	Antimicrobial ability helps stop bleeding & prevents infection.
	White oak	Powdered bark	Tightens tissues and speeds healing.
	Yarrow	Fresh leaf poultice	Acts as a natural antibiotic and antiseptic and stops bleeding.

398

HERB TERMINOLOGY

Adaptogen: Allows the body to have greater resistance to stress.

Alterative: Producing gradual change in the body, usually through blood cleansing and gentle removal of waste products.

Anaphrodisiac: Reduces sexual desire.

Anodyne: Relieves or soothes pain.

Anti-bacterial: Destroys or prevents the growth of bacterial infections.

Antibiotic: Destroys or prevents the growth of micro-organisms.

Antidepressant: Relieves symptoms of depression.

Antifungal: Destroys or prevents the growth of fungi.

Antihydrotic: Reduces or suppresses perspiration.

Anti-inflammatory: Diminishes or prevents inflammation.

Antineoplastic: Prevents the development, growth or spreading of malignant cells.

Antioxidant: Prevents free radical or oxidative damage to body tissue and cells.

Antiparasitic: Destroys or prevents the growth and development of parasites.

Antirheumatic: Prevents or relieves rheumatism.

Antiseptic: Destroys or inhibits pathogenic or putrefactive bacteria.

Antispasmodic: Prevents or relieves spasms.

Antitussive: Inhibits the cough reflex thereby helping to quiet or stop a cough.

Antivenomous: Stops or reduces the effects of venom on the body.

Anti-viral: Fights against invading viral infections.

Aperient: Mild stimulant for the bowels with the purging action.

Aphrodisiac: Stimulates sexual desire.

Appetizer: Excites or stimulates the appetite.

Aromatic: A substance with a fragrant odor which usually aids digestion and relieves gas pains.

Astringent: Constricts and tightens tissues while reducing secretions or discharge.

Bitter: Stimulates secretions of digestive enzymes while stimulating the appetite.

Carminative: Expels gas from the intestines.

Cholagogue: Increases the flow of bile into the intestines.

Counterirritant: Causes slight irritation in one part of the body to counteract or relieve pain in another part.

Demulcent: Softens and soothes inflamed tissue, especially the mucous membrane.

Depuritive: Removes impurities from the body via the bloodstream, producing a cleansing action.

Diaphoretic: Promotes perspiration to increase toxic elimination through the skin.

Digestive: Aids digestion.

Diuretic: Promotes and increases the flow of urine.

Emetic: Causes vomiting.

Emmenagogue: Promotes menstruation. (Always avoid emmenagogue herbs during pregnancy since they generally stimulate the uterine muscles).

Emollient: Softens and soothes tissue or skin.

Expectorant: Promotes the discharge of mucus from the respiratory passages.

Febrifuge: Reduces fever.

Galactagogue: Promotes the flow of milk in nursing mothers.

Hemostatic: Stops bleeding.

Hepatic: Stimulates the action of the liver.

Hypoglycemic: Reduces blood sugar in the body.

Hypotensive: Reduces blood pressure.

Irritant: Creates a local irritation or inflammation on the skin.

Laxative: Stimulates the bowels to release waste products.

Lymphatic: Stimulates the pumping action and flow of the lymph fluid through the various lymphatic vessels of the body.

Mineral Tonic: An herb which delivers organic, easily assimilated minerals to the body.

Mucilage: Creates a gummy or gelatinous protection over inflamed tissue.

Nervine: Produces a calming or soothing effect on the nerves.

Nutritive: Nourishes and feeds the body.

Pectoral: Soothes and calms diseases or illness related to the lungs and chest.

Refrigerant: Cools and reduces heat. Often used for reducing fevers.

Restorative: Brings back health and vitality.

Rubefacient: Stimulates blood flow (circulation) to the skin and causes localized reddening.

Stimulant: Excites and increases circulation and metabolism.

Stomachic: Strengthens, stimulates and tones the stomach.

Tonic: Restores and supports the body through a gentle strengthening effect.

Vulnerary: Stimulates the healing of wounds.

BIBLIOGRAPHY

Angier, Bradford. *Field Guide to Edible Wild Plants.* Harrisburg, PA: Stackpole Books, 1996 (15th printing).

Bairacli-Levy, Juliette de. *Common Herbs for Natural Health.* Woodstock, NY: Ash Tree Publishing, 1997.

——. *The Illustrated Herbal Handbook for Everyone.* London: Faber Paperbacks, 1991.

Bartram, Thomas. *Encyclopedia of Herbal Medicine.* Dorset, England: Grace Publs., 1995.

Beatty, Bill. *Bill & Bev Beatty's Wild Plant Cookbook.* Happy Camp, CA: Naturegraph Publs., 1987.

Berwick, Ann. *Aromatherapy–A Holistic Guide.* St. Paul, MN: Llewellyn Publs., 1997.

Bremness, Lesley. *Herbs (Eyewitness Handbooks).* New York: Dorling Kindersley, Inc., 1994.

——. *Pocket Garden Herbs.* New York: Dorling Kindersley, Ltd., 1997.

Brill, Steve and Dean, Evelyn. *Identifying and Harvesting Edible and Medicinal Plants in Wild (And Not So Wild) Places.* New York: Hearst Books, 1994.

Brinker, Francis, N.D. *Herb Contraindications and Drug Interactions.* Sandy, OR: Eclectic Institute, 1997.

Brown, Tom. *Tom Brown's Field Guide to Wilderness Survival.* New York: Berkley Publishing Corp., 1983

——. *Tom Brown's Guide to Wild Edible and Medicinal Plants.* New York: Berkley Books, 1985.

Buchanan, Rita. *Taylor's Guide to Herbs.* New York: Houghton Mifflin Company, 1995.

Buchman, Dian Dincin. *Herbal Medicine–The Natural Way to Get Well and Stay Well.* New York: Wings Books (Random House), 1996.

Castleman, Michael. *The Healing Herbs.* Emmaus, PA: Rodale Press, 1991.

Christopher, John R., N.D., M.H. *Natural Healing Newsletter: "American Indian Herbs"* (Volume 4, No. 11). Springville, UT: Christopher Publications, 1983.

——. *Natural Healing Newsletter: "Herbal First Aid–Part I"* (Vol. 3, No. 1). Springville, UT: Christopher Publs., 1982.

——. *Natural Healing Newsletter: "Herbal First Aid* -Part II" (Volume 3, No.1). Springville, UT: Christopher Publs., 1982.

——. *Natural Healing Newsletter: "Oak Bark"* (Vol. 2, No. 10). Springville, UT: Christopher Publs., 1981.

——. *Natural Healing Newsletter: 23 "Pain Palliatives"* (Vol. 4, No. 5). Springville,UT: Christopher Publs., 1983.

——. *Natural Healing Newsletter: "Ten Honorable Herbs"* (Vol. 4, No. 7). Springville, UT: Christopher Publs., 1983.

——. *Natural Healing Newsletter: "The Ten Most Important Herbs."* (Vol. 1, No. 3). Springville, UT: Christopher Publs., 1980.

——. *School of Natural Healing.* Springville, UT: Christopher Publs., January 1996 (11th printing).

Duke, James A., Ph.D. *The Green Pharmacy.* Emmaus, PA: Rodale Press, 1997.

Elias, Thomas S. and Dykeman, Peter A. *Edible Wild Plants–A North American Field Guide.* New York: Sterling Publishing Co., 1990.

Foster, Steven and Duke, James A., Ph.D. *A Field Guide to Medicinal Plants–Eastern and Central North America (Peterson Field Guide Series No. 40).* New York: Houghton Mifflin Co., 1990.

Foster, Steven. *Herbal Renaissance.* Layton, UT: Gibbs Smith Publisher, 1984.

Gibbons, Euell. *Stalking the Healthful Herbs.* Putney, VT: Alan C. Hood & Co.., 1966.

——. *Stalking the Wild Asparagus.* Putney, VT: Alan C. Hood & Co., 1962.

Grieve, Mrs. M. *A Modern Herbal–*Vol. I. New York: Dover Publs., 1971.

——. *A Modern Herbal–*Vol. II. New York: Dover Publications, Inc., 1971.

Heinerman, John. *Heinerman's Encyclopedia of Fruits, Vegetables and Herbs.* New York: Parker Publishing Company, 1988.

Hobbs, Christopher. *Usnea: The Herbal Antibiotic–And Other Medicinal Lichens.* Capitola, CA: Botanica Press, 1990 (3rd Ed.).

Hoffman, David. *The New Holistic Herbal.* New York: Barnes & Noble Books, 1995.

Jacobs, Betty E.M. *Growing and Using Herbs Successfully.* Pownal, VT: Garden Way Publishing, 1991.

Keller, Erich. *The Complete Home Guide to Aromatherapy–Self-Help With Essential Oils.* Tiburon, CA: H.J. Kramer, 1991.

Kloss, Jethro. *Back to Eden.* Loma Linda, California: Back to Eden Books Publishing Co., 1992 (11th printing).

Kourik, Robert. *Designing and Maintaining Your Edible Landscape Naturally.* Santa Rosa, CA: Metamorphic Press, 1986.

Kowalchick, Claire and Hylton, William H. *Rodale's Illustrated Encyclopedia of Herbs.* Emmaus, PA: Rodale Press, 1987.

Kroeger, Hanna. *Spices to the Rescue.* Hanna Kroeger Publs.

Kruger, Anna. *An Illustrated Guide to Herbs–Their Medicine and Magic.* Great Britain: Dragon's World Ltd., 1993.

Low Dog, Tieraona. *Gifts of the Earth.* Albuquerque, NM: Tieraona's Herbals, 1991.

Lucas, Richard M. *Miracle Medicine Herbs.* New York: Parker Publishing Co., 1991.

Lust, John. *The Herb Book.* New York: Bantam Books, 1974.

Mabey, Richard, et al. *The New Age Herbalist.* New York: Macmillan Publishing Co., 1988.

Marcin, Marietta Marshall. *The Herbal Tea Garden–Planning, Planting, Harvesting & Brewing*. Pownal, Vermont: Garden Way Publ., 1995 (5th printing).

McGuffin, Michael. *American Herbal Products Association's Botanical Safety Handbook*. Boca Raton, FL: CRC Press, LLC, 1997.

McHoy, Peter and Westland, Pamela. *The Herb Bible*. New York: Barnes & Noble Books, 1997.

McIntyre, Anne. *The Medicinal Garden—How to Grow and Use Your Own Medicinal Herbs*. New York: Henry Holt & Co., 1997.

McVicar, Jekka. *Herbs for the Home—A Definitive Sourcebook to Growing and Using Herbs*. New York: Viking Penguin, 1995.

Metcalfe, Joannah. *Herbs and Aromatherapy*. New York: Penguin Books, 1989.

Michalak, Patricia S. *Rodale's Successful Organic Gardening Herbs*. Emmaus, Pennsylvania: Rodale Press, 1993.

Miller, Douglas C. *Vegetable & Herb Seed Growing for the Gardener and Small Farmer*. Boise, ID: Seeds Blum, 1984.

Moore, Michael. *Herbal Tinctures in Clinical Practice*. Albuquerque, NM: Southwest School of Botanical Medicine, 1996.

——. *Medicinal Plants of the Desert and Canyon West*. Santa Fe, NM: The Museum of New Mexico Press, 1989.

——. *Medicinal Plants of the Mountain West*. Santa Fe, NM: The Museum of New Mexico Press, 1979.

——. *Medicinal Plants of the Pacific West*. Santa Fe, New Mexico: Red Crane Books, 1995 (2nd printing).

Mowrey, Daniel B., Ph.D. *The Scientific Validation of Herbal Medicine*. New Canaan, Connecticut:: Keats Publishing, 1986.

Nuzzi, Debra, M.H. *Pocket Herbal Reference Guide*. Freedom, CA: Crossing Press, 1992.

Nyerges, Christopher. *Guide to Wild Foods*. Los Angeles, CA: Survival News Service, 1997 (4th Rev. Ed.).

——. *Wild Greens and Salads*. Harrisburg, Pennsylvania: Stackpole Books, 1982.

Ody, Penelope. *The Complete Medicinal Herbal*. New York: Dorling Kindersley, 1993.

Palaiseul, Jean. *Grandmother's Secrets—Her Green Guide to Health From Plants*. New York: Viking Penguin, 1986.

Page, Linda Rector, N.D., Ph.D. *Healthy Healing*. Carmel Valley, CA: Healthy Healing Publications, Tenth Edition, January 1997.

——. *How to Be Your Own Herbal Pharmacist*. Sonora, CA: Crystal Star Herbs, 1991.

Peterson, Lee Allen. *Edible Wild Plants (Peterson Field Guide Series No. 23)*. New York: Houghton Mifflin Company, 1977.

Peterson, Nicola. *Herbs and Health (Culpeper Guides)*. New York: Seafarer Books, 1994.

Ritchason, Jack, N.D. *The Little Herb Encyclopedia–The Handbook of Nature's Remedies for a Healthier Life*. Pleasant Grove, UT: Woodland Health Books, 1995 (3rd Ed.).

Rose, Jeanne. *The Aromatherapy Book–Applications & Inhalations*. Berkeley, CA: North Atlantic Books, 1992.

Schar, Douglas. *The Backyard Medicine Chest–An Herbal Primer*. Washington, D.C.: Elliott & Clark Publ., 1995

——. *Thirty Plants That Can Save Your Life*. Washington, DC: Elliott & Clark Publ., 1993.

Scott, Julian, Ph.D. *Natural Medicine for Children*. New York: Avon Books, 1990.

Seebeck, "Cattail" Bob. *Best-Tasting Wild Plants of Colorado and the Rockies*. Englewood, CO: Westcliffe Publishers, 1998.

Tenney, Louise, M.H. *Health Handbook*. Pleasant Grove, UT: Woodland Books, 1994 (Second Edition).

Theiss, Barbara & Peter. *The Family Herbal*. Rochester, VT: Healing Arts Press, 1989.

Thomas, Ian. *How to Grow Herbs (Culpeper Guides)*. New York: Seafarer Books, 1994.

Thomas, Lalitha. *10 Essential Herbs*. Prescott, AZ: Hohm Press, 1992.

Tierra, Lesley. *The Herbs of Life–Health & Healing Using Western & Chinese Techniques*. Freedom, CA: The Crossing Press, 1992.

Tierra, Michael. *The Way of Herbs*. New York: Pocket Books (Simon & Schuster), 1990.

Tilford, Gregory L. *The EcoHerbalist's Fieldbook–Wildcrafting in the Mountain West*. Conner, MT: Mountain Weed Publ., 1993.

——. *Edible and Medicinal Plants of the West*. Missoula, MT: Mountain Press Publ., 1997.

Tisserand, Maggie. *Aromatherapy For Women*. Rochester, VT: Healing Arts Press, 1988.

Tisserand, Robert B. *The Art of Aromatherapy*. Rochester, VT: Healing Arts Press, 1977.

Treben, Maria. *Health From God's Garden*. Rochester, VT: Healing Arts Press, 1988.

——. *Health Through God's Pharmacy*. Austria: Wilhelm Ennsthaler Publishing, 1980.

Vogel, Alfred. *The Nature Doctor*. New Canaan, Connecticut: Keats Publ., 1995 (9th printing).

Weiner, Michael A. *The Herbal Bible*. San Rafael, CA: Quantum Books, 1992.

Wildwood, Christine. *Holistic Aromatherapy*. London: Thorsons, 1992.

Willard, Terry, Ph.D. *Edible and Medicinal Plants of the Rocky Mountains and Neighbouring Territories*. Calgary, Alberta, Canada: Wild Rose College of Natural Healing, Ltd., 1992.

Wood, Matthew. *The Book of Herbal Wisdom–Using Plants as Medicines*. Berkeley, CA: North Atlantic Books, 1997.

Wren, R.C. *Potter's New Cyclopaedia of Botanical Drugs and Preparations*. Essex, England: C.W. Daniel Company, Ltd., 1985 Edition.

HERBAL RESOURCES

Remember to tell these fine businesses that
you read about them in *Plant Power!*

AROMATHERAPY

LAVENDER LANE - "HARD TO FIND HERBALWARE." If you are looking for fifty of the purest essential oils, glass jars, plastic jars, glass bottles, glass jars or glass vials, we carry over 300 different containers. We also offer soap making supplies, candle making supplies, lip balm supplies, bath crystal making supplies, 10 carrier oils, 70 fragrance oils, diffusers, "how to kits," "how to books," and a whole lot more. Call toll free (888) 593-4400 for a catalog or see our web site at *www.lavenderlane.com* or write Lavender Lane at 7337 #1 Roseville Road, Sacramento, CA, 95842.

BOTTLES/CAPS/DROPPERS

PACKAGING WEST, INC. Packaging West has all of the rigid packaging components for the herbal, homeopathy, and nutritional supplement markets. We offer glass and plastic bottles (both wide mouth for solids and narrow mouth for liquids), glass and plastic jars, bulk containers, caps (regular and dispensing), dropper assemblies to fit glass bottles. We take Visa. Minimum order is $150. Full case lots only. Please call the location nearest you. Albuquerque: (505) 344-7575; Denver: (303) 375-7700; Kansas City: (816) 241-1717; Los Angeles: (562) 407-0557; Seattle: (253) 395-3610.

BULK HERBS

HERB PRODUCTS COMPANY. We stock over 300 bulk botanicals for preparing teas and capsules, culinary spices, a large selection of essential oils, aromatic oils, extracts, books, tea accessories and much more. As one of California's largest suppliers of bulk botanicals and herbal products, we are committed to obtaining and providing the best in quality and selection. Proprietors of high quality botanicals and related herbal products since 1965, our philosophy has always been to provide the highest quality products at the lowest possible price. No minimum order—4 oz. minimum quantity for botanicals and 1 oz. minimum quantity for oils and extracts. All products are shipped via UPS within 24 hours from receipt of order. Our catalog is free by calling (800) 877-3104, writing us at

Herb Products Company, P.O. Box 898, North Hollywood, CA 91603-0898 or check out our web site at www.herbproducts.com.

HERBAL BODY PRODUCTS

FLOWER CHILD HERBS. Flower Child Herbs is the realization of a dream for herbalist Jill Howard. Using organically grown herbs from her gardens such as Rosemary, Calendula and Lavender, Jill lovingly creates vegetarian soaps that pamper the skin and senses. Body oils, creams and delightfully inspired teas are but a few of the many products offered by Flower Child Herbs. For your catalog, send $2.00 (deductible from your order) to: Flower Child Herbs, 16532 Milliman, Rockwood, Michigan 48173.

HERBAL PRODUCTS & NATURAL REMEDIES

PENN HERB COMPANY, LTD. Looking for the most complete selection of herbs, herbal products and natural remedies available anywhere? Penn Herb Company is your one stop source for over 7000 natural products in stock and ready to ship within 24 hours. We carry over 500 varieties of bulk herbs from around the world. Select from whole, cut, powder and capsule forms. Our unique full color catalog also features a complete selection of Men's Products, Women's Products, Vitamins, Minerals, Essential Oils, Ginseng, products for Arthritis, Asthma, Cholesterol, Detoxification, Dieting, Energy, Immune System, PMS, Seniors and much, much more. Since 1924 Penn Herb Company has been serving satisfied customers and has earned the reputation as "America's Most Unique Source for Medicinal Herbs and Natural Remedies." Satisfaction guaranteed! Our full color, 80 page catalog is available free of charge by calling (800) 523-9971 or write to: Penn Herb Co., Ltd., 10601 Decatur Road, Philadelphia, PA 19154. P.S. Visit our web site at www.pennherb.com.

ORGANIC FERTILIZERS

NITRON INDUSTRIES. Nitron Industries has the most complete line of organic fertilizers and soil conditioners in the world. Famous for Nitron A-35 soil conditioner and many more such as sea grow, humic acid, fish emulsion, green up, pep up, green sand, soft rock phosphate, kelp meal, fish meal, bat guano, diatomaceous earth, alfalfa meal, tree magic, nature meal for vegetables, and many, many more. For our free catalog call (800) 835-0123 or visit our web site at www.nitron.com.

SCHOOLS/EDUCATION

THE SCHOOL OF NATURAL HEALING. *The School of Natural Healing* was founded in 1953, making it the oldest herbal school in America. The School's correspondence course offers students the chance to certify as a Master Herbalist and study in the comfort of their own home. The course can be completed in just under two years (studying one hour per day). The course consists of 36 video cassettes, 24 audio cassettes, and 23 high quality books (more material than any other herbal program). For more information, write *The School of Natural Healing,* P.O. Box 412, Springville, Utah 84663 or call (800) 372-8255. Fax (801) 489-8341. E-Mail: snh@avpro.com. Web site: www.schoolofnaturalhealing.com. *Dr. Christopher's Herb Shop* (800) 453-1406.

SEEDS & GARDEN PRODUCTS

GARDEN CITY SEEDS. Garden City Seeds specializes in vegetable, flower, and herb varieties for northern gardens. We conduct yearly varietal trials in Montana to determine which are the most vigorous, best tasting, and highest quality cultivars. We carry over 450 different varieties, with many from our own exclusive production. We work with independent plant breeders to develop new varieties for our customers. We carry many high nutrition vegetable varieties, including ones with newly recognized phytomedicinals. Our diverse line of culinary and medicinal herbs and wild plants includes *Echinacea angustifolia,* Feverfew, Self Heal, Milk Thistle, Blessed Thistle, Bee Balm, etc. Most of our newest herbs are from organic production in Montana. We support and promote sustainable agriculture and have a complete line of cover crops and organically approved fertilizers and pest control products. Send $1 for our highly informative 88 page catalog. Garden City Seeds, 778 Highway 93 N., Hamilton, MT 59840, 406-961-4837.

INDEX

A peaceful mind is like a rock in the ocean

on which the raging waves break and lose their strength.

Hope, faith, strength and confidence can only blossom

in a peaceful mind.

Oscar Brunler

BLANK PAGES FOR
NOTES

~